☼ *Sunlight and vitamin D help control heart disease, blood pressure and multiple sclerosis and increase muscle strength.*

☼ *Sunlight and vitamin D may put a halt to autism.*

☼ *Vitamin D and sunlight may be the answer to preventing colds and flu.*

☼ *Learn the surprising truth about tanning beds, sunscreens and melanoma.*

☼ *Vitamin D is good news for the health of African Americans and other dark-skinned people.*

Here is a list of 105 diseases and disorders or conditions, mentioned in this book, which may be diminished by regular sunlight exposure and/or vitamin D supplementation:

Twenty major internal cancers, including breast cancer, prostate cancer, lung cancer and colon cancer

Acute lower respiratory infection
Anaphylaxis
Anemia
Anxiety
Arthritis
Asthma
Atherosclerosis
Autism
Autoimmune diseases
Bacterial contamination
Bipolar disorder
Brain damage
Breast-tissue density
Chronic fatigue
Chronic pain
Cognitive ability
Colds
Craniotabes
C-reactive protein levels
Crohn's disease
Cystic fibrosis
Dental caries (cavities)
Dyslexia
Eczema
Epilepsy
Epstein Barr Virus
Falls
Fibromyalgia
Flu
Fractures
Headache
Hearing loss
Heart disease
Heart failure
High cholesterol
HIV/AIDS
Hyperactivity
Immune system
Infertility
Inflammation
Inflammatory bowel disease
Inflamation
Insomnia
Intermittent claudication
Kidney disease
Leprosy
Low-back pain
Low birth weight
Lupus
Macular degeneration
Melanoma
Meningitis (bacterial)
Metabolic Syndrome
Migraines
Mood disorders
Muscle strength (low)
Myeloma
Myopathy
Myopia
Necrotizing fasciitis
Neuroblastoma
Neuropathy
Nonspecific muscle pain
Nursing home risk
Obesity
Osteomalacia
Osteoporosis
Parasites
Parkinson's disease
Periodontal disease
Peripheral artery disease
PMS
Pneumonia
Polycystic ovary disease
Pre-eclampsia
Psoriasis
Retinoblastoma
Rickets
Sarcopenia
Schizophrenia
Seasonal affective disorder (SAD)
Sepis
Septicemia
Stroke
Tuberculosis

VITAMIN D3

AND

SOLAR POWER

FOR OPTIMAL HEALTH

Marc Sorenson, EdD.

Foreword by William B Grant, PhD.

Author: Marc Sorenson, EdD
Editorial Director: Marc Sorenson, EdD

Composition: Dimension Design & Print

DISCLAIMER: This book is not meant to substitute for the counsel of a qualified health professional or to diagnose or treat any disease. Improper use of sunlight or other ultraviolet light exposure may result in various types of skin cancer, as well as aging of the skin. Some persons may also have skin types or conditions that preclude sun exposure or other ultraviolet light exposure, and certain diseases may also preclude exposure to ultraviolet light. Other persons may be sensitive to vitamin D from supplements or food. The reader takes full responsibility for any action taken after reading this material. The reader is advised to consult a health professional before making any changes in sunlight exposure or vitamin D supplementation.

ISBN 1-4243-1387-2

Printed in the United States of America

14 13 12 11 10 09 08   2 3 4 5 6

Dedication

This book is dedicated to the millions of people whose health has been compromised by a lack of sunlight and vitamin D—a condition brought on by the misguided policies of governmental agencies, organized medicine and the pharmaceutical industry. It is especially dedicated to African Americans and other dark-skinned people whose excess of cancer, heart disease and hypertension can be explained to a great extent by insufficient sunlight exposure when living in northern latitudes. It is my intention to play a part in reversing the current sun phobia and the unwarranted sunscreen mania and to bring the people out of the shadows and back into the sunlight, that their health might be restored and their quality of life enriched.

A special dedication is also given to Dr. Zane Kime, whose early work and writings in the field of sunlight provided impetus for my study of sunlight's marvelous healing effects. Dr. Kime's untimely death in a mountain-climbing accident took away one of the great advocates of sunlight exposure for optimal health.

Table of Contents

Foreword by William Grant, Ph.D 2
Acknowledgements 4
Author's Preface 6
Introduction 10

Section 1:
Background Material 13

Chapter

1. Sunlight, vitamin D and health: history and function 14
2. Seasons and sunlight 37
3. Free radicals and antioxidants 45
4. Solar Power, dietary fat and skin cancer 52
5. Solar Power and melanoma: burned by sunscreens? 60

Section 2:
Solar Power and prevention of the Deadly Cancers 75

Chapter

6. How Solar Power prevents cancer 76
7. Solar Power, breast cancer and other women's cancers .. 79
8. Sunlight, vitamin D and prostate cancer 88
9. Solar Power, colon cancer and other internal cancers 96

Section 3:

Solar Power and other major diseases and health issues 107

Chapter

10. Boning up: Solar Power, osteoporosis, falls, arthritis and pain 108
11. Sunlight reduces the risk of multiple sclerosis 131
12. Solar Power, diabetes and autoimmune diseases 140
13. Solar power, heart disease and high blood pressure 150
14. Solar Power and a potpourri of health concerns 160
15. Solar Power fights depression and other mental disorders 183
16. Solar Power and African Americans 193
17. Tanning beds as health-promoting devices 195
18. Summary 198

Epilogue 202
Suggestions for further reading and other resources 204
A final word on the importance of Solar Power 207
References 209
Glossary 247
Index 254
A Tribute to William Grant, Ph.D 261
About the author 263

"Let there be light."

"My very dear brethren, my good friends, there are in France thirteen hundred and twenty thousand peasants' cottages that have but three openings; eighteen hundred and seventeen thousand that have two, the door and one window; and finally, three hundred and forty-six thousand cabins, with only one opening—the door. And this is in consequence of what is called the excise upon doors and windows. In these poor families, among the aged women and the little children, dwelling in these huts, how abundant is fever and disease? Alas! God gives light to men; the law sells it. I do not blame the law, but I bless God….."

From Les Miserables by Victor Hugo

Foreword

By
William B. Grant, Ph.D.,
Sunlight, Nutrition and Health Research Center (SUNARC)

Mankind has, until lately, always been in harmony with the sun, regardless of race or geographical area in which he lived. In the plains of Africa, a high degree of pigmentation is required to protect the skin from damage. In the bright tropical sun, enough solar ultraviolet B (UVB) radiation penetrates the skin to produce adequate levels of vitamin D. In Asia and Europe, lighter-pigmented skin permitted him to produce vitamin D with less solar UVB but still offered sufficient protection against the harmful effects of solar UV. Until the age of modern mass migrations to the New World and Australia, man generally lived where his skin was well-suited for the usual UV irradiance except at high latitudes, where, since it is impossible to make vitamin D in winter, populations rely on a diet rich in fish to make up the deficit.

Before the industrial age, man spent much of his time outdoors hunting, gathering, or working in agricultural production and living in harmony with the sun. However, with rising affluence in the 17th and 18th centuries, pale skin became a mark of the upper class in Northern Europe (to the detriment of their health), and as people spent more time indoors, diseases associated with vitamin D deficiency manifested themselves. In the 19th century, exposure to the sun was prescribed to prevent or treat rickets and, in the early 20th century, tuberculosis, although it wasn't until the 1919-1924 that vitamin D was isolated and identified. Then, thanks to Coco Chanel and her summer spent sailing off the Cote d'Azur of France about that time, tanning became fashionable and enjoyed widespread popularity until the early 1980s, when dermatologists began advising the public to take measures to avoid solar UV irradiance to reduce the risk of skin cancer and melanoma.

The beneficial role of vitamin D in calcium absorption and bone mineralization was realized in the 1960s. Its role in cancer risk reduction was hypothesized in 1980 by Cedric and Frank Garland and confirmed over the next 26 years, when finally a randomized controlled trial found a 77% reduction in all-cancer incidence rates. The role of vitamin D in improving the innate immune system through induction of human cathelicidin, LL-37, has only been known since the early 1990s. It now appears that LL-37 provides reasonable protection against some bacterial and viral infections including seasonal influenza, periodontal disease, and septicemia. Vitamin D's role in reducing the risk of autoimmune diseases such as multiple sclerosis was documented in the 1990s, and appears to be related to its effects on the innate immune system. The benefits of vitamin D in reducing the risk of cardiovascular and metabolic diseases have been reported in the past few years. By now, the evidence for a beneficial effect of UVB and vitamin D for a large variety of diseases has become quite strong. It appears that serum 25-hydroxyvitamin D (calcidiol) levels of at least 40 ng/ml (100 nmol/L) are required for optimal health. In the absence of ultraviolet-B irradiance, an average-sized person should take about 4000 International Units (IU) of vitamin D3 per day to achieve this level. It is also advisable to have serum calcidiol levels measured.

Why does vitamin D remain so underappreciated now? There appear to be three primary reasons. One is that there is little profit to be made in promoting the idea that everyone should have higher serum 25-hydroxyvitamin D levels; a year's supply of vitamin D at 4000 I.U. day costs about $40. A second reason is that UV irradiance is also associated with skin cancer, melanoma, and premature skin aging. A third reason is that vitamin D insufficiency generally manifests itself in long-latency diseases such as osteoporosis, cancer and autoimmune diseases, so there is generally little direct immediate evidence that vitamin D levels are low.

Given this state of affairs, I was delighted when Marc Sorenson sent me his manuscript, *Solar Power*, for colleague review and comment. This book fills an important need for a comprehensive source of information on the health benefits of solar UVB and vitamin D, as well as the risk factors for skin cancer and melanoma, while simultaneously providing extensive references for those who want to read the original papers. Dr. Sorenson's background ideally suits him for the task; as the owner/operator of a top-rated health resort, he educates the general public persuasively, and as a master of English literature he writes with scholarly precision and passion. He has also done his homework, synthesizing the important literature for each topic covered. This book will be an important step in moving the UVB/vitamin D agenda forward. If I had written a book on UVB and vitamin D, this would be it.

Acknowledgements

Gratitude is expressed to my wife Vicki (who always brings sunshine into my life) for her support, suggestions and for proofreading of this text. Also to Todd and Colleen Cummings, Robbie Howard, Dr. Gordon Ainsleigh and Dr. John Clark, I express my gratitude for help in proofreading. I also greatly appreciate Jim Catano's meticulous and professional editing. The work of these individuals gave a clarity and impact to the text that would otherwise have been difficult to achieve. William Bagnol, my illustrator, also did yeoman's work in helping to make lucid the concepts of sunlight and season.

Drs. Cedric and Frank Garland deserve thanks for their ground-breaking research on the relationship of sunlight to colon cancer. Theirs was the spark that led ultimately to the exploding interest in sunlight and health. And to their associate Carol Baggerly, whose work and enthusiasm is moving the vitamin D agenda forward, I express my gratitude.

To Pamella Asquith, the librarian at Dixie Regional Medical Center, I am profoundly grateful for the myriad full-text medical papers she procured for me—papers that were sometimes new and sometimes nearly a century old.

Appreciation is also due Dr. William Grant, formerly a scientist with NASA and now one of the most respected researchers in the fields of sunlight and vitamin D. He is the founder of the Sunlight, Nutrition and Health Research Center (SUNARC) and a full-time researcher who is also the epitome of a sound-thinking scientist and a wonderful human being. Before he even knew me, Dr. Grant responded to my emails and offered his help unreservedly. He agreed to read the text, make suggestions and provide scientific papers that strengthened the research.

I also mention Dr. Michael Holick, a dermatologist and researcher at Boston University Medical School who wrote his own book on sunlight, *The UV Advantage*, but who helpfully answered my queries. Similar gratitude is expressed to Dr. Bruce Hollis and Dr. Oliver Gillie, who have written many papers and reviews on the topics that are covered in *Solar Power*, and who promptly answered my requests for clarification and information. And to Drs. John Cannell, Gordon Ainsleigh and Philip Miller, I express thanks for suggestions that improved the text. Dr. Cannell's vitamin D newsletter was also a cornucopia of valuable information that opened the door to many research papers. Dr. Cannell and I are currently coauthoring another book, and he has been terrific to work with.

Finally, I salute Drs. Reinhold Vieth, Edward Giovannucci, Robert Heaney, Joan Lappe, Bruce Hollis and all other scientists who labored to bring forth the truth. They are the heroes who are reestablishing the importance of sunlight for human health. Without their efforts, there could have been no research to quote and no knowledge to disseminate.

SOLAR POWER
Author's Preface

Here are some headlines you may have missed:

Low Vitamin D Levels and Lack of Sunlight may be Killing African Americans: Is it Time for a Change in National Policy Regarding Sunlight Exposure?

The Risk of Prostate Cancer may be Reduced as Much as 80% by Regular Sunbathing.

Breast Cancer Risk is Reduced up to 65% with Sunlight Exposure.

Vitamin D May be the Best Form of Cancer Chemotherapy.

Low Blood Levels of Vitamin D are Closely Correlated with Obesity.

Vitamin D Supplementation May Prevent Nearly 100% of Winter Flu Outbreaks.

Sunlight is the "Drug-free" Antidepressant. Depression is Remarkably Reduced by Sunlight and Light Therapy.

Tanning Bed use Profoundly Increases Both Vitamin D Levels and Bone Strength.

Sunlight Exposure may Reduce Cholesterol and Prevent Heart Attacks and Stroke— Better Than Statin Drugs?

Ovarian Cancer is Much More Common in Northern States Than in Southern States. Is Sunlight Exposure and Vitamin D the Answer?

Multiple Sclerosis is Virtually Non-existent Among People Living at the Equator. Is Sunlight Exposure the Protective Factor?

Colon Cancer Risk is Predicted by Lack of Exposure to Sunlight.

A History of Skin Cancer Correlates to a <u>Lower</u> Risk of Developing Many Major Diseases.

Sunscreens may be Causing Melanoma; as Sunscreen use has Increased by 1800%, Melanoma Risk has Tripled.

Sunscreens Fail to Protect Against UVA Light; Manufacturers Face Lawsuit for Making False Statements about their Products.

Eighty Percent of Type-1 Diabetes in Children May be Prevented by Vitamin D Supplementation. Regular Sunlight Exposure Predicts Lower Risk of Lymphoma.

High Sunlight Exposure Reduces the Risk of 18-20 Major Cancers.

Five People Leave Wheelchairs After Six Weeks of Vitamin D Therapy.

The use of Sunlight Exposure and Ultraviolet Light from Tanning Beds may Reduce Chronic Pain and Increase Muscle Strength.

The USA Economic Burden Due to Inadequate Exposure to Sunlight, as Well as Lack of Vitamin D Supplementation, is Estimated at $200 billion in direct costs and another $400 billion in indirect costs.

Melanoma Survival is Greater Among Those who receive the Greatest Sunlight Exposure.

Sunlight May be the Best Antifungal, Antibiotic and Antiseptic.

Immune System Function May be Profoundly Improved by Treatment with Vitamin D.

So why did you miss these headlines? Could it be because they were never written even though the research upon which each "headline" is based was reported in mainstream scientific journals? If similar good news about a commercial drug were reported, that news would be emblazoned across the front pages of the nation's newspapers, featured in the health segments of television and radio news reports and prominently displayed in popular magazines.

Assuredly, there are those who prefer that this information not be made public; they make their livings by promoting the ridiculous anti-sun sentiment that is prevalent today. Nonetheless, the truth will be told. Many scientists are demanding it, many writers will publish it, many web sites will display it, and a spate of new research will continually confirm it. ***Sunlight, used correctly, is not only good for the human being; IT IS ESSENTIAL TO HEALTH.*** There is more to sunlight than skin cancer, and most skin cancer can be prevented by proper nutrition. Read on to find out exactly how SOLAR POWER—the power of the sun and vitamin D—can reduce depression, cancer, heart disease, osteoporosis, diabetes, insomnia, muscle weakness, multiple sclerosis, chronic pain and numerous other maladies.

Introduction

*"Do not anticipate trouble, or worry about what may
never happen. Keep in the sunlight."*
Benjamin Franklin

Perhaps there *is* something new under the sun—an appreciation that
sunlight is one of the greatest weapons in the arsenal against diseases
ranging from cancer to depression to the common cold. Sunlight and its
corollary, vitamin D, form Solar Power, a one-two punch that may enhance
human health more than any other factor, with the possible exceptions of
natural, nutritious foods and regular exercise. The value of sunlight was
understood by ancient societies, and many of them worshipped the sun as
a God. Sunlight exposure was used to cure diseases throughout much of
history and continued until the advent of antibiotics. Today we know that
the sun controls weather patterns, enables plant growth and keeps Earth in
orbit. Without the sun, life would shortly cease to exist.

Regrettably, the idea of sunlight as the giver of life and health has
changed. Sunlight has been pronounced "Public Enemy Number One"
by the multimillion-dollar sunscreen industry in complicity with a group
of misguided health professionals. This nonsense has produced the
current sun phobia and is taking an incalculable toll on health. The habit
of avoiding sunlight has caused vast emotional and physical suffering,
shortened human life, decreased productivity and increased the economic
burden to the individual and society for so-called "health care."

To those medical professionals who parrot the official doctrine of the
sunscreen manufacturers, and to anyone who has been deceived by anti-
sun propaganda, my pro-sun statements seem like heresy. This book,
however, is based on the best scientific research regarding sunlight,
vitamin D and disease. It will persuade the open-minded reader that the
public has been misled, and that the anti-sun groups are, as Dr. Michael
Holick says, "scaring the daylights out of people in order to scare them out
of the daylight."

The irrational advice to avoid the sun may prevent some non-lethal skin
cancers, but the increased health burden it causes costs hundreds of billions
of dollars worldwide and profoundly increases deaths from the major
internal cancers. Anti-sun propaganda is responsible for millions more

deaths and disabilities from multiple sclerosis, arthritis, osteomalacia, osteoporosis, heart disease, chronic pain, flu, dental disease and others maladies. And these statements are not just opinions; research reported in the best scientific journals confirms them. You will see that nearly every claim made in this book has one or more footnotes that refer to the scientific literature where it is verified. If it were not for such documentation, this book would be nothing more than a series of unconfirmed health opinions in a field already replete with unverified beliefs.

So how did I develop an interest in sunlight as a basic component of human health? The background follows:

Until the age of thirty-five, too much of my life was spent fighting flu and colds. My first head cold would occur in autumn around mid-November and would keep me in bed two or three days. The illness would then subside over several weeks. Then I would contract the flu that was currently making the rounds. These ailments took a toll on my school work and social life. My friends would suffer one cold in a year; I was blessed with up to half a dozen. Winter was an unhappy time, and I dreamed of leaving the cold weather of the central Nevada and Utah border and moving to warmer climes. My winter experiences convinced me that colds and flu were caused by the weather. This, of course, was not true—a fact that didn't occur to me until years later.

Finally, the summer would arrive. The sun blazed from dawn to dusk and I soaked it up. The work on our ranch was intense, and the days were long, starting with morning feeding of animals followed by irrigating, hauling hay and performing other tasks that were part of ranch life. Nevertheless, I loved the sun and it made the work worthwhile. Whenever possible, my shirt came off, and because of my deep tan, my friends called me "brown man." Those were halcyon days, though I would have preferred less work. Nevertheless, I was happy and healthy and enjoyed a vigor that was lacking in winter.

The ranch meals were ample, delicious and unhealthful: bacon and eggs, steak or lamb chops for breakfast along with rich, whole raw milk, hash-brown potatoes fried in animal fat and biscuits slathered with butter and jam. Lunch was more of the same, but we added a few fresh vegetables and fruit. For dinner, we ate the staple of the rancher's diet: rich brown gravy and mashed potatoes, followed by my mother's desserts. Our diet was laden with fat, sugar and cholesterol, yet my illnesses occurred only during winter. I was never sick when I was regularly exposed to summer sunlight. I decided very young that summer was my "healthful season."

Later, during study for my profession as a health resort owner, I began to peruse medical and nutritional journals and became convinced that my diet, as then constituted, would ultimately kill me. After reading impactful books by Nathan Pritikin and Dr. John McDougall, I transitioned to a whole-food, plant-based diet, and voila! My cold and flu episodes decreased to one or two per year and didn't even keep me from work. Later, as I began to eat more colorful vegetables and fruits, I could go all year with only a sniffle or two. But one thought was always present: in spite of the previous atrocious diet, I had never been ill under the sun. It seemed that sunlight negated the deleterious effects of bad diet, at least as far as respiratory illnesses were concerned.

About 1980, I was driving and 'radio-station surfing" to find some music to my liking, and I serendipitously happened onto an interview with Zane Kime, a California physician. He cogently explained that sunlight was essential to health, and that the advice to avoid the sun was dangerous. I immediately pulled over and wrote down the name of his book: *Sunlight Could Save your Life*. After reading it, I never again feared the sun. It was one of those fortuitous occurrences that sporadically arrive to impact one's life, and I am grateful to Dr. Kime and others who bucked the trend and did the research proving sunlight is essential to health.

The purpose of this book is to present the positive side of the sunlight story—a side hidden under an avalanche of negative press and a torrent of misinformation. Deceit about sunlight is responsible for reducing the quality of life for many individuals, and dark-skinned people are literally being killed by those who disseminate the falsehoods.

The reader will note that I frequently delve into nutrition and exercise, which go hand in hand with good habits of sunlight exposure and vitamin D repletion. The nutrition information may seem redundant, as it is mentioned in several chapters. The reason for the repetition is that some people may not read the chapters that do not relate to their particular interest and may fail to appreciate the importance of nutrition and exercise if some discussion were not contained in each chapter. The book, of course, is best read cover to cover.

My wife, Vicki, and I regularly take sun vacations in winter and hike outdoors and sunbathe in summer. Our health and mental outlook has improved immensely. We are careful not to burn, and advise all who read this book to exercise caution when sunbathing or otherwise enjoying the sun.

Now let's delve into the world of Solar Power, vitamin D and human health. May your reading be enlightening!

SECTION 1

Background Material

The discussions in this section present the basics of sunlight intensity and its relationship to skin cancers and should develop an appreciation of the sun's benefits for disease prevention. For those who would rather "cut to the chase" in terms of health concerns, please refer to the table of contents for the chapters dealing with specific health issues. However, for those who want to know the "why" as well as the "how," this first section will be of great interest.

Chapter 1

Sunlight, vitamin D and health: history and function

Sunshine is a marvelous health-giving and healing power in the world. While sunshine is death to disease-producing agencies, it is life and health to all natural forms of life. Sit in the sun, recline in the sun, walk on the sunny side of the street, avoid parasols, and ever recognize the sun as a friend and not an enemy, a promoter of health, and a destroyer of disease.

Frederick M. Rossiter, M.D. The Practical Guide to Health, 1913

Types of light pertinent to this discussion

To understand the history and function of vitamin D (whose production is stimulated by sunlight), you should know the differences among the different types of ultraviolet light:

1. ***Ultraviolet light (UV)*** is a light that is invisible because its wavelength is shorter than the violet part of the sunlight spectrum. UV is available year round in the tropics and during part of the year farther north and south. UV is also produced by sunlamps. There are three main varieties of UV: UVA, UVB and UVC. UV wavelengths are measured in nanometers (one billionth of a meter).

   a. ***UVA*** has a wavelength of 320-400 nanometers and when contacting the skin can penetrate beyond the outer layer (epidermis) into a layer called the ***dermis***. UVA does not stimulate vitamin D production.

   b. ***UVB*** light has a wavelength of 280-320 nanometers and penetrates only the epidermis when it contacts the skin. UVB stimulates the skin, which produces vitamin D.

   c. ***UVC*** light has a wavelength of 200-280 nanometers and is filtered out by the Earth's outer atmosphere.

A brief history of life-sustaining vitamin D—the sunshine vitamin

As early as the mid-seventeenth century, two scientists working independently of each other identified the disease called rickets[1-2] and observed that it occurred among children who were seldom exposed to sunlight. This illness was characterized by defective bone growth and horribly deformed bodies. By the twentieth century it was well established that rickets had something to do with lack of sunlight. It was not until 1919-1921, however, that Sir Edward Mellanby's studies on dogs helped define the substance whose absence caused rickets.[3-4] His dogs were fed only oatmeal, and they were raised without any exposure to sunlight, which caused them to develop the disease. By observing the effects of different diets, Mellanby determined that if they lacked a particular substance, rickets developed. He found that the substance was contained in cod liver oil, which he stated was an effective anti-rickets agent; the dogs were cured by adding cod liver oil to their diets. (Please note: Cod liver oil is not an ideal form of vitamin D supplementation; it may lead to osteoporosis due to its excessive vitamin A concentration.)[112]

Shortly afterward, Dr. E.V. McCollum and his team performed experiments on the substance they thought was a "fat- soluble vitamin" and differentiated it from vitamin A.[5] They had found the substance that "promotes calcium deposition" and named it "vitamin D," which was a mistake since it is not a vitamin, but the name stuck. A year later, a Dr H. Goldblatt and his team exposed cholesterol in skin to ultraviolet light and produced the exact substance that had been labeled a fat soluble vitamin.[6] Nearly simultaneously, Dr. A. Hess performed an experiment in which he exposed animal skin to ultraviolet (UV) light and then fed it to sunlight-deprived rats. The rats were completely protected from rickets.[7] Another researcher, Dr H. Steenbock, discovered that irradiating various foods with UV from sunlamps caused those foods to have anti-rickets properties.[8,9] This discovery led to the irradiation of foods, especially milk, as a means of preventing rickets. However, it was later discovered that vitamin D could be synthesized in large quantities by other methods at fraction of the cost of irradiating foods—a method that sometimes caused spoilage.[10]

In the 1930's, the chemical structure of vitamin D was established by German scientists, and they proved that the substance in cod liver oil was vitamin D.[11-12] Vitamin D was then established as a prohormone—a substance that is later converted into an active hormone. Though the interest in vitamin D's power was originally limited to the prevention and treatment of rickets, it would later be found that this substance had myriad other benefits.

In the 1970s several researchers, including Michael Holick, isolated and identified the hormone form of vitamin D.[13] It was discovered that both dietary vitamin D and vitamin D produced by the skin in response to sunlight are stored in the liver. They found that when stored vitamin D is needed, the liver releases it to the kidney, which converts it into the hormone form. Later on Dr. Holick realized that really only a very small quantity of the activated hormone form, known as 1,25-vitamin D or *calcitriol*, was produced in the kidney. ***It is important to understand that calcitriol is the only form that produces benefits. The stored form of vitamin D has no effect until it is converted to calcitriol.***

Dr. Holick states that "Until the mid-1990's it was believed that the kidneys made the body's entire supply of activated vitamin D." The next major discovery was that cells throughout the body had the ability to produce calcitriol. This was exceptionally important, as the amount of calcitriol produced by the kidneys is quite small and could not possibly have produced the beneficial effects on cancer, heart disease, bone health and diabetes that Dr, Holick had observed. The finding that cells throughout the body could produce their own calcitriol—provided there was sufficient stored vitamin D in the liver—established the importance of a ready supply of stored vitamin D.

In 1980, Doctors Cedric and Frank Garland observed that USA colon cancer rates were lowest in the Southwest and highest in the Northeast.[14] They were struck by the possibility that vitamin D could be the physiological means by which sunlight exposure lessened the risk of colon cancer. This seminal paper awakened the scientific community to the fact that sunlight and vitamin D might have beneficial influences on illnesses other than bone diseases. Then, in 1981, a group of Japanese researchers discovered that adding calcitriol to immature malignant leukemia cells caused the cells to normalize.[15] These findings were the watersheds that gave impetus to the study of the relationship of sunlight and vitamin D to internal cancers. From that time there has been an increased interest in researching the effects of vitamin D on other illnesses. An even greater impetus was given to the sunlight movement in 1993 by Dr Gordon Ainsleigh[113] and again in 2002 by Dr. William Grant;[114] both published important papers showing a greatly decreased death rate from cancer associated with UVB exposure.

The results of the above-mentioned explosion in research will be, to a great extent, the subject of the remainder of this book. It is now established that vitamin D has beneficial influences on osteoporosis,[16] diabetes,[17] muscle strength,[18] gum and dental health,[19-20] prostate cancer,[21] colon cancer,[22] lung cancer,[23] breast cancer,[24] lymphoma,[25] depression,[26] PMS,[27] kidney disease,[28] heart disease,[29] multiple sclerosis,[30] arthritis,[31] pain,[32] flu and colds,[94] pre-eclampsia,[95] anaphlaxis[96] and possibly obesity,[33] as well as many others.

Since science has now established the benefits of vitamin D, why then would so many physicians—and the general public—recoil in fear from the thought of letting the sunlight touch their bodies? After all, when it contacts our skin, it produces large quantities of this marvelous prohormone.

How did the sunlight so quickly change from friend to foe? A brief history of the rise and fall of sunlight as therapy for disease (heliotherapy)

Whereas vitamin D has been accepted as absolutely essential to human health, the source that stimulates its production (sunlight) certainly has been condemned, at least for the past forty years. Sunlight, in the view of many misguided health professionals and the patients they serve, is an enemy. Because of the injudicious (and in some cases deliberate) attack on sunlight, hundreds of thousands of people each year are afflicted with a host of completely avoidable diseases. These victims have vitamin D-depleted bodies because they live in sunless homes and work in sunless offices. As shown in the cartoon, we have become, for the first time in human history, true cave men. Our caves are our homes and offices. And when we do go outside, we dutifully cover ourselves with clothing and pour sunscreen on any exposed areas. Unfortunately, sunscreens block up to 99.9% of vitamin D production by the skin in response to sunlight.[34]

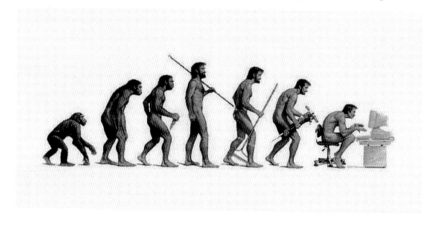

How did this vilification of sunlight develop? Following is a brief history of sunlight and health.

Part of the following history of sunlight therapy is a compendium of Dr. John Fielder's exceptionally well-written paper, *History of Heliotherapy*.[35] From this history, one easily sees that the present disparagement of sunlight exposure contrasts starkly with the acceptance sunlight therapy enjoyed in the past.

Many ancient peoples were sunbathers. The Egyptians, Babylonians, and Assyrians had sun gardens and gave the sun the status of a god. Hippocrates, the Greek physician known as the "father of medicine," recommended sunbathing and had his own large solarium—an enclosed area for sunning. This was also true of the ancient Romans, whose thermae (hot tubs and baths) were equipped with solaria. The Roman writer Pliny wrote that "the sun is the best remedy."

In the early 19th Century, scientists began to experiment with sunlight as a remedy and were so impressed with the results that they attempted to build a new system of therapeutics based on heliotherapy. In 1857 Madame Duhamel of France exposed children with TB to sunshine because it hastened their recovery. Many doctors used heliotherapy with great success, and as Dr. Fielder states, "As a general rule, the experience of all the Hygienists in their use of sunbathing was so successful that all question of doubt as to its place in the Hygienic System was ensured."

Madame Duhamel was correct about sunbathing healing tuberculosis (TB). Later on a disillusioned physician, Dr. Rollier, gave up a promising surgical practice and moved to the mountains of the Swiss countryside to practice medicine there. However, he discovered that the people needed little help, as they were seldom sick. People were always telling him, *"Where the sun is, the doctor ain't* [sic]." In fact, Dr. Rollier's fiancée had TB and would have died without intervention. He brought her to the Alpine area, exposed her regularly to sunshine, and she completely recovered. Dr. Rollier opened a sanatorium in 1903 that was really just an extremely large solarium with patient living quarters. *There were 2,167 patients under Dr. Rollier's care for TB following World War One. Of these, 1,746 completely recovered their health.* Only those in the most advanced stages of the disease failed to recover.

In 1895, Dr. Niels Finsen made use of the first artificial UV light in treating patients with a particularly virulent form of TB known as lupus vulgaris (a skin disease). Though the disease was considered incurable, 41 of every 100 patients under his care recovered. Finsen's work earned the Nobel Prize in medicine in 1903.

These researchers and physicians were not alone in their observations of the therapeutic power of sunlight. In 1877, two scientists, Arthur Downes and Thomas Blunt, discovered that sunlight was bactericidal. In 1890, the German microbiologist Robert Koch (who had isolated and described the tuberculosis bacterium in 1882), showed that sunlight killed TB bacteria.[36] The legendary humanitarian Florence Nightingale also observed that sunlight helped heal wounded soldiers and insisted that hospitals be constructed to allow the free entry of sunlight.[37]

For many years afterward, heliotherapy was the treatment of choice for bacterial infections. Unfortunately for heliotherapy, however, penicillin was discovered in 1928 and sulfanilamide in 1939. Sulfanilamide in particular was effective against TB, so the era of antibiotic drugs was born and heliotherapy virtually forgotten. People still loved the sun, however, and sun tanning became popular for several decades. Then, as more evidence accumulated that sunlight exposure correlated to common skin cancer, the attitude toward sunshine began to change.

Dr. Holick states, "In the 1920's it was recognized that farmers in Europe developed skin cancer on their most sun-exposed parts—their ears, face, nose, and backs of their hands.[13]" This news was the beginning of the war on sunlight. Still, there was early research that also indicated that sunlight might have anticancer properties, and *in 1932 an editorial in the British medical journal "Lancet" suggested that since sunlight was so effective in promoting health, the government should set aside public areas for nude sunbathing![86]*

In 1936 and 1937, Dr. Sigismund Peller demonstrated that solar UV radiation reduced the risk of internal cancer but not common skin cancer. In the first paper, he demonstrated that in outdoor occupations and surroundings where skin cancer was prevalent, other cancers diminished.[38] In the second paper, he showed that sailors—individuals who spent long hours in the sun—had about eight times the expected common skin cancer rate, but only about 40% the expected rate of deadly internal cancers.[39] Peller was impressed with the reduced mortality from deadly cancers experienced by those who had previously had skin cancers—cancers which were easily removable or "cured." He felt he had found the answer to reducing deadly cancers by 60%, but he erroneously concluded that skin cancer itself, rather than sunlight, triggered a protective mechanism that prevented the deadly internal cancers. *He went so far as to suggest that UV light be used to induce skin cancer as a method of vaccination to prevent internal cancers!* The name of his first paper was "*Carcinogenesis as a means of reducing cancer mortality.*" His methods would probably have worked, but it would have been trading a greater evil for a lesser evil—something that is absolutely unnecessary. His methods would have indeed saved many lives from major cancer while creating a pandemic of skin cancer. He was, however, completely wrong about immunity; skin cancer provides no immunity to major cancers. But, as we shall see, sunlight and vitamin D do indeed lessen the rate of major internal cancers, and that is what Peller was really observing.

In 1941, Dr. Frank Apperley stated that Peller was wrong to suggest inducing skin cancer as a method of preventing the more deadly cancers.[40] Apperley's research showed that it was sunlight—not skin cancer—that reduced the risk of the deadly caners. He studied cancer incidence at different latitudes and demonstrated the following: North American death rates for major cancers among the inhabitants of cities between 30° and 40° north latitude were 85% higher than death rates among inhabitants of cities between 10° and 30°; inhabitants of cities between 40° and 50° north latitude had cancer death rates 118% higher than those between 10° and 30°; inhabitants between 50° and 60° had death rates from internal cancers 150% higher than those between 10° and 30°. The following chart shows Apperley's findings:

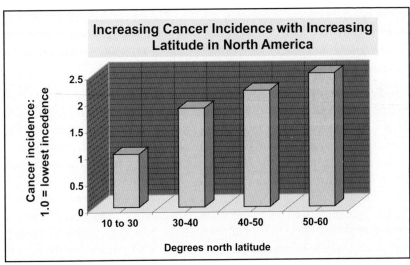

Apperley did not know how sunlight reduced the incidence of the major cancers, but stated, *"The presence of skin cancer is really only an occasional accompaniment of relative cancer immunity in some way related to exposure to ultraviolet light."* He suggested that a higher degree of common skin cancer was the price to be paid for the decreased death rate from the major cancers.[40] *Apperley was incorrect on that point. Dr. Homer Black's research makes clear that higher skin cancer incidence is not necessary if people make moderate changes in the quantity and type of fats they consume and eat foods rich in antioxidants* (see chapter 3). [115-117]

Apperley and Peller demonstrated sunlight's ability to reduce the incidence of the major "killer" cancers, but the fear of skin cancer began to sweep all other considerations aside, and the sunscreen industry was born. Sunscreen sales in 1972 were about $18 million per year,[41] and the total USA market for sunscreens in 2005 had climbed to $640 million a year.[42] In 1972 dollars that is equivalent to $320 million, an almost 18-fold increase. Sales increased despite the fact that **sunscreens may be responsible for increasing the deadliest of skin cancers, melanoma.**[43] The "powers of darkness" as Dr. William Grant calls them, are not easily overcome, especially when that much money is at stake.

A few thoughts about the above history and our present situation

Notwithstanding the positive research regarding sunlight exposure and disease, sunlight exposure—all else being equal—correlates with higher rates of common skin cancer. This one negative effect of sunlight exposure has formed the basis of the pernicious advice to avoid sunlight like the plague. I estimate that there are about 275 deaths prevented by higher vitamin D levels due to sunlight exposure—for every death caused by sunlight exposure. In 2005, Dr. Grant performed an analysis of cancer deaths caused by inadequate sunlight and concluded that each year in the USA 50,000–63,000 Americans die prematurely from major internal cancers caused by insufficient vitamin D.[44] And in 2008 he estimates that the USA economic burden from all diseases due to vitamin D insufficiency from inadequate exposure to solar UVB irradiance, diet, and supplements is $200 billion in direct costs and $400 billion in indirect costs.[120] Others would agree. Dr. Edward Giovannucci of Harvard University suggests that sunlight might prevent 30 deaths for each one caused by skin cancer.[45] He further stated that, "I would challenge anyone to find an area or nutrient or any factor that has such consistent anti-cancer benefits as vitamin D. The data are really quite remarkable."

Sunlight and race: Are they related?

Vitamin D is produced very slowly in dark skin. Indeed, it has been shown that light skin produces vitamin D six times more efficiently than does dark skin.[46] This slow rate of production, however, does not create a health hazard in hot, sunny climates, because exposure to sunlight is regular and lengthy, which is perfectly suited to dark skin's slow production. A *small, constant production of vitamin D over a long period of time is as good as a large production in a short time.* Hence, dark-skinned people who live in sunny climes produce adequate vitamin D for optimal health.

In northern geographical areas humans are exposed to less sunlight and in cold seasons must cover themselves with clothing. They can therefore produce vitamin D only when there is sufficient sunlight to stimulate its production in the skin, i.e. only in spring, summer and fall. A paper by Dr. Nina Jablonski and Dr. George Chaplin demonstrates that skin pigmentation is predicted accurately by latitude, with increasing latitudes correlating to lighter skin.[89] There are only a few exceptions to this rule, one being the Eskimos, who can obtain their vitamin D from fish. The farther north the latitude, the shorter is the season for receiving vitamin D-producing sunlight (see chapter 2). These northern people do not have the luxury of receiving ample direct sunlight year around as do their neighbors to the south. They therefore need to produce sufficiently large quantities of vitamin D to supply their daily needs and in addition store a large quantity for the winter, when the sun does not stimulate its production. These people have light skins so they can produce more vitamin D when sunlight is available.

The rapid and large production of vitamin D in light-skinned people allows large quantities to be produced and stored during sunny seasons. During winter, those stores are depleted and by spring, the body's supply of vitamin D is low and must be replenished. The sun begins to warm the Earth and people doff their winter clothing to receive the sun's rays. In early spring at these high latitudes, ultraviolet light (UVB) is not available in the early morning, and the temperature is too cool to shed warm clothing. However, toward midday when UVB became available, the temperature warms, and they begin to remove clothing, which exposes them to both the tanning rays and vitamin D-stimulating rays. Since the sun is weak in early spring, the people are not susceptible to burning. As the season progresses toward summer, the sun's rays become more direct and capable of causing sun burn, and tans form to protect against that hazard. *A tan is not a sign of injured skin as stated by those who promote sun avoidance; it is a sign of protected skin.*[98]

Then, as the sunlight subsides during the late summer and fall, the tan become lighter, so their skin "soaks up" as much UVB as possible in order to produce the maximum vitamin D achievable. As autumn comes, the early morning temperature cools, and the clothing goes back on during early-morning outdoor activity. However, at midday the temperature becomes comfortable enough to remove the warm clothes, thus ensuring that the people have the benefits of the diminishing amount of UVB. During this time of vitamin D production, the quantity produced above that needed for daily use would be stored for winter. The system is a cycle similar to that of the bees that produce honey and store it in order to live in the season when the flowers do not bloom. However, in the far north, "vitamin D winter" is several months long, and storage is not sufficient to last until the return of "vitamin D summer." Dr. Grant points out that the half-life storage time for vitamin D is only one to two months, so it is necessary for people in the very far north, such as the Inuit, to obtain a sustained source of vitamin D from fish and sea mammals. [87]

I have observed the working of this system in my own body. My tan starts light in spring and becomes dark in summer. I am wont to sunbathe every day that weather permits in our southern Utah area. It is far too hot to sunbathe for long periods at midday in summer, so I usually expose my body for only twenty minutes on each side at midday. During late autumn, mornings become uncomfortably cool, and midday sunbathing is comfortable. My total exposure to midday sunlight in that season is usually more than an hour. As winter approaches, my skin gradually loses its deep color. Obviously, my body is trying to absorb as much as possible of the tenuous UVB that remains before winter.

It is an excellent system, but we subvert it with our ill-advised avoidance of sunlight. Neither I nor anyone I know has developed cancer by following such a routine. It is ludicrous to frighten the entire populace out of enjoying the sunlight and to advise them to wear strong 'protection" whenever they venture outside. Dr. Grant's research[44] indicates that such policies create a multi-billion-dollar health disaster in the USA. A British PhD, Oliver Gillie, is also concerned about the disastrous effects of sunlight deprivation among people who live in northern climes, particularly in Britain where the sky is overcast a great deal of the time, even in the summer.[47] Such counterproductive health policies are nonsense, especially for dark-skinned individuals. It is well known that blacks in the USA have much higher rates of diabetes, high blood pressure and most internal cancers than do whites. Vitamin D helps prevent many of these maladies. Since the skin of black people requires six times more sunlight exposure to produce vitamin D, is it rational to advise them to avoid the sun and slather on sunscreen? *It is nearly impossible for dark-skinned people to produce enough vitamin D from sunlight in high-latitude countries. When USA white and black women are compared for vitamin D levels, black women are ten times more likely to be vitamin D deficient![48]* (See following graph) In one interesting piece of research on patients in Minneapolis, Minnesota (45 degrees north latitude) with chronic pain, it was found that 100% of African Americans, American Indians, East Africans and Hispanics were vitamin D deficient.[49] Dark-skinned people living in northern latitudes need supplementation with vitamin D3.

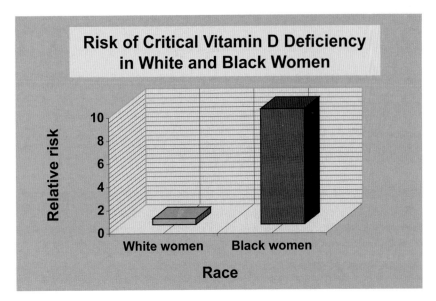

Risk of Critical Vitamin D Deficiency in White and Black Women

Relative risk (y-axis: 0, 2, 4, 6, 8, 10)

Race (x-axis: White women, Black women)

Vitamin D sources in our modern world

Sunlight exposure is the most natural way to ensure adequate vitamin D levels. However, a large area of skin must be exposed. ***Some argue that sufficient vitamin D is produced by exposing only the face and arms, but this is not true!*** For example, a Hawaii investigation established that even among people who work outdoors in semi-tropical sun, there is a high incidence of vitamin D deficiency.[97] The same is true of people living in Southern Arizona, with 55.5% of blacks, 37.6% of Hispanics and 22% of whites having serum levels below 20 ng/ml.[118]

Some fish are a source of dietary vitamin D, and most tanning beds also stimulate its production in skin. For modern people in the far north who choose not to eat fish, a tanning bed could be a life saver. Tanning beds can produce up to 10,000 IU of vitamin D in only eight or nine minutes.[88] Supplementation is another source, but always supplement with vitamin D3. Vitamin D2 is generally considered less effective than D3,[90,109,110] although one study showed equal effectiveness.[111] D2 is also not produced naturally in the body; and while it is equally effective in raising blood levels of vitamin D, when supplementation is discontinued, those levels diminish much more rapidly than when D3 is used.[110]

Vitamin D testing

Ideally, everyone should get a blood test for 25(OH)D, ***the only valid test for vitamin D level or status.*** This is especially true for dark-skinned people who are living in northern areas and for anyone who lives and works indoors and makes no concerted effort to sunbathe. In addition, those who neither supplement their diets with vitamin D, nor eat oily fish like salmon, may be deficient in vitamin D if they receive little unblocked sunlight exposure. Blood levels of vitamin D are usually given in <u>nanograms per milliliter</u> (ng/ml) or <u>nanomoles per liter</u> (nmol/l). A millimeter (ml) is one thousandth of a liter, and a nanogram (ng) is one billionth of a gram. For the purposes of this book, we will use only ng/ml to express vitamin D levels; but for those who may see vitamin D levels expressed in nmol/L, here is a conversion table:

1. **1ng/ml is equal to 2.5 nmol/l.**
2. **1 nmol/l is equal to 0.4 ng/ml.**
3. **To convert ng/ml to nmol/l, multiply by 2.5.**
4. **To convert nmol/l to ng/ml, multiply by 0.4.**

In 2005, Doctors William Grant and Michael Holick reviewed the research and made the following assessments of serum (blood) vitamin D levels:[50]

1. **Levels less than 20 ng/ml were considered *deficient* (extremely low).**
2. **Levels between 21-32 ng/ml were considered *insufficient* (too low for good health).**
3. **Levels between 33-100 ng/ml were considered *sufficient* (conducive to good health).**
4. **A level between 54-90 ng/ml was typical of residents of sunny countries.**
5. **Levels greater than 100 ng/ml were considered excessive.**
6. **Levels greater than 150 ng/ml were considered toxic (detrimental to health).**

Currently, however, 40 ng/ml is thought to be the cutoff point for the minimal healthful level of vitamin D. (See Dr. Hollis and colleagues' research below.)

Deplorably, until recently lab reports showed levels less than 10 ng/ml (severely deficient) to be normal. These levels had been established as normal because they were sufficient to prevent (barely) two bone diseases: rickets and osteomalacia. However, such levels are not nearly adequate to prevent cancer, osteoporosis or other degenerative diseases. Often, nutrient levels are assessed as optimal when they are barely adequate to prevent the most obvious symptoms of certain terrible diseases. This is known as the "lowest observable adverse effect level (LOAEL)," and anything above that level is mistakenly thought to be desirable. As you will see later in this book, the LOAEL for vitamin D may be as little as one-tenth the optimal level for preventing other diseases.

How prevalent is vitamin D deficiency?

A study done on Boston adolescents revealed that nearly one in four was vitamin D deficient. About 14% were severely deficient, having blood levels of vitamin D lower than 8 ng/ml (20 nmol/L).[51] *And a study of black teenagers (mostly girls) in 14 American cities showed that the average vitamin D level was only about 8 ng/ml (dangerously low) and that at least 87% were deficient.* [93] Another investigation showed that nearly all non-white girls in an inner city school were severely deficient.[107] Dr. David Hanley of The University of Calgary in Alberta, Canada, stated that if a level of vitamin D greater than 32 ng/ml is the cutoff point for good health, then "virtually 100% of the people are vitamin-D deficient at least part of the year"[52-53] However, Dr. Reinhold Vieth has reported research indicating that people over 70 years old may need a blood level of 40 ng/ml to hold parathyroid hormone (PTH) at proper levels.[54] When vitamin D levels are too low, PTH increases and triggers bone loss (see chapter 10). Dr. Bruce Hollis reported that when considering markers for vitamin D sufficiency such as the level at which PTH begins to increase, a minimum level of 32 ng/ml is absolutely necessary.[55]

However, Dr. Hollis and his colleagues later performed research in which they determined that no circulating vitamin D3 can be measured in the blood until 25(OH)D levels are greater than 40-50 ng/ml.[119] This means that all vitamin D3 is used by the tissues to make 25(OH)D until the level is greater than 40-50. At that point, vitamin D3 begins to be measurable, meaning that the tissues are no longer so "hungry" for D3 that they use up every molecule. *Therefore, the optimal level is somewhere over 50.* Dr. John Cannell and I, in researching our forthcoming book on vitamin D and athletics, have found that athletic performance peaks at about 50-60, which would corroborate Dr. Hollis' assessment.

In a 2005 study, researchers looked at data from the third National Health and Nutrition Examination Survey (H3) and determined that "Serum levels of 25(OH) D3 (vitamin D) are below the recommended levels for a large portion of the general adult population and in most minorities."[56] The assessment used 28ng/ml as the adequate level of vitamin D. The assessment was done on adults eighteen years of age and older. The following results were obtained:

1. **Women had an average level of 28.4 ng/ml.**
2. **Men had an average level of 31.5 ng/ml.**
3. **White women had an average level of 30.4 ng/ml.**
4. **White men had an average level of 33.2 ng/ml.**
5. **Hispanic women had an average level of 22.7 ng/ml.**
6. **Hispanic men had an average level of 27.3 ng/ml.**
7. **Black women had an average level of 18.1 ng/ml.**
8. **Black men had an average level of 20.9 ng/ml.**
9. **People over 60 years old had lower levels than younger people (18-59).**

The only group that averaged slightly above the minimum recommended by Dr. Hollis was white men. And considering that these figures are averages, it is likely that just slightly less than half of white men are also insufficient. Vitamin D deficiency is a pandemic, but one that could be resolved by a change in national health policies regarding sunlight exposure. The NHANES III assessment, of course, is based on a minimum vitamin D level that is already too low. If the level recommended by Grant, Holick and Hollis had been used, a higher percentage of the population would have been assessed as deficient. It is also likely that 90% of the Hispanic and black populations are deficient when the 32 ng/ml level is used as the lower level. This would be especially true in winter in the northern USA. Black Americans in that region have serum levels of vitamin D that are only half that of white Americans.[99] What is needed is a national health priority to educate dark-skinned populations to increase vitamin D levels for good health. Could it be, for example, that the generally high level of poor health among blacks and Hispanics (heart disease, diabetes, prostate and breast cancer, etc.) is primarily due to vitamin D deficiency? In later chapters, you will see that the answer is "yes!"

H3 also demonstrated that the elderly of all races are more deficient than are younger people, meaning that elderly minorities may be approaching 100% in terms of vitamin D deficiency. This graph illustrates the prevalence of vitamin D deficiency as assessed using data from H3. Bear in mind that H3 *understated* the rate of deficiency. The 70 nmol/l level used in the chart is only 28 ng/ml. *If 50 ng/ml or more is really the best level for health, it is easily seen that nearly every human being in the USA has suboptimal levels.*

Research also indicates that 85% of infants and toddlers in Boston have levels below 40, meaning that nearly 100% would be below the optimal level of 50.[123] The same is true for Canadians. In Quebec, 93% of youngsters have suboptimal levels, based on 30 ng/ml as the lowest "optimal" threshold.[122]

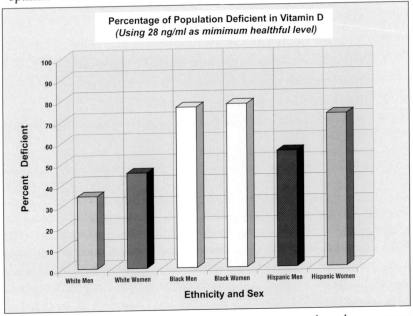

Percentage of Population Deficient in Vitamin D
(Using 28 ng/ml as mimimum healthful level)

Ethnicity and Sex

It is also important to note that among women who always wear concealing clothing, the incidence of vitamin deficiency is an astounding 99%, and the incidence of severe deficiency is 82%.[102] Other research, as yet unpublished, showed that 100% of African Canadians and 93% of Canadians of South Asian background are vitamin D deficient.[103] Four times as many babies born to these high risk women have vitamin D deficiency compared to women with lighter skin or who do not conceal their bodies from the sunlight.[105]

In view of these statistics on vitamin D deficiency, it is appropriate to mention *a study of centenarians (those 100 years old or more) showed that 99 of 104 subjects had vitamin D levels that were undetectable on the blood test, meaning that the levels were less than 2 ng/ml!*[57] The reasons for these extremely low levels are these: (1) the elderly produce far less vitamin D in response to sunlight,[100] (2) people tend to spend less time in the sun as they age, and (3) the consumption of dietary vitamin D declines as people age.[101] As you will see, throwing billions of dollars at research projects to find cures for osteoporosis, cancer, heart disease and type-2 diabetes, without addressing vitamin D deficiency, is absurd. However, there will be opposition from the powers of darkness, because such information does not sell drugs, sunscreens and medical treatments.

How much supplementation is necessary to produce optimal levels of vitamin D?

To understand vitamin D supplementation, let's first define a few terms:

1. **International Unit (IU). One IU is equal to 0.025 micrograms (mcg) of vitamin D as cholecalciferol, which is the form of vitamin D produced by the skin in response to sunlight. Or in other words, 100 IU is equal to 2.5 mcg. Most vitamin D supplements are labeled in IU's.**

2. **One microgram (mcg) is one-thousandth of a milligram (mg), which is one-thousandth of a gram.**

3. **One nanogram (ng) is one-thousandth of a microgram, or one-billionth of a gram.**

Most multivitamins contain only 200-400 IU per day—not nearly enough to maintain healthful levels. And remember that 32 ng/ml is not nearly high enough for optimal health. Maximum reductions in diseases occur around 50.

Are there toxic effects with extremely high doses of supplemental vitamin D?

Of course, maintaining optimal levels—not minimal levels—is the goal. Research indicates that no adverse effects are produced by taking 4,000 IU per day for a period of six months.[26,58] Dr. Reinhold Vieth has extensively studied the intake of vitamin D that is toxic or safe, and concluded that if there is published evidence of toxicity in adults from intake of 10,000 IU per day, he has yet to find it.[81] **Dr. Vieth also pointed out that 4,000 IU are necessary to maintain his recommended serum levels of 100 nmol/l (40 ng/ml), and he reasons that since in Caucasians 10,000 IU per day are easily produced by full-body exposure to sun in about twenty minutes, 10,000 IU of supplemental vitamin D3 should be quite safe. His logic is difficult to refute.** He and his colleagues also showed that 4,000 IU daily for six months considerably improved the wellbeing scores (measured as elevated mood, happiness, etc.) of those taking it, and that there was no adverse influence on serum calcium levels (which has been speculated by others).[82] Since no adverse effects are observed at 10,000 IU per day produced in response to sunlight, 4,000 IU or more per day is a safe supplemental intake for adults. However, you should consult a physician before deciding on a safe dosage. Children's smaller bodies need smaller quantities of vitamin D, and the level of supplementation at which any toxicity might occur would be lower. Conversely, large individuals need to take more vitamin D.[12]

As early as 1963 it was reported that vitamin D supplementation in excess of the recommended dosage might cause hypercalcemia—an excessively high concentration of calcium in the blood—in infants.[59] Usually, however, it requires massive doses to cause toxic reactions, and these doses would not occur in normal supplementation. One writer suggests that 10,000 IU per kilogram (2.2 pounds) of weight per day during pregnancy may cause birth defects; an intake of 1,000 to 4,000 IU/day may cause toxicity in infants; in children 10,000 IU/day for four months or 200,000 IU/day for two weeks is toxic, and 100,000 IU/day will cause toxic reactions in adults within a few weeks of months.[60] Massive doses of vitamin D have been used as a rodenticide (rodent poison), and studies done on animals indicate that 20,000 IU *per kilogram per day* cause signs of toxicity. This would be equivalent to a 150 pound woman taking 1,363,363 IU per day! Research performed on dogs indicated that a dose of 3,520,000 IU per kilogram would kill half of the animals.[61] *Dr. John Cannell states that this dosage of vitamin D would be about the equivalent of 440,000 (400 IU) vitamin capsules per day.*[62] Who even thinks up this research? No one should be surprised that such a ridiculously large amount of vitamin D is toxic! *Taking such high doses is crass stupidity. It would be akin to eating a box of salt daily because a few milligrams had been established as being essential for health; it would kill you!* Deficiency is thousands of times more likely than excess. *As Dr. Vieth points out, "Worrying about vitamin D toxicity is like worrying about drowning when you are dying of thirst."*[82] He and his colleagues have expressed frustration with the currently recommended intakes of vitamin D and stated that there is a dire need to recommend intakes that are effective in reducing disease.[106] That is not surprising, since Dr. Vieth established in 1999 that toxic levels causing hypercalcemia (excessive blood levels of calcium) were not reached with a dose less than 40,000 IU daily.[121]

One troubling finding is the possibility that both high and low blood vitamin D levels relate to a higher incidence of prostate cancer.[63] The study looked at subjects from Nordic countries and found that the optimal blood-vitamin D level was 16-24 ng/ml for best protection against prostate cancer. However, Scandinavians take cod-liver-oil supplements, and supplements from such animal sources may contain excessively high levels of vitamin A, which has been shown to cause cancer. *Here is what we do know: A study done by Dr. Esther John and her colleagues assessed sunlight exposure among men living in the San Francisco Bay area and correlated that exposure to the incidence of prostate cancer. Those who received the greatest sunlight exposure had a 49% reduction in prostate cancer compared to those who received the least.*[64] There is little doubt that those receiving the most sunlight also have the highest vitamin D levels, so there is a disparity in these two studies. Several additional studies cited in chapter 8 show that increasing sunlight exposure correlates with reduced rates of prostate cancer.

It is simple to conclude that the best way to receive vitamin D is by sunlight or tanning-bed exposure. No research has ever indicated a toxic effect from the vitamin D produced by the skin in response to ultraviolet B light (UVB).[74] Yet the skin, in response to peak summer sunlight, can produce and release up to 20,000 IU in a period of only 10-15 minutes.[55] Since sunlight exposure also destroys vitamin D when it reaches excessive levels, long-term exposure does not create excessive vitamin D. Those levels are self-adjusting and self-limiting. Whether a person is exposed to thirty minutes or eight hours of direct equatorial sunlight, the quantity of vitamin D produced is the same.[73] It is far more efficient to expose one's skin to the appropriate quantities of sunlight than to rely on taking supplements. However, supplements *are necessary* for those who cannot access the sun or a tanning bed or for those who choose not to use those methods. Remember it is unlikely that even barely adequate blood levels of vitamin D will be achieved with anything less than 1,000 IU per day.[50]

Tanning beds and vitamin D production

The use of tanning beds is an excellent way to increase vitamin D content in the blood. Early research on older model beds demonstrated that a ten-minute session stimulated the skin to produce 2000 to 4,000 units of vitamin D, and a full session (around fifteen minutes) that caused minimal pinkness of the skin produced about 15,000 IU.[77-78] However, Robert Wagner and Dr. Grant recently tested a modern bed and informed me that in one minute, the upper lights produced 2,300 IU and the lower lights produced 1,300 IU. He also stated that his figures would extrapolate to 10,000 IU in six minutes and as much as 15,000 IU in ten minutes.[88] Now that's efficiency! What a boon such a tanning bed would be to dark-skinned Americans, who take longer to produce vitamin D. Even if it took 40 minutes to produce the same quantity of vitamin D, that would be a good investment in time.

In a study that compared tanning bed users to non-users, weekly users had a 90% greater concentration of serum vitamin D[65] and significantly greater bone density than non-users. Chapter 10 establishes UVB exposure as an excellent way to check the osteoporosis pandemic. Note that there is a proper ratio of UVA to UVB light that should be emitted by a tanning bed: three to five percent UVB and 95-97 percent UVA.[50,65] Of course, due to the "sunscare" campaign, many people worry about melanoma. Interestingly, two studies in 2004 and in 2005 showed very little association between tanning bed use and melanoma.[75,76] In chapter 17, this is fully discussed.

Vitamin D supplements: how much is necessary?

One investigation showed that vitamin D supplements given to postmenopausal black women were ineffective in either preventing or reversing bone loss.[66] Forty percent of the women studied did not reach a level of 35 ng/ml after supplementation, so it is no wonder that the supplementation did not help. However, Dr. Grant has informed me that the likely reasons for these findings are that (1) black women in general have very low levels of vitamin D. (2) black women typically have high percentages of body fat, which absorbs vitamin D and prevents it from acting on other areas of the body. Both factors indicate a higher supplementation requirement to make a difference. In fact, supplementation with 4,000 IU per day is needed to achieve vitamin D levels of 40 ng/ml.[108] Could it be that black women need 6,000-10,000 IU per day for sufficiently high blood levels to prevent bone loss? The idea is fertile ground for further research. Chapter 10 shows that in most studies, supplements do indeed help prevent osteoporosis.

Supplementing vitamin D by nursing mothers helps increase vitamin D to desirable levels in their breast-fed infants. *One study showed that forty-six percent of mothers and eighty percent of infants had serum vitamin D levels below 25 nmol/L (10 ng/ml).[68] That level indicates severe deficiency.* The American Academy of Pediatrics now recommends supplementing vitamin D in all breastfed infants, stating that "exclusively breastfed infants are at increased risk of vitamin D deficiency and rickets.[69]" *Of course, this is not an indictment of breast milk, as it is impossible for human breast milk to contain enough vitamin D if the mother is deficient.* A supplement of at least 4,000 IU of daily is necessary to increase blood vitamin D in infants to healthful levels (in 90 days).[70] Another study shows that during wintertime, when vitamin D levels are low, 1,000 IU daily of vitamin D does little to raise levels in infants, whereas 2,000 IU brings levels to normal.[71] But was the vitamin D supplementation as beneficial as sunlight exposure? The researchers don't know. *What we do know is that a 2006 study reports that children born to mothers with low vitamin D levels during pregnancy had weaker bones at age 9.*[72] Sensible sunlight exposure for the mother and/or infant, when adequate UVB is available, is the best method to ensure sufficient vitamin D, but vitamin D supplementation is advisable when one's levels are low and UVB exposure is not available.

Dr. Robert Heaney and associates assessed the Food and Nutrition Board (FNB) recommendations for vitamin D intake and found them wanting.[84] Its recommendations for total intake—600 International Units (IU) per day—provide less than 15% of the amount required to achieve the "ideal" level of 28-32 ng/ml. The researchers stated, *"Thus, the recommendations of the FNB with respect to oral vitamin D input fall into a curious zone between irrelevance and inadequacy."* These researchers also established that 3,000-5,000 IU per day is necessary for men who have achieved healthful summer levels of vitamin D to maintain them throughout winter.[84]

Dr. Heaney and colleagues stated that taking 600 IU daily would result in severe deficiency in the elderly. Other experts suggest that the upper limit for supplementation be increased to 10,000 IU daily for those who do not get sufficient UVB exposure.[103] *However, they found no indication that supplementation above that level was toxic.* Certain medical organizations are beginning to pay attention to the research. The Canadian Pediatric Society, for example, now recommends 2,000 IU for pregnant and lactating mothers.[104] Unfortunately, the American Pediatric Society refuses to make the same recommendation. Perhaps they can't read, or perhaps dollars are involved.

Nevertheless, truth will finally push aside misinformation. As an example, *the "discovery" in modern times that vitamin D is an effective therapy for tuberculosis shows that we have come full circle; history is repeating itself.*[79-80]

Given the American population's limited sunlight exposures, it is obvious that the current recommended level of supplementation is inadequate.[85] Sunlight exposure is the best method to attain adequate levels, and among those who have optimal levels, the small quantity of recommended supplemental D does nothing to increase those levels.[84]

How does the vitamin D system work?

How does the skin produce vitamin D in response to UVB, and how does vitamin D from sunlight exposure, food or supplementation change to a potent hormone—calcitriol—that produces beneficial effects? I express appreciation to Philip Miller, MD for help in preparing this section.[92] Dr. Miller founded the Los Gatos Longevity Institute, and lectures on anti-aging medicine. For more information on Dr Miller, see the "Suggestions for further reading" section.

Here are the terms needed to understand this short discussion:

1. Vitamin D2 or ergocalciferol: a form of supplemental vitamin D. It is not the form that functions well as a supplement is not recommended.

2. Vitamin D3 or cholecalciferol: a "prohormone" form produced by the skin after sunlight exposure or taken in the diet. Vitamin D3 is the preferred form for supplementation.

3. Calcidiol or 25-hydroxycholecalciferol: this is the stored form. The liver converts D3 to calcidiol. Calcidiol the only form that should be measured in Vitamin D tests. It has a half-life of several weeks, and is also known as 25(OH)D.

4. Calcitriol or 1,25-dihydroxycholecalciferol: the active form produced in the kidney and many other tissues. It is also known as 1,25(OH)D, and has a very short half-life—only a few hours.

5. Vitamin D receptor (VDR): a hormone receptor found in most tissues. It specifically links with and binds calcitriol. Calcitriol then interacts with the tissues to produce a variety of beneficial effects.

Here are the steps through which vitamin D3 is produced and the steps through which vitamin D3 taken as food or supplements is converted to the hormone form, calcitriol.

1. **The skin contains cholesterol known as 7-dehydrocholesterol. When UVB light contacts the skin, some of the cholesterol converts to vitamin D3. Vitamin D3 also enters the blood through food or supplements.**

2. **Vitamin D3 is transported to the liver where it is further converted to calcidiol.**

3. Calcidiol is then changed to calcitriol in the kidneys and other tissues.

4. Calcitriol then binds to the vitamin D receptor (VDR) of the various tissues, where it performs its remarkable functions in enhancing human health.

5. Calcitriol works in concert with parathyroid hormone (PTH) to regulate calcium absorption and control serum calcium levels. PTH levels rise when vitamin D is insufficient, and cause loss of calcium from the bone. High PTH levels also relate closely to an increase in most of the diseases discussed in the remainder of this book. The production and use of vitamin D is represented in figure 1.

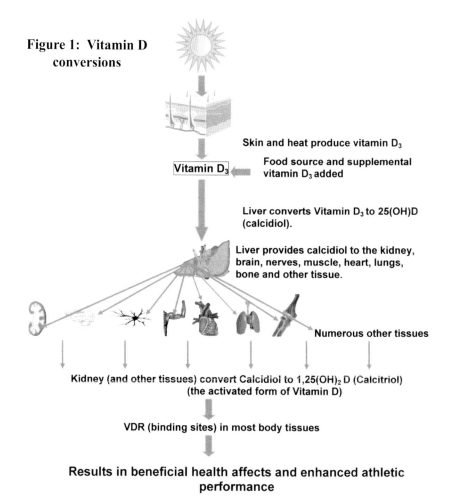

Figure 1: Vitamin D conversions

Skin and heat produce vitamin D₃

Vitamin D₃ ← Food source and supplemental vitamin D₃ added

Liver converts Vitamin D₃ to 25(OH)D (calcidiol).

Liver provides calcidiol to the kidney, brain, nerves, muscle, heart, lungs, bone and other tissue.

Numerous other tissues

Kidney (and other tissues) convert Calcidiol to 1,25(OH)₂ D (Calcitriol) (the activated form of Vitamin D)

VDR (binding sites) in most body tissues

Results in beneficial health affects and enhanced athletic performance

We have provided a history and background on vitamin D and have defined the necessary serum levels for optimal human health. We will now discuss how the intensity of sunlight in different times, seasons and geographical areas determines the quantity of vitamin D that can be produced by sunlight.

Chapter 2

Seasons and sunlight

"Whoever wishes to pursue the science of medicine in a direct manner must first investigate the seasons of the year and what occurs in them."
Hippocrates

To appreciate the healthful influence of sun exposure, we must understand the influence of the seasons on ultraviolet B light (UVB). UVB stimulates the skin to produce vitamin D, but if the sunlight is not sufficiently direct, or if it has been filtered extensively by the atmosphere, UVB will not be present in sunlight, and vitamin D will not be produced.[1]

Our planet rotates on its axis, but that axis is not parallel to the sun. It is tilted at a 23.5% angle, the tilt that causes the change in seasons (figure 1). Figure 2 shows the physical relationship of the Earth to the Sun during Earth's orbit around that fiery orb. Earth tilts toward the sun during summer in the northern hemisphere and away from the sun during winter. The exact opposite is true for the southern hemisphere. That tilt sun causes the northern hemisphere to receive more sunlight in summer. The sunlight is also more direct and less filtered than that received in winter.

Figure 1.

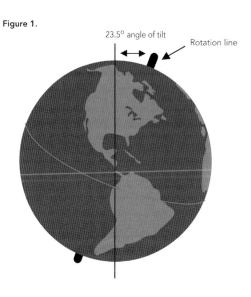

23.5° angle of tilt

Rotation line

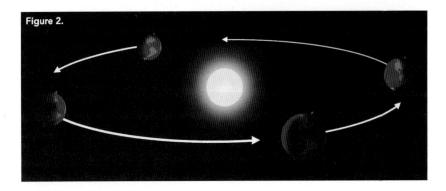

Figure 2.

In figure 3 the globe on the left represents the position of Earth in summer in the northern hemisphere and in winter in the southern hemisphere. After revolving around the sun for six months, the Earth reaches the position represented on the right. This is the position of Earth in winter in the northern hemisphere and summer in the southern hemisphere.

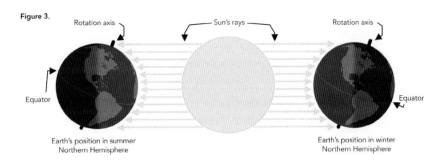

Figure 3.

Latitude lines measure the distance from the equator to the north or south poles, with the equator being represented by 0° and the poles being represented by 90°. Saint George, Utah is located at 37.1° north latitude, meaning that our little city is located 37.1° north of the equator. The Tropic of Cancer, which is the northernmost line of latitude where the sunlight hits the Earth vertically on June 21 (the first day of summer), is located at 23.5° north latitude. The Tropic of Capricorn at 23.5° south latitude is the corresponding line in the southern hemisphere where the sun is perfectly vertical on December 21 (the first day of summer there). The rays of the sun in the northern summer are still fairly direct up to about 60° north latitude (Juneau, Alaska is 58.3° north latitude). At 60° south latitude, however, it is winter because the Earth is tilted away from the Sun, making the sunlight indirect and sparse.

Figure 4. Latitudes

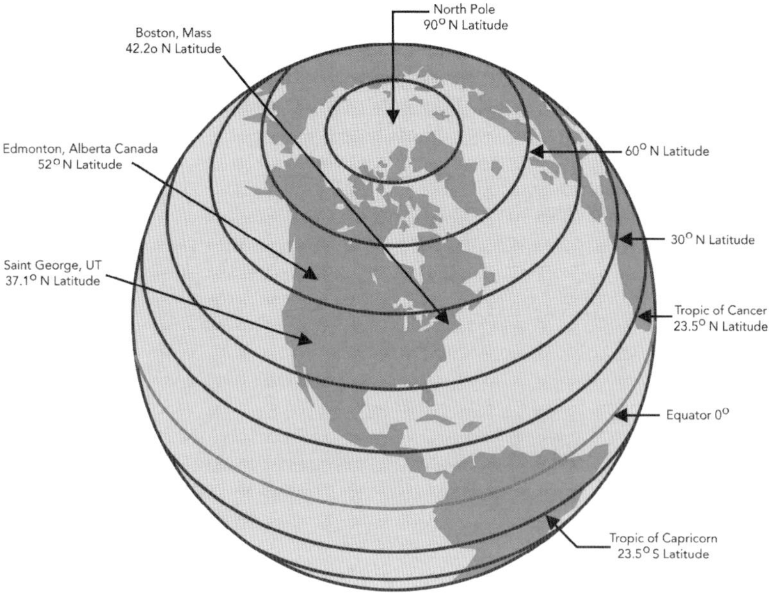

For greater understanding of this concept of "tilt," you can perform the following experiment: Concentrate a horizontal flashlight beam directly on a vertical book. You will observe a round spot of bright, direct light (figure 5). Now tilt the book away from the beam while keeping the flashlight stationary. Note that the formerly round spot of light elongates into an oval and covers a bigger area. (Figure 6). The larger spot also becomes dimmer. This experiment shows that the same amount of light is spread over a larger area when it shines on a slanted surface. For ease of illustration, let's suppose the flashlight projects 100 units of light on the round spot. We will refer to area of the round spot of light as a "unit area." When the book is tilted away from the light, let us suppose that the elongated spot is twice the area of the bright, round spot. The amount of light per unit area covered is only 50 units, and the concentration of light at any point on the tilted book is only half that of the vertical book.

Figure 5.

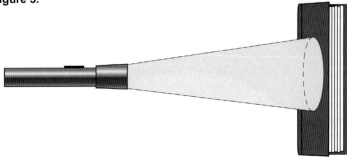

Figure 6.

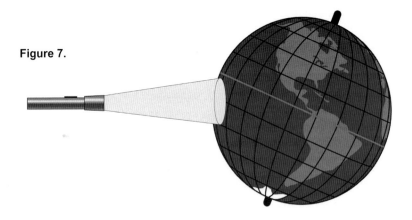

Now let's consider the sun's rays. This time, concentrate the beam perpendicular to the line that represents the tropic of Capricorn on a globe. You will note that the light covers a small, round area (figure 7).

Figure 7.

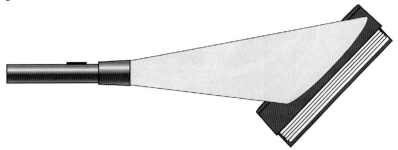

Figure 8.

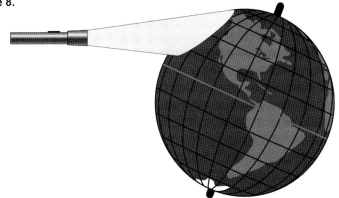

Now, raise the beam vertically so that it shines on the northern part of the globe. You will note that the same amount of light spreads out over a much larger area (figure 8). You can see that the more directly the rays from the sun contact a particular area of the Earth, the greater will be amount of light received and heat produced. We can also conclude that UVB light, which is present in sunlight during summer, will be greater on those areas that receive the most direct sunlight. Conversely, when the sunlight touches the Earth at an indirect angle, the lesser will be the heat, light, and UVB in that area. The lower beam in figure 9 illustrates the directness of sunlight at the Tropic of Capricorn on the first day of winter in the northern hemisphere and summer in the southern hemisphere and contrasts it with the indirect sunlight (in the upper beam) that reaches the upper part of the northern hemisphere during the same season. Note how much more diffused the sunlight is in the northern hemisphere.

Figure 9.

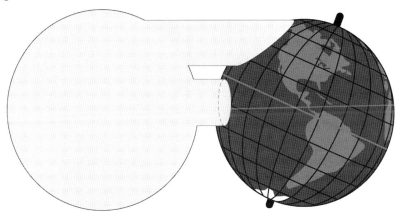

The sunlight does not always contain the quantity of UVB light necessary to produce vitamin D. UVB light is filtered by the atmosphere, and that filtration is much greater in winter than in summer. Figure 10 shows the globe surrounded by a circle that represents the atmosphere, which is greatly exaggerated. For purposes of illustration, we will arbitrarily say that the sunlight passes through 100 units of UVB-filtering atmosphere at its most direct contact with the Earth—a point located in the southern hemisphere. In the northern hemisphere, the light passes on an angle through more of the atmosphere, especially farther north than 60° latitude where it is filtered by 200 units of atmosphere. At that latitude, all of the UVB light is filtered out during the winter. It has been established that in Boston, Massachusetts (latitude 42.2° north), there is insufficient UVB available to produce any vitamin D from November through February.[1] At Edmonton Alberta, Canada (52° north latitude), the "vitamin D winter" extends from October through March.

Figure 10.

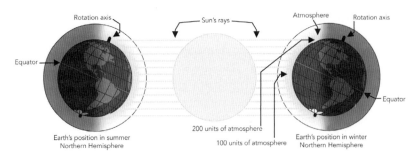

Another factor is time of day. At dawn, sunlight comes to Earth at an almost horizontal angle and passes through miles of filtering atmosphere. All UVB is filtered out, even on summer's first day. At midday, however, the sun is directly overhead and passes through little atmosphere, so much more UVB reaches the Earth. (Figure 11).

Figure 11. Filtration of sun at different times of day

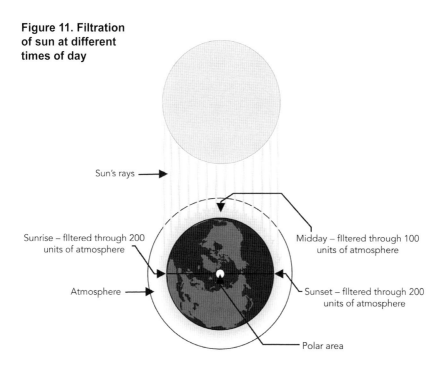

Sun's rays ⟶

Sunrise – flltered through 200 units of atmosphere

Midday – flltered through 100 units of atmosphere

Atmosphere ⟶

Sunset – flltered through 200 units of atmosphere

Polar area

Other factors that influence the quantity of Vitamin-D-producing UVB available at any season or time:

1. **Altitude:** The atmosphere is denser at sea level, and therefore more UVB is filtered out at the beach than on a high mountain. The National Weather Service in Flagstaff, Arizona states that the increase in UVB per 1,000 feet elevation gain is 4%-5%.[3] Let's use an example to illustrate the influence of altitude on UVB. Phoenix is located at an altitude of about 1,000 feet. Flagstaff is located at an altitude of 7,000 feet. Therefore, if all other factors were equal, the intensity of UVB light at Flagstaff would be about 27% greater than in Phoenix.

2. **Surface reflection:** Light colors reflect sunlight. Snowy areas reflect the most light, meaning that people enjoying outdoor winter sports at high altitude receive more UVB than they would where there is no snow. Let's use the Arizona example again. Snow is about four times more reflective than desert, and snowfall is substantial during the Flagstaff winter but only rarely seen in the Phoenix desert. UVB intensity is already 27% higher in Flagstaff due to altitude, and with snowy ground, it would be 100% more intense at Flagstaff than at Phoenix.[3] Be careful at high altitudes

when doing summer hiking; you will often not realize you are sunburned, because the coolness of the weather.

3. **Cloud cover:** Clouds quite obviously filter out sunlight and UVB. However, in seasons of direct sunlight, some UV light penetrates clouds. Caution should be exercised during cool, cloudy days to avoid burning.

4. **The ozone layer:** The layer of O3, or ozone, that surrounds most of the Earth, acts as a filter for UVB. Where the layer is thicker, more UVB is filtered out.

5. **Pollutants:** Ozone produced by industrial processes is a pollutant at lower altitudes. It and other pollutants filter UVB. For example infants and toddlers in most polluted areas of Delhi, India, have less than half the serum vitamin D levels of those who live in its least polluted areas.[4] Since vitamin D is produced in response to UVB, this indicates the dramatic effect of pollution in filtering it out.

6. **Sunscreens:** The use of sunscreens greatly reduces the quantity of UVB available for producing vitamin D.

The following chapters discuss the many benefits and the relatively few dangers of UVB so you will be able to derive the greatest benefit from healthful sunlight exposure. We begin by explaining the role of free radicals in producing skin damage by showing the relationship of sunlight exposure and antioxidant nutrients on these destructive molecules.

Chapter 3

Free radicals and antioxidants

"Pleasant the sun when first on this delightful land he spreads his orient beams on herb, tree, fruit and flower."
John Milton

As we discuss skin cancer and sunlight, you should understand the profound influence nutrition has on skin cancer and all other aspects of human health. Because antioxidants are critical to good nutrition, we first consider what they do to prevent cancer. We will begin with a very elementary summary of the basic chemistry of the ubiquitous free radical and its influence on health. We will also illustrate how these nasty little fellows are extinguished by antioxidants. Then, in the next chapter, we will tie together the relationships among fats, antioxidants, free radicals and skin cancers.

The notorious free radical

A free radical is a highly unstable atom capable of independent existence, and that has at least one unpaired electron in its outer shell.[1] Atoms are stable when they have at least two electrons in their outer orbit that balance each other.

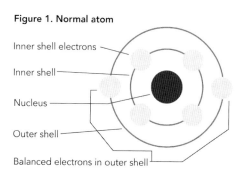

Figure 1. Normal atom

Inner shell electrons

Inner shell

Nucleus

Outer shell

Balanced electrons in outer shell

When an atom loses an electron, it becomes unstable and seeks to reestablish balance. Figure 2 represents an atom that lacks the "balancing electron" on the left side of its outer shell.

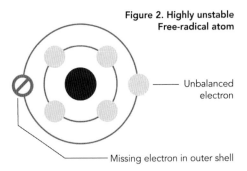

Figure 2. Highly unstable Free-radical atom

Unbalanced electron

Missing electron in outer shell

Because this atom "craves" to have its balance restored, it will "steal" an electron from another atom to achieve the desired balance. When it has snatched the electron, it becomes stable. However, the atom from which the electron is stolen becomes another free radical. This causes what Dr. Gordon Ainsleigh calls the "random rearrangement of molecules," as the process repeats innumerable times,[2] in a chain reaction that continues until a substance with an extra electron to "give away" steps in and furnishes the electron that stops the reaction. (Figure. 3) Of course, that substance must be able to give away its electron without becoming a free radical itself. Antioxidants have many extra electrons to give away. Figure 4 shows a free radical receiving an electron from an antioxidant, which loses an electron. Figure 5 represents the newly stabilized atom and shows the antioxidant atom with one less electron.

Figure 3.

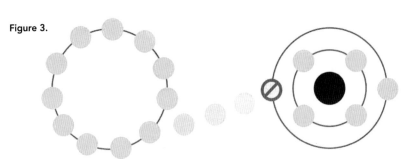

Antioxidant substance "gives away an electron"   Free radical atom lacking an electron

Figure 4.

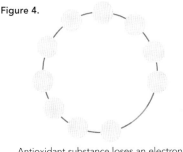

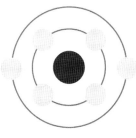

Antioxidant substance loses an electron

Free radical receives an electron

Figure 5.

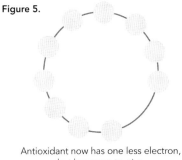

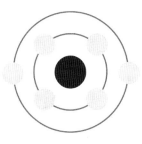

Antioxidant now has one less electron, but has more to give

Atom is now stable

The role of oxygen in free-radical formation

The process of free-radical formation is known as oxidation, because free radicals are usually formed due to oxygen molecules, which are unstable. Oxygen easily combines with other substances. *It gives us life, but its byproducts, if not controlled, can quickly end life*. As an iron pipe rusts, it is succumbing to the free-radical attack of oxidation. When anything burns, free radicals form. A single cigarette puff creates about one quadrillion free-radical attacks.[16]

So the process of "oxidation" gives rise to the term "antioxidant." The body produces some of its own antioxidants, and others must be consumed and absorbed through the digestive process. Without antioxidants, our own metabolic processes, which give us energy for life, would quickly kill us. All processes such as heartbeat, breathing, digestion, etc., require oxygen, and they produce free radicals. Exercise itself requires large quantities of oxygen, and a great deal of that oxygen generates harmful molecules.[3] In fact, as much as 2-5% of the oxygen taken in during exercise or even during rest has the ability to form free radicals.[4] Since exercise can increase oxygen consumption by as much as 20 fold,[3] it is easily seen that vigorous physical activity greatly increases free radicals. ***But don't stop exercising!***

Provided there are sufficient antioxidants available, free-radical production is balanced, and no harm takes place due to exercise. However, when the free-radical load exceeds the body's ability to neutralize it, there are terrible consequences: tissue is damaged, DNA (the genetic headquarters of cells) is altered, and degenerative diseases are produced. It is no wonder that cigarettes inflict such harm; unless there are vast quantities of antioxidants coursing through the tissues, the free radicals produced by cigarettes are unopposed and lead to cancer, heart disease and other degenerative maladies. The fact that smoking kills so many people attests to the reality that most people have insufficient levels of antioxidants to handle the free-radical load it produces. In fact, smoking is a major cause of non-melanoma skin cancers (NMSC); the greater the number of cigarettes smoked, the greater is the risk of skin cancer.[15]

Cigarettes, however, are only one source of free radicals. Environmental pollutants such as paint fumes, carpet glue, exhaust smoke, chlorine, petroleum products and many others bombard us with free radicals. X-rays and other sources of radiation cause free radical damage. Radiation from the sun causes free radicals when it strikes the fats in the cell membranes of our skin, which can lead to skin cancer if nutrition is also poor. (***Note: sunlight is only one factor in skin cancer! As you continue reading you will understand that poor nutrition relates very closely to the disease.***) Even foods, particularly fats, often go through processes that make them free-radical producing poisons.

Two ways to reduce the damage of free radicals (oxidation)

There are two ways to balance the free-radical load: (1) Decrease the number of free radicals that the body must deal with. (2) Increase the quantity of antioxidants in the body. Be careful with this second piece of advice—some antioxidants—produced in a lab and taken in massive doses—may actually cause cancer.[5-6] Our immune systems need some free radicals to destroy foreign invaders,[7] but mega-doses of certain antioxidants interfere with immune function. ***The very best way to get antioxidants is by eating large quantities of dark-green vegetables and colorful fruits***. However, supplementation with ***natural***, properly ***balanced antioxidants in reasonable amounts*** may be of value.

48

Decreasing the load of free radicals may not be as complex as you might think, but it will require taking some lifestyle modification measures. If you smoke, stop. If your work exposes you to toxic chemicals, try to find other employment. And for goodness sake, stop eating at "fast fat" restaurants, where most foods contain a load of free radicals. However, by picking and choosing foods carefully at some restaurants, the damage may be minimized. Some of the most lethal sources of free-radical attack are processed vegetable oils known as polyunsaturated fatty acids (PUFA). The remainder of this chapter deals with the dangers of these ubiquitous poisons.

Understanding lipid peroxidation

All cells have membrane walls that are composed mostly of lipids (fats) and a waxy, lipid-like substance called cholesterol. These membranes protect the inner parts of the cell and selectively allow nutrients to enter and wastes to exit. When subjected to excessive free-radical attack, membrane structures degenerate and become unable to perform their vital functions.[8] This degeneration includes structural breakdown and an increased permeability to chemicals that should never enter the cell. This in turn leads to DNA damage that may result in cell mutation,[9] which may lead to various cancers. A process known as cross-linking of lipids and proteins also occurs[10-11]—a process that is implicated in aging and wrinkling of the skin. The attack on the cell membranes by free radicals is called *lipid peroxidation*. As we will see in the next chapter, excessive quantities of fat in the diet lead to a greater incidence of skin cancer. It is indisputable that the type of fat consumed by most citizens of Western society is itself a contributor to lipid peroxidation. Let us now consider the deadly, processed polyunsaturated fat.

The processing of PUFA (polyunsaturated fatty acids)

French fries are normally cooked in boiling oil. Typically, this oil is produced by concentrating vegetable oil (such as corn oil) and processing it to concentrate its PUFA, a process that also removes anything of nutritional value such as fiber, vitamins, minerals and antioxidants. The seeds, or corn kernels, are first crushed or mixed with a chemical solvent to remove the oil from the grains. Lye and bleach are added to clarify and lighten the color, and then the oil is heated to a temperature of 330-380° Fahrenheit for up to twelve hours.[12] During this process the natural antioxidants that protect corn oil are destroyed or removed, so a chemical antioxidant is

49

added to prevent further oxidation and rancidity. The byproducts formed in heated oils are called peroxides, hydroperoxides, aldehydes (have you heard of formaldehyde?), ketones, polymers and cyclic monomers.[13] Now really, does this sound like something you want to eat? If these fats are further processed with hydrogen to partially solidify them, then they become the infamous partially-hydrogenated fats (trans fats)—fats that can lead to hardening of the arteries and heart disease.

These processes occur prior to when the oil is used to cook the foods for public consumption. Furthermore, boiling the oil in the presence of oxygen to cook French fries, chicken and other foods, produces another load of lipid peroxides that is added to the free-radical load already created during the process of manufacturing the oil itself.[14]

According to Dr. Walter Vieth, animal fats, which are saturated fats (meaning they are solid at room temperature), also undergo tremendous lipid peroxidation when they are used to fry foods. This is due to their lack of natural antioxidants. Yet, PUFA sustain the most free-radical damage during heating—as much as 10,000 times the damage sustained by monounsaturates such as almond oil, avocado oil and olive oil.[13] It is unlikely that you could eat enough vegetables and fruits—with their accompanying antioxidants—to ever balance out the destruction produced by the vast quantities of unhealthful fats in fried foods, especially in fast-fat restaurants.

Here are some important questions: Could ingested oxidized fats find their way to the skin and create skin cancer? If so, could the exposure to sunlight and oxygen inside the skin further exacerbate the carcinogenic potential of these killers? Could reducing the quantity of fats in the diet diminish the amount of oxidized fat and decrease the likelihood of developing common skin cancer? Could supplementation with—or topical application of—antioxidants decrease the risk of sun damage and common skin cancer? The following chapter considers those possibilities.

What have we learned?

1. Free radicals are unstable atoms that lack an electron in an outer shell.

2. Free radicals are formed by oxygen combining with other molecules, a process called oxidation.

3. Free radicals often damage DNA and become the precursors to cancer and heart disease.

4. Antioxidants from vegetables and fruits can inhibit or put a halt to free-radical processes.

5. Animal fats and processed polyunsaturated fats (PUFA) easily combine with oxygen to create free radicals in a process called lipid peroxidation. When these fats are eaten, some end up in the skin. If subjected to sunlight, they may create the damage that causes skin cancer.

6. Cooking PUFA increases the damage they do.

7. By lowering the fat content of the diet and avoiding PUFA, free-radical damage is diminished.

Chapter 4

Solar Power, dietary fat and skin cancer

Most skin cancers can be prevented, even when sunlight exposure is habitual. But before debunking the falsehoods regarding skin cancer, here are a few terms important to this and subsequent chapters.

Types of skin cancer and precursors:

1. *Common skin cancer,* also known as *non-melanoma skin cancer (NMSC),* is the most common, yet least dangerous of all cancers and is easily removed. Common skin cancer has two forms: basal cell carcinoma and squamous cell carcinoma.

2. *Basal cell carcinoma* (BSC) occurs in the lower layers of the epidermis, the outer layer of the skin. It does not spread rapidly and is not considered dangerous except in persons with compromised immune systems. It is characterized by pale, waxy gray nodules or distinct, red, scaly patches.

3. *Squamous cell carcinoma* (SCC) occurs in the upper layers of the epidermis and is characterized by rough, scaly patches. It is less common than basal cell carcinoma, but grows faster and is more likely to spread.

4. *Malignant melanoma (MM or CMM)* is a dangerous cancer that attacks the pigment (melanin) producing cells of the skin. It usually appears as a brown, irregularly-shaped patch. Melanoma is easily treated if detected early but can become deadly if left to develop, because it spreads so easily to other body parts.

5. *Actinic keratosis (AK)* is a slightly raised scaly area that forms on the skin surface. AK's are considered precursors to some skin cancers. Left untreated, some AK's may become squamous cell carcinomas.

Different oils (fats, lipids) that influence skin cancer

1. *Polyunsaturated fatty acids* (PUFA), previously mentioned, are a class of fats that are liquid at room temperature and are found primarily in corn, soybean, safflower, nut, flax and fish oils. They are called essential fatty acids since they form an

integral part of every cell membrane, help to insulate nerves, and produce hormones called prostaglandins. However, they are easily oxidized. When they are processed, used in high-heat cooking or irradiated by sunlight, they become harmful lipid peroxides. With the exception of fish and flax oils, their increased consumption may be a key reason for the dramatic increase in skin cancers. We are concerned primarily with two types: Omega-6 and Omega-3.

2. *Omega-6 fatty acids* are the type usually used in frying. They produce inflammatory prostaglandins. Small amounts of Omega-6 fats are essential, but consumed as cooking oils, can be extremely harmful.

3. *Omega-3 fatty acids* are considered to have health benefits, but are easily oxidized and may be harmful when oxidized. They are essential and are also known as alpha-linolenic acid, EPA and DHA. They produce anti-inflammatory prostaglandins.

4. *Saturated fatty acids* are solid at room temperature and come primarily from animal sources. They are easily oxidized and may contribute to the dramatic increase in skin cancer.

5. *Monounsaturated fatty acids* are found chiefly in olive oil, almonds, peanuts, avocados and canola. They are far more stable than PUFA or saturated fats and less likely to oxidize when used to cook or fry.

Common skin cancer: it isn't just from sunlight!

More than a million new cases of basal cell or squamous cell cancers occur annually.[1] These cancers, known as common skin cancers or non-melanoma skin cancers (NMSC) are highly curable and the death rate is very low. Nevertheless, they are associated with skin aging. *Simple dietary changes can prevent most of these cancers, and common sense lifestyles can prevent most of the rest.* The advice to stay out of the sun in order to prevent an already preventable cancer is misguided, and it is costing thousands of lives annually by increasing the incidence of the deadly internal cancers as well as heart disease, osteoporosis, multiple sclerosis and other diseases.

There is little doubt that–all else being equal–exposure to sunlight increases the likelihood of developing common skin cancer and accelerates the aging processes of the skin.[2] However, all else does not need to be equal!

Sunlight has one relationship to common skin cancer and quite another to melanoma, the sometimes deadly skin cancer that can spread to other parts of the body. Melanoma will be discussed in chapter 5. In this discussion we will consider only common skin cancers (NMSC)–cancers that have multiple causes.

The profound influence of fat

Due to the sun phobia that has gripped the world in the past few decades, valuable research regarding other skin cancer contributors has been ignored. In 1930 researchers demonstrated that the consumption of butter greatly accelerated the development of skin cancers in mice treated with carcinogenic tar. [3] Animals fed on high-fat diets had coats described as *"straight and greasy" and their appearance was "as if they had been dipped in fat."* [3-4] Obviously, some oils are absorbed into the skin, where they are susceptible to lipid peroxidation (see previous chapter). We thus see that dietary fats may have a carcinogenic effect on skin—at least in rats. The researchers suggested that fats serve as a medium through which carcinogens are absorbed into skin. That is probably true, but it is also likely that both the fats and carcinogens create tremendous free-radical damage that leads to cancer. *Could it be possible, then, that diets containing too much of the wrong kinds of fat act in concert with sunlight to increase skin damage?*

Another study of dietary fat and skin cancer was performed in 1939.[5] The researchers exposed five groups of albino mice to intense radiation with ultraviolet light for one hour daily and then fed each group a different diet. *Cancerous tumors were produced most rapidly on a diet high in hydrogenated fats*. These fats, now ubiquitous in foods, are used to retard food spoilage. Could they be one reason for the rapidly increasing skin cancer incidence—an increase that has taken place despite the increasing use of sunscreen? Did you or your doctor know there are multiple causes of skin cancer? Did you think it was caused only by exposure to sun?

Long after the 1939 research, a series of animal experiments were performed by Dr. Homer Black and his colleagues at Baylor University. They used ultraviolet light (UV) to induce cancerous changes in the animals and then placed them on either a low-fat or high-fat diet. The results: "a high level of dietary fat markedly shortened the time between UV exposure and tumor appearance and increased the number of tumors that developed."[6-7] The researchers also noted that "*switching from a high-fat to a low-fat diet immediately after administering the UV initiating dose negated the exacerbating effect of the high-fat intake." In other words, a certain quantity of UV was sufficient to initiate cancer in the animals consuming a high-fat diet. However, the same quantity of UV did not initiate cancer when the animals were switched to a low-fat diet directly after the exposure.* If similar results could be produced in humans, the implications for health would be great. Perhaps skin cancers wouldn't develop in sunbathers eating a low-fat diet.

Dr. Black tested that hypothesis. Two studies, performed over two years and reported in 1995 and 1998, showed the following: the simple measure of putting subjects on a diet consisting of 21% of calories from fat reduced the rate of actinic keratoses (AK) by 73% when compared to those who maintained a typical USA diet (37% of calories from fat).[7-8] AK are precursor lesions that occur prior to the onset of skin cancer. *More impressive, however, was the fact that those on the "low-fat" diet were 94% less likely to develop skin cancer at all.* It makes me wonder if a truly low-fat diet—one having only 10% of calories in fat—could have prevented even more AK and common skin cancer.

The restriction of total calories also has a beneficial effect. Therefore it has been suggested that reducing fats (a dense source of calories) did nothing more than reduce total calories, and that calorie restriction was the real factor that reduced skin cancer. However, the researchers noted that the experiments proved conclusively that *fat per se was the factor that led to the increased skin cancer. There were no significant differences in caloric intakes or body weights between the high-fat and low-fat subjects, but the reduction in cancer in the low-fat group was extraordinary.*

All fats are not created equal

The type of fat also makes a difference. Omega-6 fats such as corn oil and other commercial vegetable oils seem to be the most carcinogenic, and Omega-3 fats such as those contained in fish, flax oil and walnuts inhibit the formation of skin cancers.[9-11] As a society we ingest far too many Omega-6 fats compared to Omega-3 fats;[12] the ratio of Omega-3 to Omega-6 should be about 1:2 and no greater than 1:5 to produce beneficial health outcomes. Lamentably, in western societies the ratio is about 1:16.[12] The best way to improve the ratio is to remove Omega-6 "junk" fats from the diet while bringing the total fat content to 21% or less of calories consumed. Eating a diet containing dark-green vegetables and colorful fruits reduces fat intake while simultaneously adding important antioxidants.

Our population's typically poor ratio of Omega-6 to Omega-3 is harmful enough, but it is likely that the source of most Omega-6 fat in the western diet is even more destructive. You will recall from Chapter 3 that lipid peroxidation occurs during the heating and processing of oils, which produces free-radical atoms by the quadrillions. Those nasty little atoms wreak havoc in DNA and are the precursors to many cancers. Can you imagine the harm done by consuming vegetable oils heated repeatedly in deep-fat fryers to cook French fries? The cigarette has been properly labeled a "cancer stick," and that appellation may also be appropriately applied to the deadly French fry. In addition to plugging arteries, these oils find their way into the skin where the sunlight further damages them. It is no wonder that in Dr. Black's research, lowering the fat content to 21% of calories lowered the incidence of skin cancer by as much as 94%.[7-8] Sunlight exposure becomes dangerous when there is too much fat and too few antioxidants in the diet.

If a person insists on eating toxic fats, the skin will be damaged by sunlight! Sunlight is a vigorous promoter of overall human health, but it leads to common skin cancer (NMSC) if poor dietary habits are followed.

The death rate for NMSC is *estimated* at about 1,500 people per year in the USA out of the million or more who contract the disease.[13] That is less than ½% of all cancer deaths, although these cancers amount to more than half of all cancers. Those who die of NMSC usually do not receive treatment soon enough, and sometimes their immune systems are compromised by receiving anti-rejection drugs after organ transplants.[13] By adhering to a diet containing 21% or fewer calories from fat, and by having any lesions treated immediately, nearly all deaths from NMSC could be prevented. The reason given by governmental agencies and medical professions to avoid the sun is based on the premise that sunlight causes skin cancer regardless of lifestyle choices. That premise is patently false!

Dr. Black's group also demonstrated that antioxidants were protective against skin cancer in rats fed high amounts of corn and soy oils, but not in those fed low amounts.[14] *The primary dietary method of protecting against skin cancer is to lower the toxic-fat content of the diet*. Obviously, if fat content is low, the need for antioxidants is lower, because there is less damage to prevent. The research also suggests that lipid peroxidation caused by the sunlight contacting PUFA within skin tissue is immense, which dramatically increases the skin's need for antioxidants. In Dr. Black's research on fats and skin cancer, PUFA were used. Could it be that a different result might have occurred if monounsaturated fats, which are less susceptible to oxidation, were used?

You might ask yourself, "why not just give up sunlight rather than fat? The answer is that sunlight exposure promotes health in numerous ways. Sunlight avoidance may prevent an easily-removed NMSC, but at what risk? Lack of sunlight promotes prostate, breast, ovarian and colon cancers, as well as hypertension, heart disease, diabetes, multiple sclerosis and other illnesses. Toxic fats contribute to all of those diseases; sunlight does not.

A hundred years ago sunlight exposure while working outdoors was a part of daily living for the majority of the culture. We gradually moved indoors, and the rate of skin cancer increased dramatically. How then, is sunlight the primary cause of skin cancer? To rationally draw a conclusion that some factor (sunlight exposure) caused an increase in the incidence of a disease (skin cancer) during a time period, that factor (sun exposure) must also increase during the same time period. If sunlight exposure caused the increase in skin cancer, sunlight exposure must have increased along with the increase in skin cancer. It did not. Before anyone blames sunlight exposure for the increased incidence of skin cancer, he should answer this question: *Why has skin cancer increased as sunlight exposure has decreased?* Sunlight exposure is certainly a plausible causative or promoting influence, but it is neither the only factor nor the most important. Sunlight has been an innocent bystander. Sunlight causes lipid peroxidation in the skin when it comes in contact with PUFA, and if PUFA consumption increases, then more oxidative damage occurs. To blame the sunlight is ludicrous.

Conversely, if skin-cancer-protective nutrients (like antioxidants and omega3 fats) have *decreased*, then we would expect a parallel *increase* in skin cancer incidence. *Research reported by Dr. Hughes and colleagues in the __International Journal of Cancer__ indicated that of those people who had previously had at least one squamous cell carcinoma (SCC), those who also had the highest intakes of green leafy vegetables had only 45% of the risk of developing another.*[15] *Furthermore, those with the highest intake of dairy had two-and-one-half times the risk*.

Here are the factors that we expect increase skin-cancer incidence. All are plausible contributors to the disease:

1. **A dramatic increase in the use of PUFA in preparing foods, particularly fried foods.**

2. A decrease in consumption of vegetables and fruits and a decrease in the consumption of the anti-cancer antioxidants they contain.

3. A decrease in Omega-3 fats and a simultaneous increase in Omega-6 fats.

The advice to stay out of the sun is costing hundreds of thousands of lives per year due to increased cancer, osteoporosis, diabetes, heart disease, multiple sclerosis and a host of other diseases. If cutting dietary fat to 20% of total calories negates nearly all of the harmful effects of moderate sunlight exposure, the advice to treat the sun as an enemy makes no sense. Yet, the American Cancer Society's publication, *Cancer Facts and Figures 2005* makes the statement that "many of the more than one million skin cancers that are expected to be diagnosed in 2005 could have been prevented by protection from the sun's rays."[16] In view of the research that is readily available to these "experts," they should have said this: *"most of the million skin cancers that will be diagnosed this year could have been prevented by a diet low in fat and high in dark-green vegetables and colorful fruits.*

The following chapter will surprise many lay readers and astound many medical professionals who counsel us to avoid sunlight exposure. We examine the evidence that regular sunlight exposure leads to *decreased risk of the deadly skin cancer known as melanoma* and may increase the chance of survival from that disease once it is contracted. We have shown that common skin cancers are preventable by sensible changes in diet. Could it also be true for melanoma? Must we stay out of the sun or risk dying of a cancer that easily metastasizes (spreads) to other parts of the body? Chapter 5 will discuss melanoma and its relationship to sunlight and vitamin D.

What have we learned?

1. Sunlight is only one of many factors that may produce common skin cancers.

2. Removing harmful fats from the diet is much more important than avoiding sunlight; without these fats in the diet, common skin cancer is unlikely to occur.

3. Both processed polyunsaturated fats and animal fats other than fish oils should be greatly limited or avoided in order to protect against skin cancer.

4. One should strive to reduce Omega-6 fats in the diet while increasing Omega-3 fats.

5. Over the years, as sunlight exposure has *decreased* in the USA population, skin cancer has *increased*. Therefore, sunlight exposure cannot be the primary cause of skin cancer.

6. Sunlight protects us from many deadly diseases.

7. Common skin cancers (NMSC) are seldom fatal and easily removed. Therefore it is unwise to avoid the sun at the risk of death by diseases that are far more dangerous than skin cancer.

8. Colorful vegetables and fruits furnish antioxidants that protect the skin against NMSC.

Chapter 5

Solar Power and melanoma: burned by sunscreens?

"The windows of my soul I throw wide open to the sun."
John Greenleaf Whittier

The February 2005 issue of the *Journal of the National Cancer Institute* reported the stunning results of two studies: One by Dr. Marianne Berwick and colleagues showed *an increased survival rate for melanoma patients with histories of high sunlight exposure.*[1] *The other showed identical results in patients with non-Hodgkin's lymphoma.*[2] The papers caused some head scratching among the anti-sun group, although previous research indicated that sunlight exposure was protective against prostate cancer, breast cancer and colon cancer. *Amazingly, melanoma and lymphoma patients who had experienced more sunburns also had better survival rates from both diseases.*

Getting sunburned is still dangerous and should be avoided.

I will make this point many times: sunburn in these studies was really nothing more than a marker for a high quantity of sun exposure, even if that sun exposure was not ideally done. With prudent sunning, these benefits are achieved without burning. *Burning definitely contributes to melanoma.* A review of all research on sunlight and melanoma up to 1997 showed that burning at any age increased melanoma risk 70%-95%.[3] *However, the same review showed that regular sunlight exposure decreased the risk of melanoma by 14%.* Obviously, a key to avoiding melanoma is to avoid burning. Burning, however, is only one of many factors that lead to melanoma. Painful sunburns prior to age 20 increases the incidence of melanoma, *yet, lifetime sun exposure is associated with a reduced risk.*[4]

Perhaps the results of these studies should have been expected; other research had already shown that *melanomas occurred more frequently on areas of the skin that had seldom been exposed to sunlight*, and that those who worked almost exclusively indoors were more likely to develop melanoma than those who worked both indoors and outdoors.[5] In fact, *those who worked indoors had 50% more melanomas than those who worked both indoors and outdoors.* When assessing the incidence of melanoma occurring at various sites, this research found higher rates on the trunk (seldom exposed to sunlight) than on the head and arms (commonly exposed to sunlight). Children and adults who regularly play and work outdoors are less likely to develop melanoma.[6,7] Melanomas in women occur primarily on the upper legs, and in men more frequently on the back—areas of little sunlight exposure.[8] In blacks, melanomas are more common on the soles of the feet and on the lower legs, where exposure to sunlight is almost nil.[9]

Dr. Warren Christophers conducted a meta-analysis of case-control studies that examined the relationship between melanoma incidence and total accumulated sun exposure.[38] He found that 22% of melanomas occur on the more exposed areas and that 78% occur on the less exposed areas. Clearly, there is more to melanoma than sun exposure.

We established that NMSC is preventable by a low-fat diet combined with high intake of colorful vegetables and fruits, and that NMSC is lessened by maintaining a proper ratio of Omega-3 to Omega-6 fats in the diet (see chapter 4). Does sun avoidance prevent other more deadly cancers? No. Dr. William Grant's 2005 analysis indicates that 50,000-63,000 cancer deaths per year are due to insufficient ultraviolet light exposure—a health disaster that carries an economic burden of $40-56 billion.[10] However, he recently updated that assessment and has determined that the economic burden for all diseases is a staggering $200 million in direct costs and $400 billion in indirect costs.[61]

In 2006, Dr. Edward Giovannucci and colleagues determined that low vitamin D levels cause 85,550 cancer deaths per year among men alone![35] Obviously, *cancer prevention is not a valid reason to avoid the sunlight!*

Even if sunlight exposure raised the risk of melanoma (which it does not), sunning would still be advisable.

Suppose that sunlight did cause skin cancers regardless of dietary habits. Then consider the following: according to Dr. Giovannucci, *for every death caused by excessive exposure to ultraviolet light, at least thirty are due to insufficient exposure to ultraviolet light.*[11] If we were to play the odds, the best bet would be to get regular sunlight exposure. Prudent people would risk NMSC or melanoma rather than risk dying from the deadly cancers of the colon, breast and prostate. But you wouldn't really be gambling; you don't need to "play the odds." The correct diet helps to prevent NMSC, and sunlight exposure (without burning, of course) *lessens* the risk of melanoma. Remember that melanoma can be safely removed if detected early, so it is a good idea to check the entire body regularly, especially if you do not get into the sun regularly. It is also advisable to have regular dermatological checkups.

The idea that sunlight is the only cause of melanoma can be a deadly misconception.

An interesting paper on melanoma was written by Dr. Arthur Rhodes,[4] a professor of dermatology at Rush Medical College. *He states that the dermatology profession's message—that sunlight is the only cause of melanoma—is killing many people.* He gives several examples of death that resulted due to that deadly misconception:

1. A dermatology trainee died of melanoma at age 28. He watched a mole change in his armpit for years, but because that area never received UV light, he assumed it was not melanoma and delayed seeking help.

2. A 40-year-old woman had a sore on the bottom of her heel, and believing only sunlight caused melanoma, she had no idea that it was melanoma. She died three years later.

3. A Harvard-trained lung specialist ignored a sore on his upper back. He and his fiancée, a Harvard-trained pediatric resident, observed the change for several years without having it examined. They didn't know that melanoma could occur in an area that never received sunlight. He died six months after diagnosis at age 29.

Here is a quote from this enlightened dermatologist:

> *If a medical resident can misinterpret public health messages about sun exposure and melanoma, and two Harvard-trained physicians were ignorant about the most important risk factors for developing melanoma, then the general public will tend to make the same potentially fatal mistakes. Those mistakes lead to delayed diagnosis of this potentially lethal cancer—particularly when we pound out the message that the culprit in melanoma is sun, sun, sun, and we are not sufficiently emphasizing the most important risk factors for developing melanoma.*

A diet replete with antioxidants cuts the risk of melanoma.

A recent study of the correlation between dietary habits and melanoma showed that:

1. Individuals with the lowest intake of alpha-carotene, beta-carotene, cryptoxanthin, lutein, and lycopene (all carotenoid antioxidants) had a 50% increased risk for melanoma.

2. Those who consumed the most alcohol had a 65% increased risk.[12]

Another study indicated a 2.5 times increased risk for melanoma among those who consumed two or more alcoholic drinks per day.[29] Melanoma and NMSC are to a greatly preventable by good lifestyle choices. Lifestyle trends during the past 100 years are partially responsible for the increase in skin and many other cancers. These trends include:

1. The decrease in green vegetable and colorful fruit consumption
2. The increased exposure to chemicals
3. The proliferation of prescription drugs
4. The obesity pandemic
5. The consumption of fast foods
6. Increased sedentary living
7. *Decreased* sunlight exposure.

The change from outdoor, agrarian living to indoor living correlates to the spectacular increase in skin cancer. Yet, as we became more urbanized, and sunscreen use increased, melanoma rates skyrocketed. Between 1973 and 1999, they increased from 7.4 per 100,000 to 20.1 per 100,000[13]—a near tripling.

If sunburning causes melanoma, shouldn't we use sunscreens?

The answer is "no," although many disagree. Be sure to consult a physician before making any changes to your habits, and give him or her a copy of this book. Caution is the best prevention for sunburn. You should never stay out until the skin turns red, and in the beginning stages of sun exposure, gradually increase it until a tan develops. A tan is a sign that the skin is protecting itself against burning. In a landmark paper published in 1993 in the journal *Preventive Medicine*, Dr. Gordon Ainsleigh stated, *"As melanoma research has demonstrated, the best prevention is regular exposure, thereby maintaining a protective tan and high vitamin D blood and tissue levels."*[36]

Up to 99% of vitamin D production is stopped by sunscreen,[14] rendering many of the health benefits of sun exposure null and void.

Sunscreens also provide little free-radical protection.[15] **Sunscreen manufacturers have claimed a free-radical protection factor ten times greater than that afforded by their product!** Such overblown claims have led to lawsuits. **Furthermore, sunscreens protect only the outer layers of skin from burning while leaving the inner layer (where melanoma is initiated) vulnerable to damage**[15] (See Figure 1). Sunscreen use increased because governments and physicians promoted it. Unfortunately, the rate of melanoma increased in lockstep,[16] and there is even a possibility that the estrogenic compounds and other chemicals found in sunscreen may actually themselves be carcinogenic.[37]

Queensland, Australia has vigorously promoted sunscreens for decades, and Queensland now has one of highest rates of melanoma in the world,[16] **along with a rate of vitamin D deficiency that is becoming critical.**[40] In the period between 1980 and 1987, skin cancers doubled. Sunscreens, as explained below, remove the warning signal for excessive sun exposure.[17] Therefore, sunscreens (ironically) promote melanoma. Research was conducted in Italy on sunscreen use among children.[18] The researchers interviewed parents to determine if sunscreen use, protective clothing and other precautions were used to prevent sun damage. They counted the moles on the children, since high mole count is correlated to a high risk of melanoma. Protective clothing was associated with a 41% reduction in the number of moles when compared to the average, but **sunscreen use was associated with a 68% INCREASE in mole count, regardless of skin type or eye color.** Interestingly, the number of sunburns was not correlated to mole number, and the children who had the highest mole counts had never had sunburns. The probable explanation is that the children who wore the most sunscreen never felt the hot sensation produced by UVB on the epidermis (outer layer of skin) and missed nature's warning signal for excessive sun exposure. Meanwhile, UVA light penetrated deeply into the dermis (the lower layer of skin) causing damage to the melanocytes and producing precancerous changes (moles).

It is worth repeating that sunscreens may prevent external burning by UVB but permit UVA to burn the lower layers of skin and initiate melanoma. The body's protective mechanism may be rendered useless by sunscreens, which lull users into a false sense of security while UVA wreaks havoc with their skin. This is more than conjecture. **Research on sunscreen use and the amount of time spent in direct sunlight shows that**

the stronger the rating of the sunscreen, the longer people using it tend to expose themselves.[19]

Taking vacations to sunny areas correlates to increased melanoma incidence[34] and higher accessibility to air travel correlates strongly with the increasing incidence of melanoma, presumably due to taking sunny vacations that lead to sunburn.[35] Most of those vacationers are probably applying plenty of sunscreen that blocks UVB. They therefore do stay out in the sun too long, especially if they have not built up a protective tan. Others may simply stay out too long and burn themselves, which can lead to melanoma. Occasional orgies of sun exposure damage the skin, so the key is to carefully and *regularly* enjoy the sun. Several studies make a case that UVA penetration allowed by sunscreens may lead to melanoma.[62-65]

Figure 1 shows a cross section of skin, and the way that it is affected by UVA and UVB.

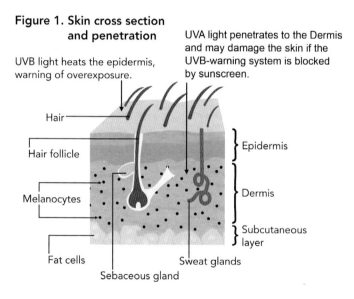

Figure 1. Skin cross section and penetration

UVB light heats the epidermis, warning of overexposure.

UVA light penetrates to the Dermis and may damage the skin if the UVB-warning system is blocked by sunscreen.

Hair

Hair follicle

Melanocytes

Fat cells

Sebaceous gland

Sweat glands

Epidermis

Dermis

Subcutaneous layer

A comprehensive review done between 1966 and 2003 revealed absolutely no correlation between sunscreen use and Melanoma.[20] In other words, sunscreens don't work. One science writer concluded that the review confirmed it is still safe to "protect" our skins with sunscreens. My question is, "Why—so we can waste money on a product that does nothing to protect us? How can anyone in good conscience recommend what doesn't work? It is also possible that the original reviewers missed an important study from the *International Journal of Cancer* in 2000 that compared 571 people with a first diagnosis of melanoma with 913 healthy control subjects. Those who used sunscreens were 1.8 times <u>more likely to contract melanoma</u> than those who did not, and *among those who always used sunscreens so they could stay out longer in the sun, the risk of melanoma was 8.7 times greater than those who did not use them.*[34]

If we assess the question differently we indeed see that more sunscreen use equals more melanoma. We need only compare the increasing sale of sunscreens during the past three decades with the change in melanoma incidence. Sunscreens sales increased from $18 million to $640 million between 1972 and 2005. If sunscreens really help prevent melanoma, we would observe a drop in melanoma rates rather than the tripling that occurred. Figure 2 juxtaposes two graphs: one shows the increase in sunscreen sales from 1972-2005, and the other shows what *should have been* the decrease in melanoma incidence from 1973 to 1999 if sunscreen did what its proponents promise. The dollar figures are adjusted for inflation. *Sunscreen sales in 2005 were almost eighteen times higher than in 1972.* Undeniably, if the dramatic increase in sunscreen use were effective in reducing melanoma, actual data would show a dramatic *decrease* in melanoma. *However, the second chart below is a fairy tale; exactly the opposite happened.*

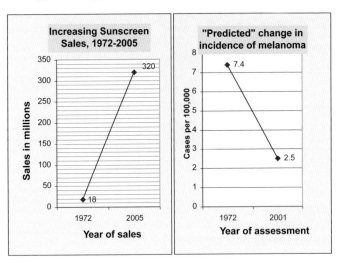

Figure 2: This might be the expected correlation between sunscreen use and melanoma—if sunscreens actually prevented melanoma.

The lifetime risk of developing melanoma in 1935 was 1 in 1500. It climbed to 1 in 75 in 2000, and the risk increases by 5% to 7% per year.[30]

Melanoma rates among Caucasians more than tripled between 1980 and 2003 alone.[31] Did this increase not parallel the mammoth and successful advertising blitz by the sunscreen industry? It is likely that as sunscreen use continues to rise, melanoma incidence will rise too. People were outside in the sun much more in 1935 that they are today because we have moved into offices and been scared out of the sunlight. Despite contrary evidence, one writer says that says that exposure to UV causes melanoma.[31] If so, then why has melanoma increased so dramatically as we have moved indoors, and why does increasing sunscreen use have such a direct correlation to increasing melanoma rates? Don't sunscreen buyers use it? Isn't it interesting that the conclusion reached by the "scientific" community is "therefore, we need to avoid the sun even more?" There is no science at all in that conclusion.

This is a summary of the counterintuitive argument they are trying to get us to accept: "As we have moved out of the sunlight and have covered ourselves with sunscreens when we do go outside, the rate of melanoma has dramatically increased. And those who receive the greatest sunlight exposure have profoundly lowered rates of major cancers, multiple sclerosis and heart attacks. Therefore, we must continue to avoid the sun and increase our use of sunscreens." They are defending the indefensible, continually selling us a bill of goods about sunlight and melanoma. Figure 3 illustrates the ***REAL*** correlation between sunscreen use and melanoma incidence. They move in the same direction.

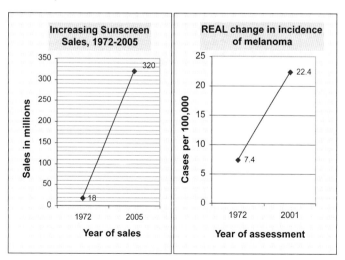

Figure 3: The true correlation of rising sunscreen use to increased melanoma incidence

So what is result of the "sunscare" tactics and the "protection" against melanoma? Melanoma has tripled! Can it be that health policies regarding sun exposure have been not only ineffective, but profoundly counterproductive? *One must conclude that sunscreens are a complete waste of money at best, and at worst they cause melanoma!*

Some people are awakening. Reuters News Service reported a lawsuit filed in the Los Angeles Superior Court accusing sunscreen manufacturers of exposing millions to cancer and other dangers through false and misleading product claims.[32] The class-action suit stated that sunscreen makers "inflate claims about their products' qualities, lulling consumers into a false sense of security over prolonged sun exposure." The defendants include some very big names: Johnson & Johnson, Schering-Plough Corp., Playtex Products, Tanning Research Laboratories and Chattem. The lawsuit further states that the sunscreens "may protect against harmful UVB rays with shorter wavelengths, but the skin remains exposed to harmful UVA rays with longer wavelengths that penetrate deep within the skin."

Also quoted in the Reuters article: "The suit also alleges that parents have been misled into believing their children are protected as a result of claims in labels for products aimed specifically at children, such as Coppertone Water Babies. *Schering-Plough misled ... the general public by representing that their Coppertone Water Babies UVA/UVB sunblock Lotion provided 45 times a child's natural protection against both UVA and UVB rays," according to the suit. It says the product only provides that level of protection against UVB, and cites scientific studies showing that the sunscreen ingredients do not provide the same level of UVA protection."* The defendants might be in for a rough ride since it has been shown that the stronger the sunscreen, the longer the users will stay out in the sun.[19]

The FDA, amazingly, is getting in on the sunscreen act. After reviewing sun-protection comments and claims made by manufacturers, it stated: "the available evidence fails to show that sunscreen use alone helps prevent skin cancer or premature skin aging. Thus, the antiaging, skin cancer, and sun damage claims proposed by the comments would be false or misleading due to lack of sufficient data in support of these claims. For example, the statement proposed by one comment that sunscreen use 'may help prevent sun-induced skin damage, such as premature skin aging' would be inherently misleading to consumers by suggesting that sunscreen use alone may help prevent premature skin aging."[50]

Even with all the research done and the lawsuits filed, many in the pharmaceutical and medical fields still just don't get it. A pharmaceutical company laments that in spite of all the information about skin cancer, people are still "baking themselves in the sun." Another preaches, "The disease is largely preventable when sun protection is consistently practiced." Is the medical/pharmaceutical industry so harebrained that it ignores the simple correlation between sunscreens and increasing melanoma? Could it be that dollars are involved?

Other dangers of sunscreens

The Environmental Working Group (EWG) has compiled an interesting number of studies regarding the potential harm done by the chemicals in sunscreen. I am indebted to them for the following information:

The Center for Disease Control (CDC) in 2008 released a study showing that 96.8% of Americans at age six are contaminated with a major sunscreen ingredient called oxybenzone and that women were 3.5 times as likely to have high concentrations as men. [51] The authors suggest that the greater use by women of personal-care products, most of which contain sunscreens, is the reason for their higher degree of contamination; oxybenzone is used in 588 sunscreens and in 567 other personal-care products.[53] *An incredible 9% or more of the applied amount is absorbed through the skin.*[57]

Pregnant mothers exposed to oxybenzone gave birth to babies with low birth weights,[52] which "programs" the developing child for greater risks of heart disease, hypertension, type-2 diabetes and other diseases in adulthood.[54] Furthermore, sunlight causes the chemical to become a potent allergen[55,56] and to form free radicals.[53]

Other dangers of sunscreen chemicals are their potential "gender-bending" characteristics; they increase estrogen and decrease testosterone in men[53,59] and may be partly responsible for the nearly 50% reduction of sperm count in the last few decades.[60] Sunscreen chemicals are also known to cause the feminization of fish,[58] and environmental pollution by these and similarly-structured chemicals are now thought to cause feminization in alligators and the gradual extinction of Florida panthers due to failure to breed.[60]

Sunscreens also increase the absorption of pesticides through the skin..[66,67] Think carefully about this information when you next see a sunscreen ad.

Melanoma and the ozone layer

Some choose to believe the increase in melanoma is due instead to the thinning of the ozone layer, which allows more UV to reach the Earth's surface. However, researchers in Norway reported that yearly melanoma incidence increased 350% in men and 440% in women between 1957 and 1984—a period when there was absolutely no thinning of the ozone layer.[21] What *had* increased was advice to use sunscreen and avoid the sunlight, and a tendency to spend time indoors rather than obtain the regular, moderate sunlight exposure that protects against melanoma.

A final word about the relationship among common skin cancers, melanoma and deadly internal cancers

We established in Chapter 4 that common skin cancers (NMSC) are seldom dangerous and easily treated. We also established that while sunlight exposure does increase the risk of these benign lesions, low-fat, high-nutrient nutrition profoundly diminishes the risk.

It is interesting to note that NMSC have an inverse relationship with melanoma; when NMSC incidence is high, indicative of high quantities of sun exposure, the incidence of melanoma is low.[45,46] Dr. William Grant, after analyzing data from the Atlas of Cancer Mortality in the United States,[47] noted that between 1950-1969 and 1970-1994, death rates from NMSC decreased by 31% for white males and by 47% for white females. However, during those same periods, melanoma rates increased by 89% in white males and 42% for white females.[48] *Therefore, if you accept the rate of NMSC as a measure of the cumulative exposure to sunlight, you must also accept that exposure to sunlight reduces the risk of melanoma and that its lack increases the risk of melanoma.* Of course, other factors such as sunscreen use, skin aging, latitude and UVA/ UVB percentages also have a bearing on skin cancers.

I repeat: occasional intense sunlight exposure, especially if it causes sunburn, increases melanoma risk.[22] Regular, moderate exposure to sunlight without burning decreases it. And remember, even with chronically sun-damaged skin, the mutations that lead to melanoma are rare.[23]

Even the dermatology profession is beginning to understand the relationship between vitamin D and melanoma. Dermatologists in England warned that sun avoidance may deplete vitamin D and thereby increase the risk of developing melanoma.[68]

Melanoma and fluorescent lighting

A study published in the British medical journal *Lancet* in 1982 showed that melanoma risk increases proportionate to the time of exposure to fluorescent lighting.[24] Women who worked under fluorescent lighting had over 200% of the risk for melanoma as those who did not work under such lights. *Among women exposed to fluorescent lighting for 20 years or more, the average risk for melanoma increased by more than 250%.* The test subjects who were heavily exposed to sunlight as children while playing outdoors, and those who sunbathed as adults had *lower* rates of melanoma. *In men, exposure to fluorescent light for more than ten years predicted a 440% increase in the chance of contracting melanoma. Those who spent the least time in the sun as children had an increase of 730%!* Another study showed that malignant (cancerous) changes to mice embryo cultures could be caused by exposing them to fluorescent light.[25]

How to safely enjoy the sun:

1. Never burn and never expose yourself until the skin reddens. If you do not tan, reddening may occur in a very few minutes. Cover up or seek shade immediately at the first sign of pinkness.

2. If you begin your sunning program during summer, be sure to start with only a few minutes and gradually work up to more time as your skin adjusts.

3. Whenever your skin feels uncomfortably hot, seek shade or cover up. Remember that on a cool spring day, you may burn before you feel uncomfortable. Reddening means you have had too much exposure.

4. Once tanned, you may enjoy the sun until you feel uncomfortable or until you begin to redden over the tan.

5. Even dark-skinned people must be careful to gradually increase sunlight-exposure times.

6. Though you often hear the advice to sunbathe only before 10:00 AM and after 2:00 PM during summer and to avoid the midday sun, it may be best for some most people to expose most of the body to sunlight for a short time at midday. The ratio of UVA to UVB is much higher in mornings and afternoons than at midday, meaning that the sun is more likely to produce UVA-induced melanoma before 10:00 AM and after 2:00 PM.

   It also requires 50% more time to produce a given quantity of vitamin D two hours before or after midday than at midday.[41,43,44] A short period (20-40 minutes for light-skinned persons) will produce all the vitamin D that the body can make in one day. If one relies on haphazard exposure of the face, hands, and arms only, insufficient skin is exposed to produce enough vitamin D for immediate health benefits and for future storage. In addition, staying long enough to receive the health-producing dose by exposure only of the face, arms and hands may cause overexposure and burning on those areas. Sunbathing at midday (perhaps during a lunch break) makes sense for those who have limited time and has been recommended by Dr. Ann Webb of England as the most efficient method of producing vitamin D.[41] For people who have type-1 skin or very light skin that does not tan, vitamin D can be produced at midday by sitting in the shade outside and thereby avoiding direct ultraviolet radiation.[42] There is sufficient UVB light reflected by surrounding objects to stimulate some vitamin D production. The key, at any time of day or for any skin type, is to avoid burning.

7. Consider that sunscreens may cause you to overexpose your skin to UVA light and thus make you more susceptible to melanoma.

8. Remember that it is neither prudent nor healthful to bake yourself in the direct summer sun for hours on end. Different seasons allow for more or less sunlight exposure, and the darker your skin, the more time you can spend in sunlight.

9. It is important to eat a diet low in fat, particularly processed polyunsaturated fatty acids (PUFA). It is also advisable to consume a large quantity of green vegetables as well as colorful fruits to increase carotenoid antioxidants in the skin. I try to eat one-half pound of dark green vegetables per day and a pound of fresh, colorful fruit such as oranges, cherries, blueberries, marionberries and raspberries.

   I try to eat at least two tomatoes daily and use some tomato sauce on my low-fat dishes. By consuming forty grams of tomato paste daily for ten weeks, you can increase sunburn-resistance time by 40%.[26] Eating other tomato-based products has also been shown to significantly reduce sunburn,[27] and topically applied lycopene (a powerful antioxidant found in tomatoes) is also effective in preventing skin damage by UV.[28]

Dr. Michael Holick's book, *The UV advantage,* has helpful charts that link latitude, skin types and time of year to the body's ability to produce vitamin D. For those who wish to be precise in their sun exposure times, I highly recommend the book; it will add much to your knowledge of sunlight and vitamin D for health.

Now that we have discussed the influence of sunlight on skin cancers, let's move on to research that correlates increasing sunlight exposure to decreases in other diseases. The following chapters deal with the major internal cancers and are followed by chapters on heart disease, multiple sclerosis and other diseases that plague the sedentary people of the toxic Western world.

What have we learned?

1. Sunburning may increase risk for melanoma. Regular sunlight exposure, however, decreases the risk of melanoma.

2. A history of sunburns lessens the risk of lymphoma and other cancers; nevertheless, sunburns should be avoided. Regular sunlight exposure reduces the risk of melanoma without burning.

3. As people have moved indoors and out of the sunlight, the incidence of both common skin cancer and melanoma has dramatically increased. The risk of contracting melanoma increased from 1 in 1,500 in 1935 to 1 in 75 in 2,000.

4. As sunscreen use has increased approximately 18 times, melanoma risk has tripled.

5. Sunscreen may increase melanoma risk by blocking only UVB light while increasing exposure to melanoma-causing UVA.

6. Melanomas occur primarily on areas of the body that are seldom exposed to sunlight.

7. People who are work outdoors have fewer melanomas than those who spend their time indoors.

8. A low-fat, high nutrient diet, replete with colorful vegetables and fruit, is absolutely essential as a protection against melanoma and all other cancers.

SECTION 2

Solar Power and prevention of the Deadly Cancers

Chapter 6

How Solar Power prevents cancer

*"I think you might dispense with half your doctors
if you would only consult Dr. Sun more."*

Henry Ward Beecher

To understand the reasons that sunlight has such a strong anti-cancer effect, the following documented information lists some of the mechanisms by which vitamin D works. Dr. Edward Giovannucci explains that many cell types contain specialized vitamin D receptors (VDR), which when activated by vitamin D, turn on the genes that regulate many cell processes, some of which are potent anti-cancer mechanisms,[1] which we will now explain.

Vitamin D promotes apoptosis

Apoptosis is defined as natural cell death. When a cell has grown old or unhealthy, it needs to be replaced. ***Apoptosis is a programmed sequence of events that leads to the old or abnormal cell's death and elimination. Apoptosis is sometimes called "cell suicide."*** The body is composed of trillions of cells, and through apoptosis, the body daily replaces multi-billions as they age or display abnormalities. When apoptosis does not take place, cells may become "immortal;" they do not die off. Instead, they multiply out of control, and that is exactly what cancer is—the uncontrolled growth of abnormal cells. ***Vitamin D promotes apoptosis so that cells die normally.***[2-5]

Vitamin D promotes differentiation

Differentiation is the process by which cells take on the characteristics of the tissue surrounding them. In other words, they become a specific type of tissue: breast tissue, heart tissue, bone tissue, etc. Cancer cells, however, resist differentiation. They exhibit out-of-control growth, cell division and multiplication (proliferation) and they do not resemble the cells surrounding them. Vitamin D helps cancer cells differentiate.[6-8]

Vitamin D retards proliferation

Proliferation is the rapid growth and multiplication of cancer cells. If proliferation can be stopped, then cancer is stopped. Although vitamin D does not always stop proliferation, it does retard it, thereby slowing cancer growth.[4,8-12]

Vitamin D inhibits angiogenesis

Angiogenesis is the formation of blood vessels. It is a process that provides blood and nutrients to newly formed tissue. If angiogenesis in cancer cells can be stopped, the cells die. Vitamin D acts a selective angiogenesis inhibitor—it retards the growth of new, undesirable "feeder" blood vessels into cancer cells.[13-15] The beautiful thing about vitamin D is that it retards angiogenesis only in cancerous tissue. It is truly a miraculous chemical that knows the good guys from the bad guys.

Vitamin D slows invasiveness

Invasiveness is the spreading of cancer cells into healthy tissue. Normal cells respect borders and do not pass into other tissue. Cancer cells invade healthy tissue. Vitamin D inhibits the invasiveness of cancer cells.[12,16]

Vitamin D inhibits metastasis

Metastasis is the spreading of cancer cells from the initial location of the disease to another location, usually by way of the blood vessels or lymphatic system. For instance, breast cancer cells may be transported to bone and create a new tumor. Vitamin D inhibits metastasis, which keeps cancer localized and renders it less dangerous.[17-21]

Vitamin D works as an antioxidant and pro-oxidant to reduce cancer:

We discussed earlier that antioxidants from colorful vegetables and fruits help prevent free-radical damage to cells—a precursor to cancer. *Excessive antioxidants from supplements, however, may actually increase cancer.* The body uses free radicals in some cases to help destroy foreign invaders and to kill cancer cells. *Thus, pro-oxidant activity is sometimes desirable.* If we overwhelm the body with supplemental antioxidants, we run the risk of reducing its ability to cope with cancer cells. Vitamin D helps the body to kill cancer by enhancing the action of free radicals against cancer cells while reducing oxidative damage to normal cells.[22-23] Therefore vitamin D acts as both a selective pro-oxidant and selective antioxidant.[26]

Before we discuss the influence of vitamin D on individual internal cancers, let's consider two studies that assessed overall cancer risk. One was a four-year study that involved 1,179 women who were assessed as cancer-free at the beginning or the research.[24] Each was randomly assigned to daily take a (1) a placebo (a pill that has no physiological effect), (2) a typical calcium supplement with vitamin D or (3) a typical calcium supplement with vitamin D *plus* another 1,100 IU of vitamin D3. Such a double-blind, placebo-controlled, interventional study is considered the "gold standard" of research. At the end of the four-year period, those who took the calcium/vitamin D supplement had approximately a 50% reduction in risk of all cancers when compared to the placebo group, and those who took the same supplement plus 1,100 IU of vitamin D3 had approximately a 60% reduction. The results were even more impressive during the last three years. *Those who had taken 1,100 IU of vitamin D3 had a 77% reduction of all cancer risk when compared with the placebo group! This reduction in is about twice what could be expected if all the subjects had been smokers and then quit.*

The second study showed that those in the highest quartile (fourth) of serum-vitamin D levels had 55% less risk of death from all cancers than those in the lowest quartile.[25] The research also indicated that each increase of 10 ng/ml in serum levels of vitamin D lowered the risk of cancer by about 33%. The researchers also noted that among the more than 3,000 subjects in the study, only one died with a level of 80 ng/ml or more. However, the average level in the highest quartile was only about 31, meaning that on average, all four groups were well below optimal levels.

Now that you have a basic understanding of the mechanisms by which vitamin D prevents, reduces or retards cancer growth, let's discuss relationships among sunlight, vitamin D and internal cancers. You will now see the value of Solar Power for the prevention of these frightening and prevalent diseases, and you will discover definite steps to reduce risk. First, we consider the scourge of women in our sedentary, overfed, under-sunned society: breast cancer.

Chapter 7

Solar Power, breast cancer and other women's cancers

"A truly beautiful woman has a radiance of sunlight from her inner glow."

A Horrific Disease

No women's disease causes more fear than breast cancer. The burden on self-esteem, particularly for those who require surgery—is immense, and the medical cost is staggering. Many feel they are the victims of their genetics because female relatives have had the disease, but nothing could be further from the truth.

The American Cancer Society states that one in seven women will contract breast cancer, up from one in eleven in 1975. There are more than 211,000 new cases of breast cancer and more that 40,000 deaths each year.[1] ***The early-to-mid seventies were when the promotions of sun avoidance and sunscreen use began in earnest.*** However, melanoma and breast cancer incidence, as well as the incidence of many other cancers, have increased significantly since that time. While those facts do not prove that breast cancer is caused by sunlight avoidance and low-vitamin D levels, the following information indicates that they may indeed be important factors. Women are not doomed to breast cancer; lifestyle changes, including more sunlight exposure, may profoundly reduce the risk.

Does sunlight have a preventive effect on breast cancer?

Let's compare the breast cancer rates of women living in sunny areas with the rates of those living in areas with little sun or shorter sunny seasons. In 1989 Doctors Cedric and Frank Garland compared the rates of breast and colon cancer in twenty Canadian cities and the degree of acid-haze air pollution in each. Women in cities with the most acid haze had a greater chance of developing breast cancer.[2] Acid haze, of course, filters out some of the UVB that would otherwise stimulate production of vitamin D in the body. It also increases the length of the vitamin D winter.

Some might argue that more acid haze would also indicate more pollution, and that would be the real reason for the increased rate of breast cancer. That point would be well-taken. However, the Garlands in 1990 reported another study that clearly showed sunlight exposure was a factor in lowering the incidence of breast cancer.[28]   They compared breast cancer rates in geographic locations in the USA and showed that it is much more prevalent in the cloudier, darker Northeast than it is in the Southwest.[3] Other research also demonstrated a geographical difference that favored areas with greater exposure to UVB.[4-5]

The following cancer mortality (death) map is produced by the National Cancer Institute.   Note the significant differences in the incidence of cancer in the Northeast as compared to the South, Southwest and West (the West also typically has a higher altitude, so more UVB is available). Also note that urban areas, where sunlight is less available due to pollution, and where people stay indoors more, have a much higher breast-cancer rate than the more rural areas.

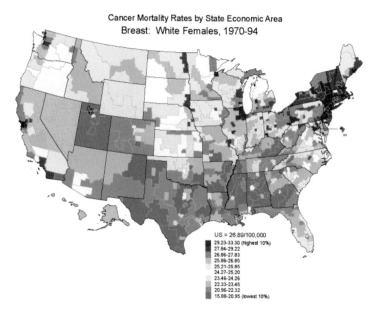

Cancer Mortality Rates by State Economic Area
Breast: White Females, 1970-94

US = 26.89/100,000
29.23-33.30 (highest 10%)
27.84-29.22
26.86-27.83
25.86-26.85
25.21-25.85
24.27-25.20
23.46-24.26
22.33-23.45
20.96-22.32
15.88-20.95 (lowest 10%)

Breast-Cancer Mortality Rates (Available at National Cancer Institute's Cancer Mortality Maps & Graphs and at SUNARC.org)

Numerous other studies show that the greater the sunlight exposure, the lesser is the rate of breast cancer. It might be argued that dietary habits, which are known to correlate to breast cancer rates, vary by locales, which explains the differing rates of cancer. However, it has been well established that there is very little difference in dietary habits from region to region in the USA,[6] so the most plausible explanation for the lower incidence of breast cancer in the South as compared with the Northeast is greater sunlight exposure in the South. Dr. William Grant authored an excellent paper on different risk factors for breast cancer and concluded that sunlight exposure stands alone as a protective factor when the data are adjusted for urbanization, pollution, dietary habits and other factors that might influence the findings.[6]

Sunlight exposure in youth predicts a lower risk of breast cancer in adulthood.

Considering the concerted effort by "experts" to ensure that children avoid that most natural of childhood activity—playing outdoors in the sun—it is no surprise that *girls who have the greatest exposure to sunlight during the ages of 10-19 have a 35% decreased risk of cancer as adults when compared to those who had the least exposure.*[35]

I found no research that indicated that the rate of breast cancer or any other major internal cancer increases due to sunlight exposure. Yet, it is common to see web-site and printed materials claiming that women who fear breast cancer should avoid "known carcinogens" like sunlight exposure. These are unfounded statements and there are never any references given for such pronouncements. In fact, such ideas are dangerous to women's health.

Dr. Esther John and her colleagues performed a study on the relationship of breast cancer rates, sunlight exposure and dietary vitamin D. They analyzed the data from a large national study called HANES 1 (H1). Dr. John studied more than 5,000 white women who had completed a health survey between 1971-1974, and who were reassessed in 1992, and found that those with higher sunlight exposure and higher supplemental vitamin D intake reduced their risk of breast cancer by 15% to 33%.[7]

Perhaps their most important finding was that those who lived in the sunniest areas and had the highest exposure to sunlight had a 65% reduction in breast cancer rates compared to those who had the least sunlight exposure. Dr. John stated, "These data support the hypothesis that sunlight and dietary vitamin D reduce the risk of breast cancer." Scientists can be masters of the understatement, perhaps to not come off as too excited about their research or to raise the ire of the medical/pharmaceutical complex. *If a pill were discovered that produced a 65% reduction in breast cancer, the news would be emblazoned across the Internet, the newspapers and every news channel.* It would cause a sensation and rack up sales in the billions of dollars. Lamentably, only people looking for research on sunlight and vitamin D are likely to find Dr. John's life-saving information.

The chart demonstrates the spectacular reduction in risk of breast cancer produced by increasing sunlight exposure for those living in areas of high solar radiation.[7] Relative Risk (RR) indicates the risk of breast cancer observed in women with differing degrees of lifetime sunlight exposure. The lowest sunlight exposure is given score of 1, which is the highest risk category for breast cancer. The other fractions represent the risk observed among those with greater sunlight exposure.

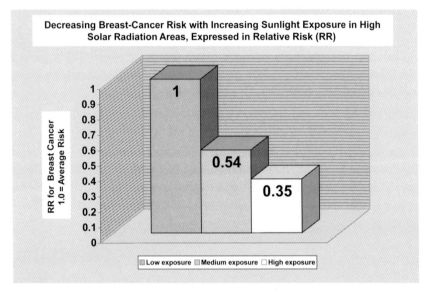

Let's repeat the statistics on NMSC and melanoma: NMSC are easily removed, and regular sunlight exposure helps *prevent* melanoma. It is estimated that about 1,500 yearly deaths are attributable to common skin cancers. More than 40,000 yearly deaths are caused by breast cancer. Which is preferable, an easily-treated common skin cancer or a deadly breast cancer? The counterintuitive advice to avoid the sun kills thousands of women each year in an attempt to prevent common skin cancer, a disease that kills very few.

Melanoma, on the other hand, kills about 2,800 women per year,[1] and occurs most frequently on areas of the body that are seldom exposed to the sun. Melanoma is easily treated if discovered in its initial stages, and is dramatically reduced by proper nutrition. Therefore, the "sunscare" has cost the lives of hundreds of thousands by increasing breast cancer. It is also likely that tens of thousands more have died of melanoma due to lack of regular, moderate exposure to sunlight. Even if melanoma were caused by sun exposure, a woman would have better chances with a cancer that claims 2,800 lives per year as opposed to one that takes 40,000. Fortunately such a choice is not necessary; sunlight exposure reduces both cancers.

Is vitamin D the key to the sun's healthful influence on breast cancer?

Let's now consider some of the research that assesses the direct influence of vitamin D on breast cancer. Low blood levels of vitamin D (less than 20 ng/ml) are associated with increasing breast-cancer rates. *Research shows that women with a combination of a genetically susceptible tendency to breast cancer and a low blood level of vitamin D (less than 20 ng/ml) had nearly seven times the breast cancer rate as those without a family history of susceptibility genetics and a blood level above 20 ng/ml.*[8] The researchers concluded that low-vitamin D, levels both alone and in combination with less favorable genetics, may increase risk of breast cancer. Another study showed that women with the highest blood levels of vitamin D had about 27% lower risk of breast cancer than those with the lowest levels.[9]

A study in 2006 showed that *the highest serum levels of vitamin D (over 52ng/ml) correlated to a 50% reduced risk of breast cancer.*[29] Other research noted that women with the greatest intake of vitamin D or the greatest sunlight exposure between the ages of 10 and 29—the most typical age of breast cancer development—reduced their risk of breast cancer by 40-55%.[30] Another study in 2007 showed that women with the highest serum levels of vitamin D had a 69% reduced risk when compared to those with the lowest levels.[36] There was a striking dose-response relationship between higher vitamin D and lower breast-cancer risk, as illustrated in the graph.

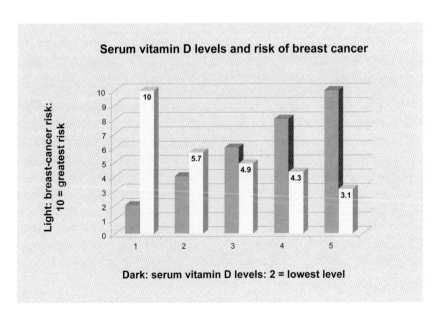

83

This research led to another study that assessed how much supplemental vitamin D was necessary to produce the 52 ng/ml needed to reduce breast cancer rates by 50%.[37] A daily intake of 2,000 IU of vitamin D3 combined with moderate exposure to sunlight did the job. Other scientists, using pooled analyses of available research, estimated that *maintaining a vitamin D blood level of 55ng/ml would prevent the breast-cancer deaths of 85,000 women yearly and that the deaths prevented worldwide would be 350,000.*[34]

The use of vitamin D in preventing breast cancer is also supported by lab studies. In one, vitamin D was added to human breast-cancer cells growing in mice. Growth was inhibited by 50% as compared to similar cells not subjected to vitamin D,[10] and without toxicity. There was significant anti-tumor activity, and the researchers suggested that vitamin D therapy be used as a form of "chemotherapy" to treat breast cancer. Another experiment arrived at similar conclusions; it showed that the proliferation of mammary cancers in mice was reduced by 35% when treated with vitamin D, and that the growth rate of hormone-induced tumors dropped by 50%.[11] *There was also a regression of tumors in some of the animals.*

Even more important than the use of vitamin D as a chemotherapeutic agent is its use as a chemopreventive agent. If regular sunlight exposure can reduce the chance of breast cancer by 50%, it seems that such information should be presented to women by physicians and by the government along with advice on how to safely and effectively sunbathe. Is it not being publicized because it would profoundly reduce profits from treating breast cancer?

One might forgive the fact that sunlight and vitamin D therapies are not being widely used as cancer-preventive measures if there were only a few isolated studies mildly hinting at their efficacy. But such *is not* the case. The literature is replete with examples of breast cancer being prevented, lessened or treated by vitamin D,[12-17] and it is also known that when a cancer is diagnosed in summer or fall (times of greatest serum levels of vitamin D), the prognosis for survival is considerably improved.[18,31] This demonstrates that vitamin D works against breast cancer even when the cancer is already detectable.

Some artificial lights may also induce breast cancer. Breast cancer implanted in mice grows vigorously when they are exposed to night light.[19] Melatonin metabolism is disrupted by evening light—perhaps the reason for the increased growth. A meta-analysis of studies done on breast cancer and shift work showed a convincing increase with increasing hours of shift work,[26] *especially after twenty years, which correlates to an 80% increase in breast cancer.*[27]

Vitamin D levels and breast-tissue density

Excessively dense breast tissue is a risk factor for breast cancer. In an investigation into the relationship of breast density as measured by mammography to serum-vitamin D levels, it was found that there was a strong inverse correlation; the higher the density, the lower the vitamin D levels.[38]

Vitamin D levels and breast-cancer survival

Does the blood level of vitamin D at the time of diagnosis of breast cancer make a difference in a woman's time of survival? Yes, it does. *The cancer is much more aggressive in those whose serum vitamin D levels are low; they are 94% more likely to have the cancer metastasize and 73% more likely to die within ten years of diagnosis.*[39] Thus, vitamin D acts to both prevent cancer and to lessen its severity once diagnosed.

Sunlight, vitamin D and other reproductive cancers

Less research has been done on ovarian, uterine and cervical cancers than on breast cancer, but there is some compelling evidence to suggest that their incidence is diminished by regular sunlight exposure[20-23] and/or high intake of vitamin D.[24] In a study done in Mexico, women who had the highest vitamin D intakes had a 57% reduced ovarian cancer risk when compared to those in the lowest intake category. Even more impressive was a later study done on uterine cancer. *The highest intake of vitamin D predicted a 62% reduced chance of uterine (endometrial) cancer.*[25]

In 2007, an inverse correlation was shown for UVB exposure and endometrial cancer when using data from 107 countries located at different latitudes.[32] The rates were much higher at higher latitudes (where there is less UVB available) in both the Northern and Southern hemispheres than at latitudes closer to the equator. Here is another map that shows the distribution of ovarian cancer in the USA. Although the distribution is not identical to that for breast cancer, the similarities are striking. Major urban areas are especially prone to high ovarian cancer incidence.

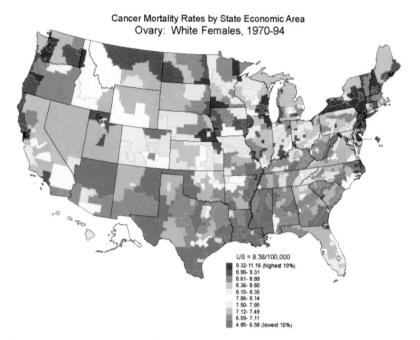

Cancer Mortality Rates by State Economic Area
Ovary: White Females, 1970-94

US = 8.38/100,000
9.32-11.16 (highest 10%)
8.90- 9.31
8.61- 8.89
8.36- 8.60
8.15- 8.35
7.86- 8.14
7.50- 7.85
7.12- 7.49
6.59- 7.11
4.85- 6.58 (lowest 10%)

Ovarian Cancer Mortality Rates (Available at National Cancer Institute's Cancer Mortality Maps & Graphs and at SUNARC.org)

Research on vitamin D supplementation and cancer in women

The most compelling study on the influence of vitamin D on cancer risk in women was conducted by Dr. Joan Lappe and her colleagues at Creighton University.[33]   The four-year study involved 1,179 women who were assessed as cancer-free at the onset. Each was randomly assigned to daily take (1) a placebo (a pill that has no physiological effect), (2) a typical calcium supplement with vitamin D or (3) a typical calcium supplement with vitamin D *plus* another 1,100 IU of vitamin D3. Such a double-blind, placebo-controlled, interventional study and is considered the "gold standard" of research. At the end of the four-year period, those who took the calcium/vitamin D supplement had approximately a 50% reduction in risk of all cancers when compared to the placebo group and those who took the same supplement plus 1,100 IU of vitamin D3 had approximately a 60% reduction. The results were even more impressive during the last three years. ***Those who had taken 1,100 IU of vitamin D3 had a 77% reduction of all cancer risk when compared with the placebo group! This reduction in is about twice what could be expected if all the subjects had been smokers and then quit.***

86

Are we seeing the pattern here? You might conclude, "Go south young woman." At least be sure that your blood levels of vitamin D measure at least 40 ng/ml. Eat a diet low in fat and high in nutrients, and use a tanning bed twice weekly when sunning is not possible—with your doctor's permission of course. A tropical vacation each winter might also be a good idea, but be sure not to burn.

Breast and reproductive cancers create fear in women, and prostate cancer scares men. Is there any evidence that sunlight reduces prostate cancer among men? That is the subject of the next chapter.

What have we learned?

1. **Breast cancer and reproductive cancers are least common in the areas of greatest sunlight exposure.**

2. **High sunlight exposure correlates with up to a 65% reduced risk of breast cancer.**

3. **Sun avoidance may cause thousands of unnecessary deaths from breast cancer.**

4. **Vitamin D may be an effective chemotherapeutic and chemopreventive agent for female reproductive cancers, without patient trauma.**

5. **Vitamin D supplementation over four years has been shown to correlate to a 60-77% reduction in the risk of *all* cancer in women.**

6. **Shift work, and exposure to some types of artificial light may promote breast cancer.**

7. **5.   Low-fat, high nutrient nutrition is absolutely essential for the prevention of all cancers.**

Chapter 8

Sunlight, vitamin D and prostate cancer

"Sunlight could save your life"
Dr. Zane Kime

Increased sunlight exposure means decreased prostate cancer.

In 2005, Dr. Esther John and colleagues reported on research in which they compared the lifetime sun exposure of 450 white men with advanced prostate cancer that of 455 white men who did not have cancer.[1] The men were divided into five groups (quintiles) according to the amount of sun exposure they had received. *The results were impressive. The men in the highest quintile of sun exposure had only 51% of the risk of prostate cancer as did those in the lowest quintile.* A similar result had been obtained in a much earlier study.[2]

Several studies have shown that high sun exposure over a lifetime relates to a considerably lower rate of death from prostate cancer.[4-7] The last study[7] showed that those living in the South had a reduced risk of prostate cancer of 32% compared to the expected rate of prostate cancer. Those who had lived longest in the South had a 34% reduced rate, and *those who were born in a state with high solar radiation had a reduced risk of 49%—results that were nearly identical to the study mentioned in the first paragraph of this chapter.*

It is also interesting that a paper written on the history of sunlight exposure—comparing it to the risk of prostate cancer later in life—revealed that numerous childhood sunburns are protective against later prostate cancer; *those men who had sunburned as children had only about one-fifth the risk of contracting prostate cancer as those who had not sunburned.[8]* Figure 1 illustrates the risk of prostate cancer compared with four measures of childhood sunlight exposure: sunburns, foreign holidays, sunbathing history and low measures of exposure to UV. Note that sunburns are the best predictor of low prostate cancer risk, and that low UV exposure predicts more than triple the average risk.

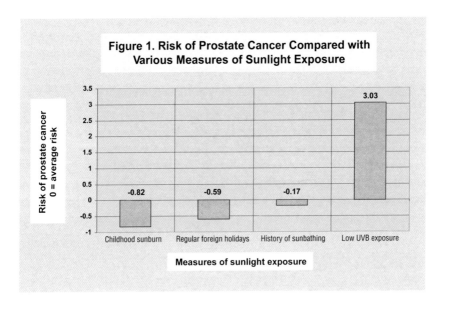

Figure 1. Risk of Prostate Cancer Compared with Various Measures of Sunlight Exposure

Nevertheless, burning *per se* is never a good thing. Burning in this study was nothing more than an indicator of high sunlight exposure during childhood and subsequently high vitamin D levels. The research also showed that among men who did have prostate cancer, the onset of the disease was delayed among those who had had the greatest sun exposure compared to those with low sun exposure.[8] The study did not differentiate between regular and occasional sunbathing, so it does not appear to be very significant for reducing prostate cancer risk, lowering the risk by only 17%. However, we will see that regular sunbathing is indeed a big boon to warding off prostate cancer.

One of the most pernicious pieces of advice for children, is that they should not play in the sunlight. ***Should they be denied the benefits of UVB that might reduce by half their risk of prostate and breast cancers by half when they are adults?*** It would be far better to keep them away from fast-fat restaurants and to instead feed them healthful, low-fat foods. Parents should resolve to teach their children to eat dark greens and plenty of colorful fruits and then send them out to play in the sun! ***Of course, it is wise to make sure they do not burn.*** Red-haired, light-skinned children or others who do not tan should protect themselves with hats and clothing after brief exposure. Remember that burning is dangerous, but plenty of sunlight may be enjoyed without damage to the skin.

Sunbathing and prostate cancer

A review of studies by Dr. S Moon and colleagues, which compared sunlight exposure and prostate cancer risk, showed an inverse relationship.[9] The researchers cite two of their studies showing that the less the exposure to sunlight, the greater the risk of cancer. The subjects in two of studies were divided into four groups (quartiles) according to the lifetime sunlight exposure they had received. ***Those in the lowest quartile of sunlight exposure had more than three times the risk of developing prostate cancer as those in the highest quartile.*** Figure 2 describes the stair-step relationship observed between sunlight and prostate cancer in the second of the two studies. It is interesting to note the profound difference between the third and fourth "steps." Those in the lowest (fourth) category of sunlight exposure were twice as likely to contract cancer as those in the third category.

Dr. Moon's group noted that when sunbathing was compared with prostate cancer, ***men in the lowest exposure quartile of sunbathing had 5.33 times the risk of prostate cancer as those in the highest quartile.*** Other research has indicated that "higher levels of cumulative exposure, adult sunbathing, childhood sunburning and regular holidays in hot climates were each independently and significantly associated with a reduced risk of this cancer."[10]

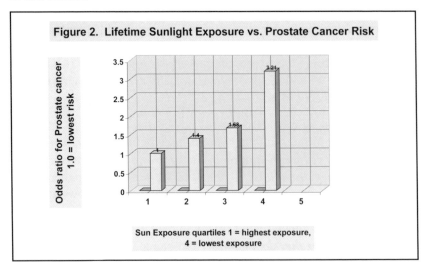

Norwegian studies further corroborated the inverse correlation between prostate cancer and sunlight when death rates from prostate, breast and colon cancer were compared to the season in which the cancer was diagnosed.[11,41]

Over 36 months, study subjects diagnosed during summer and fall had much lower death rates than those diagnosed in winter and spring.

Finally, researchers have analyzed the rate of prostate cancer by latitude in the USA and found a direct correlation between low UVB exposure in northern latitudes and the incidence of prostate cancer.[42] This correlation was particularly evident in areas above 40 degrees north latitude, where the vitamin D winter is quite long.

PSA studies

PSA (prostate specific antigen) measurements are used to assess a man's chance of contracting, or possibly already having, prostate cancer. The higher the PSA level in the blood, the greater the chance of cancer. When the prostate gland is undergoing changes that may lead to cancer, PSA levels generally rise. PSA is usually high when a man already has prostate cancer, and usually become higher as it progresses. In men who already have the cancer, *the time it takes for the PSA value to double determines how aggressively the disease is progressing.* Men with the lowest levels of lifetime sunlight exposure have the highest PSA levels.[3] Chapter 6 discussed how vitamin D thwarts cancer by promoting differentiation and apoptosis and by reducing angiogenesis, metastasis, proliferation and invasiveness. For prostate cancer we may add to that list the inhibition of increasing PSA levels or the actual lowering of PSA. This result is probably due to increased vitamin D, as shown in an investigation that considered only supplementation. The researchers administered vitamin D to fifteen men with prostate cancer and measured the time it took for the doubling of PSA. The men were treated for eight months. *PSA doubling time increased in fourteen patients, and eight of them had a drop in PSA levels.*[23] Other studies also showed benefits vitamin D on PSA levels and doubling time.[24]

Does vitamin D reduce the risk of prostate cancer?

In 1990, Dr. Gary Schwartz and colleagues observed that prostate cancer was more common among older men, black men and men who lived in northern latitudes. They saw that vitamin D deficiency closely paralleled the incidence of prostate cancer in these groups and suggested that the deficiency could increase the risk of prostate cancer.[12] Since then it has become obvious that vitamin D has a protective effect against prostate cancer, although one study indicated that high vitamin D levels might have a deleterious effect.[13] It has been suggested that since the study was done in

Scandinavia, where fish-liver oils are often used as vitamin D supplements, the high vitamin A content of these oils may inhibit the positive influence of vitamin D[13] and cause a considerable increase of osteoporosis.[14,48]

Nevertheless, the research by Dr. John and the review by Dr. Moon show that *the highest sunlight exposure is accompanied by the lowest incidence of prostate cancer.* Since sunlight in high doses produces vast quantities of vitamin D and correlates to a reduced risk of nearly all other internal cancers, the best odds for survival favor plenty of safe and sane sunlight exposure. *If sunbathers have only one-fifth the chance of contracting prostate cancer, it is obvious that the high levels of vitamin D produced by sunbathing are not a problem.*

Experiments have also shown that Vitamin D has the ability to inhibit the proliferation of prostate cancer cells.[15-16] It also decreases metastasis[17] and inhibits invasiveness,[18-19] slows angiogenesis[20] and promotes differentiation[21] and apoptosis.[22] Vitamin D retards the activity of two enzymes that prostate cancer needs to metastasize, [4] and it has been shown to stimulate the release of an antioxidant enzyme, G6PD, that quenches free-radical molecules in healthy prostate tissue. Without G6PD, free radicals might attack and cause cancerous changes.[49] *Amazingly, vitamin D does not stimulate G6PD in cancerous tissue, because the body needs free radicals to oxidize and kill cancer. Vitamin D "recognizes" the difference between healthy and cancerous prostate tissue!*

Aggressive" and "dormant" prostate cancers

Dr Gary Schwartz has produced an excellent review on the research done on vitamin D and its relationship to prostate cancer.[25] Many of the citations here are taken from that review.

Dr. Schwartz *explains that the disease can be identified in two categories: clinical and subclinical.* Clinical prostate cancer has been diagnosed and is being treated; subclinical cancer is dormant, and when observed microscopically appears identical to clinical cancer.[27] But if it becomes clinical, it becomes aggressive and life-threatening. When men who have died from causes other than prostate cancer are autopsied, 27% in their 40's, 30% in their 50's and 60% in their 80's have subclinical prostate cancer and the percentage continues to increase with age.[26-27] There is little difference in the rate of subclinical prostate cancer regardless of geographic differences or racial background.[28] Clinical prostate cancer, however, varies greatly in its geographical and racial incidence, and

92

death rates also vary greatly. As Dr. Schwartz states, there is a "striking variation by place." *There is a 20-fold variance in death from areas of highest rates to areas with the lowest rates, with African Americans and northern Europeans having the highest death rates.* The similarity in death rates in those two groups indicates a common factor that promotes the disease. That factor is probably vitamin D, since both groups have low levels. And as Schwartz notes, levels in blacks are usually less than half those in Caucasians living at the same latitudes.[29]

Vitamin D may prevent harmless, subclinical prostate cancer from developing into the full-blown, virulent and deadly form. In the 1960s, the death rate for prostate cancer among Japanese Americans was 15 times that of native Japanese men.[25] It is obvious that there has been a lifestyle change among Japanese who have moved to the USA, and that it has had a detrimental influence on their health. It is likely that part of the difference is vitamin D consumption. There is little vitamin D in the American diet, but vitamin D-rich fish is heavily consumed in Japan.[30] Tuna and skipjack, consumed regularly by the Japanese, have 16,000 and 57,000 IU in one gram of their oils,[31] and serum vitamin D levels among Japanese are among the highest in the world.[32-33]

A recent investigation showed that men who were below average in their serum vitamin D levels had about 250% greater risk of the deadly, aggressive prostate cancer than those who were above average.[43]

In another study, two groups of men were compared for fish consumption. Those in the first group all had prostate cancer. The second group was cancer-free. No one in the cancer group reported any fish consumption, but in the cancer-free group, fourteen ate fish—a remarkable finding.[34] Vitamin D was most likely the mechanism that protected the fish eaters. But before we praise fish, note that oily fish consumption correlated *positively* with another cancer—breast cancer. Those who ate such fish had about 13% more breast cancer than those who did not eat it.[35]

Since such a large segment of the world's male population has subclinical prostate cancer, the most important role vitamin D plays in thwarting prostate cancer is in preventing dormant prostate cancer from developing into the life-threatening, aggressive version. Men who are susceptible to prostate cancer due to their genetic makeup have a 250% increased risk of developing the aggressive form,[45] *but even in men who have a genetic susceptibility and above-average vitamin D levels, there is no increased risk of either the aggressive or dormant form.*

93

Metabolic syndrome, vitamin D and prostate cancer

Metabolic syndrome is a cluster of physiological measurements such as high blood pressure, abdominal obesity, high triglyceride levels, low HDL ("good cholesterol") levels, high blood-sugar and insulin resistance. Men in the top quartile (fourth) of metabolic syndrome measurements have 3.36 times risk of prostate cancer when compared to the men in the bottom three quartiles,[44] *but when the men in the top quartile also have low vitamin D levels, their risk increases to 8.03 times that of the men in the bottom quartiles!* (Read more on metabolic syndrome in Chapter 14)

What does this mean for American men?

If we exclude common skin cancers (NMSC), prostate cancer is by far the most common cancer in men.[36] There are approximately 235,000 new prostate cancer cases per year in the USA, representing 33% of all new cancer cases. Nearly 30,000 men die yearly from this disease, which represents 10% of all cancer deaths in men. That percentage is exceeded only by lung cancer. Regular sunlight exposure could prevent thousands of those deaths per year.

Even if we assumed *incorrectly* that sunlight caused melanoma, it would still be clear that we should sunbathe regularly to prevent prostate cancer. Among men, there are about 5,000 deaths yearly from melanoma. It is nonsensical to avoid sunlight to prevent a cancer that kills 5,000 men yearly while increasing the risk of prostate cancer that kills 30,000. *And don't forget that prostate cancer is only one of twenty plus major internal cancers whose incidence is dramatically lowered by sunlight exposure. Multi-thousands of people die prematurely from cancer each year due to low levels of vitamin D.*[37,38] Dr. Giovannucci and colleagues have established that 85,500 men per year in the USA die from cancer because of vitamin D insufficiency,[40] and a disproportionately high number are African Americans.[39]

In spite of these and other studies, I know of only a few physicians who prescribe vitamin D, sunlight or sunlamps to prevent cancer. What I found instead were a few doctors who said that drug companies were busy producing new vitamin D analogues. Analogues have a slightly different chemical structure (to make them patentable and profitable), and they will be frightfully more expensive than vitamin D supplements.

Next, we will discuss a cancer that devastates both sexes: colon cancer.

What have we learned?

1. Prostate specific antigen (PSA) is a marker for potential or existing prostate cancer. Men who have been exposed to more sunlight during their lifetimes have lower PSA levels.

2. Treatment with vitamin D slows the increase in PSA levels and in some cases lowers PSA.

3. Men who were sunburned as children have only about one-fifth the chance of contracting prostate cancer as those who were not sunburned.

4. Men with the least lifetime sunbathing exposure had more than five times the risk of prostate cancer as those who sunbathed most.

5. Vitamin D inhibits the proliferation of prostate cancer cells.

6. Men diagnosed during summer and fall, when vitamin D levels are highest, have much lower risks of prostate cancer death than those diagnosed in winter and spring when D levels are low.

1. There is a 20-fold difference in death rates from areas of highest prostate-cancer death to areas with the lowest levels of death, with African Americans and northern Europeans having the highest death rates. Both groups have chronically low vitamin D levels.

2. Vitamin D's major benefit for prostate cancer may be in preventing the harmless dormant type from changing into the deadly, aggressive type.

Chapter 9

Solar Power, colon cancer and other internal cancers

"Love comforteth like sunshine after rain."
William Shakespeare

It is apparent that ample sunlight exposure and optimal vitamin D levels are protective against breast and prostate cancers. ***They are decreased by at least 50% or more—when comparing the highest sun exposure groups to the lowest.*** As we consider the next major killer, we find a situation that is just as compelling. ***"Sunlight," as Dr. Zane Kime once said, "could save your life."***

The discussion now shifts from the reproductive tissue cancers—breast, ovarian, and uterine in women and prostate in men—to a deadly killer of both sexes. Ten percent of all cancer deaths in the USA are due to colon and rectal cancers, or "colorectal cancer." There are approximately 71,000 new cases per year in men and about 73,000 in women.[62]

Vitamin D and the development of polyps

A benign (non-cancerous) growth in the colon known as a polyp or adenoma is usually the precursor to colon cancer. Unless these polyps are present in the colon, cancer is unlikely to develop. Therefore, anything that prevents polyps will also likely prevent colon cancer. Some research shows that low blood levels of vitamin D are associated with an increased incidence of polyps.[1] Women with serum levels below 26 ng/ml have a 58% greater chance of developing polyps than those above 26 ng/ml. Also, ***research shows that with each 10 ng/ml increase in blood vitamin D levels, the risk of polyps decreases by 26%!***[2] Also, ***women with the highest serum vitamin D levels have only 27% of the risk of developing adenomas as those in the lowest quartile***[3] Another study showed a 29% decreased risk among men with the highest vitamin D intake compared to those with the lowest intake.[4]

Vitamin D and colorectal cancer

Men whose vitamin D levels are below 20 ng/ml have twice the risk of those with higher levels,[6] and colon cancer decreases consistently with increasing vitamin D blood levels. An even more dramatic decrease is observed for rectal cancer when evaluated separately.[6] Figure 1 illustrates the decrease of rectal cancer risk with increasing blood levels by quartile. Quartile 1 is the lowest level of serum vitamin D; quartile 4 is the highest.

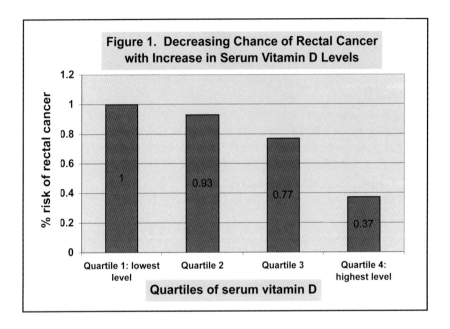

Figure 1. Decreasing Chance of Rectal Cancer with Increase in Serum Vitamin D Levels

Note the impressive drop in risk for those with very highest levels when compared to those in the second highest level. A level of 40 ng/ml and above is essential. In fact, Dr. Edward Gorham and colleagues showed that *a level of 34 ng/ml reduced colorectal cancer 50% and estimated that 46 ng/ml would reduce the risk by two-thirds compared to those who had the lowest levels.* [73] Keeping serum vitamin D levels high is exceptionally important. *Another study, showed that men with the lowest levels of vitamin D had 4.6 times the risk of rectal cancer as men with the highest levels, and women with the lowest levels had 2.7 times the risk.*[68] Many other studies show similar findings.[7-10, 14]

How many colon cancer deaths might be prevented by keeping vitamin D levels high? *In 2007, Doctor Cedrick Garland and colleagues, using pooled analyses of available research, estimated that maintaining a vitamin D blood level of 55ng/ml could annually prevent 250,000 deaths worldwide,*[67] *including 60,000 in the USA*

Vitamin D and the anti-cancer protein, bax

Bax is a protein that promotes apoptosis in the colon. Apoptosis (chapter 6), is a programmed sequence of events that leads to the natural and desirable death of old or improperly-functioning cells. Cancer cells resist apoptosis and replicate themselves uncontrollably, never dying naturally. Vitamin D and calcium supplementation increase bax and thereby may reduce colon cancer.[74]

Animal studies

Vitamin D-deficient rats experience accelerated cancer growth.[11-12] Over ten weeks, one group was fed a vitamin D-deficient diet and another a vitamin D-sufficient diet.[11] Cancer tumors were then induced in their colons and tumor growth measured. *After eighteen days, tumors in the vitamin D-deficient rats were 56% larger than in the D-sufficient group.* In a follow-up study the vitamin D-sufficient rats were given even larger quantities to determine if it would further slow tumor development. *After nineteen days, tumor growth was further reduced by 41%-52%.*

Sunlight and colon cancer

In 1980, the Garlands published a seminal paper showing the relationship between colon cancer and geographical location.[15] They observed dramatically higher rates of colon cancer in the Northeast compared with the South and West. Some might wonder why northern states in the west have low rates compared to states at similar latitudes in the Northeast. Much of the western population lives at considerably higher altitudes than people in the Northeast, and the air in the West is generally cleaner—both factors that increase the quantity of UVB available. Dr. Grant has also pointed out that the stratospheric ozone layer is thinner in the west due to the prevailing westerlies, which push air across the Rocky Mountains, and, in doing so, push the tropopause up, thereby thinning the stratospheric ozone layer and lessening the filtration of UVB.[75]

Figure 2 shows the death rates for colon cancer among men in different areas of the USA.

There is a very high rate of colon cancer in the Northeast. Of course, the area is low in altitude and high in latitude, which creates an extended "vitamin D winter." There is also more UVB-filtering pollution and people tend to spend more time indoors. Note that urban areas of the West, Northwest, Southwest and Southeast have higher rates of colon cancer than more rural areas.

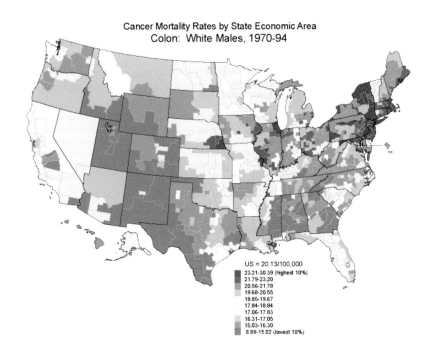

Cancer Mortality Rates by State Economic Area
Colon: White Males, 1970-94

US = 20.13/100,000
23.21-30.39 (highest 10%)
21.79-23.20
20.56-21.78
19.68-20.55
18.85-19.67
17.84-18.84
17.06-17.83
16.31-17.05
15.03-16.30
8.89-15.02 (lowest 10%)

Figure 2: Colon Cancer Mortality Rates. Available at SUNARC.org

Other studies have corroborated the correlation between high sunlight exposure and low cancer rates. In Japan, people in the areas of highest solar radiation exhibit the lowest rates of colon cancer, with those living in the areas of highest UVB having about half the colon cancer rate as those living in the lowest.[16] Dr. T Mizoue, a coauthor of this study, found that cancers of the esophagus, stomach, colon, rectum, pancreas, gallbladder and bile ducts were less common in high-sunlight areas. *A significant aspect of this research is that sunlight had protective effects on cancers even where vitamin D consumption was high.* It appears that sunlight may have beneficial affects on cancer beyond its stimulation of vitamin D production.

Sun exposure also helps people who are diagnosed with colon cancer. When patients are first diagnosed with colon cancer in summer or fall—when blood levels of vitamin D are highest—their death rates in the next several years are 30% lower than those whose cancers are initially diagnosed in winter or spring.[17]

Lifestyle factors influence colon cancer

Keep in mind that vitamin D and sunlight are two major factors in preventing colon cancer, but they are certainly not the only ones. Research shows that those in the highest third of red-meat and processed-meat consumption have 50%-70% greater risk of developing colon and rectal cancer,[18] and women who consume 94 grams of red meat per day have 122% greater risk compared to those who consume less than 50 grams .[19] Ninety-four grams is only three and one-half ounces of meat! Other studies consistently link higher red-meat consumption to colon cancer,[20-22] and white-meat intake is associated with an even higher risk. In an assessment of Seventh-Day-Adventists, those who ate one helping or more of red meat per week had a 90% increased risk of colon cancer compared with those who ate no meat. *Worse yet, one helping of white meat per week predicted an increased risk of 229% compared to no meat consumption.[31] In an assessment of risk factors, general animal-food consumption predicted a 6-10 times increased risk.[23]*

Those who want to know more about the relationship between animal foods and cancer should read Dr. T. Colin Campbell's bestselling landmark book, *The China Study*. Among other information, he and his team found, through a series of experiments, that milk protein (casein) could be used like an electric switch to turn liver cancer on and off in rats.[24-29] Campbell's studies in China, the most massive nutrition studies ever undertaken, also showed that degenerative diseases increased in a dose-response fashion with animal-product consumption.[30] The New York Times called The China Study the "Grand Prix of epidemiology."

It is indisputable that colon cancer can be quite accurately predicted based on the quantity of vegetable foods that are consumed. The higher the consumption of vegetable foods, the lower is the risk of cancer.[32] *Diseases are seldom due to one cause; they result from a combination of many factors. Conversely, diseases are seldom prevented by one lifestyle change; many factors work in concert.* That is why I cite research on nutrition and its role in colon cancer.

Another factor is exercise, which reduces the risk of colon cancer. Improving exercise and nutrition habits is difficult, but essential for those who seek vibrant health. At least sunlight and vitamin D consumption can be easily changed. Sunbathing each day is enticing, especially when one can read a good book, conduct business by phone or write while doing it. To save time, you may wish to multi-task healthful habits by walking in the sun while wearing shorts and carrying a sack full of vegetables and fruits. That would be the best of all worlds, right?

Lifestyle really does make a difference. Utah is one of the "healthiest" states in the USA. People there generally consume less alcohol and tobacco and get outdoors for exercise more than people in many other states. Next door to Utah is Nevada, which consistently ranks as one of the most "unhealthy" states. All one has to do is visit St. George, Utah and then neighboring Las Vegas, Nevada to see the contrast between lifestyles. Colon-cancer risk is higher In Nevada, although UVB availability is nearly equal in the two states.

We have shown that sunlight and vitamin D have major roles in the prevention of three major cancers: breast, prostate and colon. We have also demonstrated that the risks for other reproductive cancers such as uterine, ovarian and cervical cancer are diminished by sunlight/vitamin D. Dr Mizoue established that along with colorectal cancer, several other digestive system cancers were diminished in areas of higher sunlight and vitamin D.[16] Are other cancers prevented or retarded by regular sunlight exposure and/or high vitamin D levels? The answer is an emphatic "yes!"

Solar power and vitamin D inhibit other major internal cancers.

Pancreatic cancer

Several studies indicate a protective influence of sunlight/vitamin D on pancreatic cancer. A comparison of that cancer's incidence to sunlight exposure showed a decreasing rate with increasing sunlight availability.[33] Other research showed that vitamin D dramatically inhibited pancreatic-cancer cell growth in a laboratory.[34-37] Still another investigation demonstrated that those who consumed the most vitamin D reduced their risk of pancreatic cancer by 40% compared to those who consumed the least.[70] Impressive, but the amount of vitamin D consumed was minimal— only 600 IU daily. It would be interesting to see that would happen at 2,000-5,000 IU daily.

Bladder Cancer

Bladder cancer also diminishes as sunlight exposure increases,[33] and vitamin D inhibits bladder-cancer cell growth in dogs.[38] Whether it would work in humans is unknown, but the best advice would be to put oneself on the side of caution with high vitamin D levels. Vitamin D also inhibits cell growth and increases apoptosis in bladder cancer cells from humans and rats.[39]

Brain cancer

People born in colder seasons have greater brain cancer risk as children[40-41] and as adults. Adults born in the months of January and February have especially high rates of brain cancer compared to those born in July and August, which could be due to low vitamin D levels in pregnant mothers[42] It has also been shown that low vitamin D levels in prenatal mother rats cause alterations in the brains of baby rats[43] and reduce apoptosis and differentiation of cancer cells as those brains develop.[44] Vitamin D also causes the death of brain-cancer cells taken from both humans and rats. Even a short exposure to vitamin D (24 hours) causes an impressive cell death.[45]

Kidney (renal) cancer

One study showed that vitamin D is a strong inhibitor of kidney cancer,[46] and another showed a strong inverse correlation between sunlight exposure and kidney cancer.[63] Still another showed the same correlation in an assessment of kidney cancer and sunlight exposure in 175 countries.[72]

Leukemia

Leukemia is an often fatal disease of the blood and blood-producing organs and is yet another type of cancer that may also be inhibited by vitamin D. Lab experiments show that vitamin D inhibits the proliferation of leukemia cells and promotes differentiation or otherwise has a therapeutic effect.[47-52]

A search of PubMed on the effects of vitamin D on leukemia revealed dozens of reports that show a positive benefit and none that show negative influences. None studied the influence of sunlight on leukemia, but it does not take a great leap of faith to predict that sunlight exposure generates the vitamin D that performs anti-leukemia functions.

Lung Cancer

The season of lung-cancer surgery makes a difference in survival rates. One study states, "Patients who had surgery during summer had better recurrence-free survival (RFS) than patients who had surgery during winter."[53] The same relationship exists when lung cancer season of diagnosis is compared with the fatality rate. Those diagnosed in the fall, when vitamin D levels are higher, have a lower death rate than those diagnosed in winter.[70] Also, Black Americans, whose smoking habits are uniform throughout the country, have a lower rate of lung cancer in the southern states than northern states,[63] and an investigation that assessed the risk of lung cancer in 111 countries demonstrated that risk decreased as sunlight availability increased.[69] In addition, lung cancer patients who have the highest serum vitamin D levels have better survival rates than those who have low levels.[71]

Two research papers also indicate that vitamin D analogs (vitamin D-like chemicals) have an influence on lung cancer growth in a laboratory setting.[54,55] *They showed a substantial inhibition of angiogenesis in mice when treated with a vitamin D analog—an analog that also markedly diminished metastasis in their lung-cancer cells.*[5] It would be of incalculable value if a portion of this number-one cancer killer were prevented by regular sunlight or tanning bed exposure and vitamin D supplements.

Lymphoma (cancer of the lymph nodes)

Lymphoma is profoundly and positively influenced by sunlight exposure. In 2005, Dr. Karin Smedby and colleagues, established that greater sunlight exposure resulted in a diminished risk.[56] The subjects in this study who took regular "sun vacations" abroad had a 30%-40% reduced risk for lymphoma compared to those who did not, and those who sunbathed four times weekly also had a 30% reduced risk. *Even sunburns predicted a diminished risk of lymphoma*. I have repeated this many times: *sunburning is never recommended*; the same benefits can be achieved by careful exposure that lets the body adjust to increasing amounts of sunlight.

The season of diagnosis also makes a difference in the survival rate of lymphoma patients. Those diagnosed in the autumn, when vitamin D levels are highest, have a 20% greater survival rate than those diagnosed in winter.[57]

We know that though sunlight exposure can be a factor in causing skin cancer, it certainly is not the only cause. Could the high-fat, animal-food diet we previously discussed be a factor in causing both skin cancer and lymphoma? The non-fat portion of milk is possibly a factor in 70% of all lymphoma deaths,[58] *and although it has been hypothesized that excessive calcium in cow's milk leads to lymphoma,*[58] *we should remember Dr. Campbell's findings that milk protein activates liver cancer in rats.*[24-29] Perhaps lymphoma behaves similarly in humans. Why chance it?

Myeloma

Myeloma is a cancer of the bone marrow, and several studies have indicated that vitamin D has the ability to inhibit it.[59] In fact, the greater the dose of vitamin D, the greater is the inhibitory effect.

Neuroblastoma

Neuroblastoma is a cancerous tumor of immature nerve cells that most often affects young children. Animal experiments show that neuroblastoma cell growth is inhibited by activated vitamin D and its analogs.[76],[77]

Retinoblastoma

Retinoblastoma is a cancerous tumor of the retina of the eye that occurs mostly among infants. Both vitamin D[78] and its analogs[79] have been shown to have positive affects on the disease.

Summary statement

We have discussed the relationship of sunlight and vitamin D on many major cancers, including breast, ovarian, uterine, cervical, prostate, colon, esophageal, stomach, colon, rectal, pancreatic, gallbladder, brain, bladder, bile duct, kidney, leukemia, lung, lymphoma, myeloma and melanoma. Research by Dr. Grant demonstrates that Black Americans have only 50% to 75% of the serum levels of vitamin D as white Americans, and that they also have a greater risk of dying from many cancers. Solar radiation exposure is also greater in Black Americans who have better survival rates for cancer.[60] It is obvious that lack of sunlight is even more disastrous for blacks than for whites.

Dr. Edward Giovannucci and colleagues have recently completed an assessment of 48,700 men whose rates of cancer and cancer deaths were compared with their rates of vitamin D intake and their production of vitamin D by sunlight exposure.[61] Those with the highest vitamin D levels as predicted by sunlight exposure had a greatly reduced risk of cancers compared to those with the lowest predicted D levels. *The researchers determined that for every increase in of 10 ng/ml, there was a 45% reduction in deaths from colon cancer and a 29% decrease in death from all cancers. As mentioned in chapter 5, the researchers calculated that among men, 85,550 fewer cancer deaths would occur by increasing levels by 10 ng/ml! If the same holds true for women, then more than 170,000 lives could be saved yearly by increasing vitamin D levels by 10 ng/ml.* And what might happen with an increase of 20-30 ng/ml?

Dr. Giovannucci's group stated that 1,500 IU daily of vitamin D supplementation was necessary to achieve a 10 ng/ml increase in serum levels. That much supplemental vitamin D costs about $15 per year. *Perhaps Dr. Giovannucci and his colleagues have discovered the*

$15-per-year answer to cancer. Just imagine how much protection might be afforded by 10,000 IU per day produced by sunbathing or by tanning beds. Dr. Reinhold Vieth, after analyzing the Giovannucci paper and comparing the health problems caused by low levels of vitamin D to the health problems caused by tobacco—delineated in other research[65]—determined that low levels of vitamin D were at least as dangerous as a one-pack-per-day smoking habit.[66]

My wife, Vicki, raised her serum levels from 21 ng/ml to 55 in eight weeks by taking about 7,000 units per day of supplemental vitamin D. Based on the research just referenced,[61] how much has she reduced her risk of colon cancer? ***According to the formula given by Dr. Giovannucci, my calculations show that her risk of death by colon cancer alone has been decreased close to 73%,*** provided the influence of vitamin D is equal in men and women.

Raising serum vitamin D levels is simple and inexpensive and has profound positive implications for human health. Nothing could do more for human health than the promotion of moderate sunbathing and vitamin D supplementation. Of course, the term "moderate" depends on the skin type, the intensity of the sun and a person's recent sun-exposure history. Dr. Gordon Ainsleigh states "one or two minutes of sun at meridian in Santa Fe, NM (elev. about 7,000 ft) on June 21 are about all that a person with translucent Irish skin and no recent sun exposure history could handle. Six hours of sun throughout the midday in Memphis, TN (250-350 ft elev.) on September 21 would be a moderate exposure for a black man who was used to working on construction sites without a shirt."[64]

Since high vitamin D levels work to prevent angiogenesis, proliferation and metastasis and promote apoptosis and differentiation, it is likely that sunlight exposure/vitamin D will reduce the risk of nearly all types of internal cancer.

Now we leave our discussion of cancer and move on to the effects of sunlight and vitamin D on other maladies.

What have we learned?

1. Colon polyps are precursors of colon cancer. Women in the lowest fourth of blood-vitamin D levels have a 58% greater chance of developing polyps than those in the highest fourth.

2. With each 10 ng/ml increase in serum vitamin D levels, the risk of polyps decreases by 26%.

3. Those with the highest blood levels of vitamin D reduce their risk of rectal cancer by 67%.

4. Vitamin D-deficient rats with colon cancer have accelerated colon-tumor growth.

5. Men and women whose serum levels are below 20 ng/ml have three times the risk of colon cancer as those with levels above 30 ng/ml.

6. For every increase in serum vitamin D levels of 10 ng/ml there is a 45% reduction in deaths from colon cancer and a 29% decrease in death from all cancers.

7. People who live in the sunniest areas have a dramatically reduced risk of colon cancer compared to those living in the least sunny areas..

8. Increasing vitamin D levels may save the lives of 85,550 men yearly.

9. Even where vitamin D consumption is high, sunlight exposure further reduces the risk of colon cancer.

10. A low-meat, high-vegetable nutritional pattern lowers the risk of colon cancer.

11. In one assessment of risk factors for colon cancer, high-animal-food consumption predicted a 6-10 times increased risk compared to those who ate few of these products.

12. Sunlight and/or vitamin D also have protective influences on the following cancers: pancreatic, brain, bladder, kidney, leukemia, lymphoma, myeloma, lung, esophagus, stomach and bile duct.

SECTION 3

Solar Power and other major diseases and health issues

Chapter 10

Boning up: Solar Power, osteoporosis, falls, arthritis and pain

"There is a muscular energy in sunlight corresponding to the spiritual energy of wind."
Annie Dillard

The needless osteoporosis pandemic

You now understand that "Sunlight in any amount is harmful" is a whopper of a lie. Nowhere is this absurd belief manifested more clearly than in the topic of our next discussion.

Osteoporosis (weak, fracture-prone bones) is a disease that should never happen; it is easily preventable, and to a great extent, reversible. Unfortunately, most health-care professionals know little about the proper therapy for reversal of this malady. Instead they use drugs with side effects that may make the treatment worse than the disease. Unfortunately, the mainstream advice for prevention is to consume excessive amounts of calcium—advice that is at best slightly helpful and probably harmful if it is not consumed with sufficient vitamin D, which is essential to the intestinal absorption of calcium.[1]

If it is not absorbed, no amount of calcium can prevent bone loss. We will see that only a small amount of calcium is sufficient if vitamin D, exercise and good nutrition are present. *Weak bones result when calcium that regularly leaves the body through excretion is greater than that absorbed by the bones.* It is a question of balance.

Osteoporosis is pandemic in Western societies. It can cause severe spinal curvature due to vertebral collapse, and is responsible for more than 1.5 million fractures annually in the USA, including 300,000 hip fractures, 700,000 vertebral fractures, 250,000 wrist fractures and 300,000 others. Forty to fifty percent of all women in the USA will have an osteoporotic fracture in their lifetimes.[2] Twenty-four percent of those who fracture a hip die within one year, and 25% will require long-term care.[3] The cost to government, business and individuals is about $17 billion per year.

Nutrition and osteoporosis

Calcium is essential to human health, but only a small amount is necessary. The advice to saturate ourselves with dairy products and calcium supplements is disastrous in terms of any meaningful decrease in osteoporosis. Without adequate vitamin D, loading the diet with calcium is an exercise in futility. If calcium were the answer to porous bones and fractures, countries with the greatest calcium consumption would experience the lowest rates of fractures. This graph (figure 1) is produced from data in 1992 in the medical journal *Osteoporosis International.*[4] It shows an *inverse* correlation between calcium consumption and fractures; *the higher the consumption, the greater the fracture rate.*

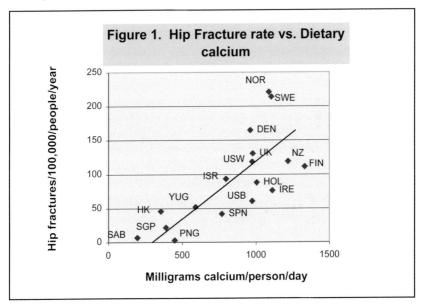

Figure 1. Hip Fracture rate vs. Dietary calcium

Note that people such as South African Blacks (SAB) and Papua New Guineans (PNG) have very low calcium intakes and very low fracture rates. Conversely, people in Sweden, Denmark, Norway, the USA (USAB = USA Blacks, USAW = USA whites) and New Zealand, whose calcium consumption is very high, have high fracture rates.

This is not to say that calcium causes osteoporosis; nothing could be further from the truth. *However, for calcium to be effective in keeping bones strong, it must be maintained by them, not lost.* High calcium intake in the above chart is simply a marker for other factors that weaken bones—factors that inhibit calcium absorption.

The first factor is animal protein, a substance replete with sulphur amino acids—acids that acidify the blood during their metabolism. To neutralize that acidity, the blood requires an alkaline substance to maintain the body's proper PH (acid-alkaline) balance. One such alkaline buffer is calcium, which is leached from the bones into the blood to counter the acidity. The calcium used as a neutralizer is excreted through the urine. Bone calcium is lost and bone strength is compromised. There is no doubt that this takes place; I researched the subject extensively in my earlier book, *Megahealth*. Now consider another graph, also produced from data in *osteoporosis International*.[4] Figure 2 compares animal protein consumption with osteoporosis rates in the same countries as in Figure 1. The relationship is nearly identical.

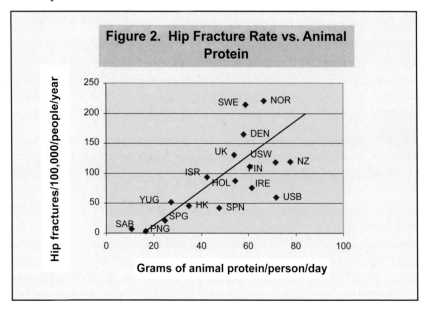

Figure 2. Hip Fracture Rate vs. Animal Protein

The authors of this research concluded exactly what I stated earlier: that extreme acidosis (acidic blood) produced by the sulfur amino acids in animal proteins causes calcium to be leached from the bones and excreted through the urine. These 1992 findings were corroborated in 2002 by Dr Lynda Frassetto and her colleagues.[5] They found that whereas animal proteins related closely to hip fractures, vegetable proteins were inversely related to fractures; the greater the vegetable consumption, the lower the fracture rate. Many others have found that animal proteins induce calcium excretion.[6-7] This was known in 1920, when meat consumption was showed to cause a net loss of calcium.[8]

Excess acidity inhibits the conversion of vitamin D to calcitriol and thereby causes a decrease in the quantity of active D produced. This also inhibits calcium absorption.[9-10] The body must be in an alkaline state to properly absorb calcium.

Calcium from dairy products is accompanied by the same amino acids that are partially responsible for osteoporosis. Furthermore, the people who consume dairy are usually the people who consume a great deal of red meat, fish, eggs, poultry, pork and other acid-producing foods. Vegetables, which are high in bicarbonates that neutralize acid, protect against fractures, and that correlation may be due in part to the fact that people who eat more vegetables tend to eat fewer animal foods. The message: eat little or no animal proteins. Dr. Frassetto's research also compared vegetable consumption to animal consumption in the various countries and found *vegetable proteins were profoundly protective: the higher the ratio of vegetable proteins to animal proteins, the lesser the risk of fracture.[5]*

Why are we discussing nutrition?

As pointed out in other chapters, there are two reasons: (1) it is important to understand that sunlight and vitamin D, while indispensable for good health, are not panaceas against disease. One must adopt other prudent healthful habits. There is no "magic bullet" that can wipe out all disease. To live healthfully, one must not only get sunlight exposure, but also follow a prudent nutrition and exercise program. People cannot ignore two laws of good health and expect the third to save them. (2) Good health habits go hand in hand. In this case, vitamin D gives the body an assist in absorbing calcium from food if the food does not contain too much animal protein, and maybe even if it does! Sensible diets also reduce the risk of common skin cancers and melanoma, making is safer to enjoy the sun.

Now let's discuss sunlight and osteoporosis. Look at Figures 1-2 again. Do you notice something about the graphs that tie nutrition to sunlight? The countries with comparatively low-animal-protein consumption, low-calcium consumption and low rates of fracture are also generally those that also receive the greatest quantity of sunlight.

Sunlight/vitamin D and osteoporosis

Historically, the interest in sunlight and health began when it was observed that bone diseases were common among sunlight-deprived people. Observations were made that children who got little sunlight were vulnerable to rickets, a horrible, crippling and deforming bone disease (see chapter 1). In the early 20th Century, researchers found that rickets was prevented by sunlight or by cod-liver oil (later found to contain vitamin D). It has since been established that sunlight and vitamin D reduce osteomalacia—the adult equivalent of rickets—as well as osteoporosis and its resultant fractures. Let's review some of the research on vitamin D and bone strength.

We will start with the youngest human—an unborn child.

Vitamin D-deficient mothers give birth to vitamin D-deficient babies, since the fetus relies solely on its mother for vitamin D. The child will then be at greater risk for bone fractures as it grows older. *Children born to mothers with low blood levels of vitamin D during late pregnancy have smaller bones at age 9 than those whose mothers have adequate levels.*[11] It is especially important in the third trimester of pregnancy that the necessary bone-building factors be available in the mother's blood for that critical period when 80% of the fetal bone mass is built. Vitamin D and calcium are both important,[12] but vitamin D is critical. Anyone who eats lots of green vegetables has more than enough calcium for good health. However, pregnant mothers who avoid the sun may be deficient in vitamin D unless they take a potent vitamin D3 supplement.

And what about babies born early? *Premature infant girls who are vitamin D supplemented during the first year of life have stronger bones at age 8 than those who are not.*[13] The same is true of *maturely* born infants.[14] This is also important to adults. Those who have lower bone mass as children have a greater risk of fracture.[11-15]

Children generally do not suffer from brittle bones unless they are so vitamin D deficient that they are verging on rickets. Most have sufficiently strong bones to carry them through adulthood, provided they have a minimal quantity of vitamin D. But as the aging process begins, those who have built the densest bones as children will have an advantage, so the importance of adequate sunlight exposure during the formative years cannot be overemphasized. Every expectant mother should make sure her levels are maintained above 40 ng/ml.

The importance of parathyroid hormone (PTH)

When vitamin D levels are low, parathyroid hormone levels rise, which triggers bone loss. According to Dr. Reinhold Vieth, a blood level of 40 ng/ml is necessary to keep parathyroid hormone (PTH) at proper levels,[16] and Dr. Bruce Hollis has indicated that blood levels less than 32 ng/ml cause a rise in PTH.[17] *Consider that among older hospital patients with hip fractures, high PTH is associated not only with accelerated bone loss, but also with a doubling of injury to the heart (see chapter13) and an 18.5 times increase in the risk of hospital death![84]* The graph below illustrates the remarkable increase in hospital deaths among those whose PTH levels are very high.

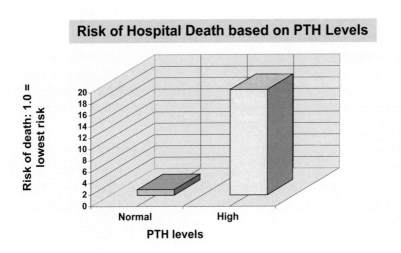

Risk of Hospital Death based on PTH Levels

How does vitamin D halt bone loss?

Vitamin D inhibits bone loss. Bones are in a constant state of breaking down and rebuilding to maintain strength. Specialized cells called osteoclasts are responsible for bone breakdown, and cells called osteoblasts are responsible for rebuilding. When osteoclasts break down bone faster than osteoblasts rebuild it, calcium diminishes and bones weaken. A protein known as c-Fos stimulates osteoclasts, and animal experiments have shown that vitamin D suppresses c-Fos and the development of osteoclasts and thereby prevents too-rapid bone breakdown. [79] In a single day, one osteoclast can break down the amount of bone produced by 150 osteoblasts,[80] so it is obvious that vitamin D's ability to prevent excessive osteoclast activity is vital in the prevention of osteoporosis.

Reversal of Bone Loss

Can sunlight help reverse osteoporosis and reduce the risk of fractures?

The answer is "yes." I had long known that osteoporosis was at least partly reversible in patients on a program of weight-bearing exercise. But it was surprising to learn that even without exercise, an impressive increase in bone density occurs with sunlight exposure. Japanese researchers studied the effects of sunlight—or the lack thereof—on the bone mass of elderly women who were either exposed to sunlight or were kept inside a care facility. Over twelve months, 129 women were exposed to regular sunlight and another 129 received no sunlight exposure. *The results were startling: in these sedentary women, the sunlight group increased bone mass by an average 3.1%; in the non-sunlight-exposed group, it decreased by 3.3%*[18]. *That is a difference of 6.4%. This is important because high bone mass prevents fractures. One assessment showed that the risk of fracture increases two to three times for every 10 percent drop in bone density,*[19] *and another showed that for every loss of 0.12g (.043 oz) per square centimeter (.15 square inch) of bone mass, the risk of a fracture increased by 360% in women and 340% in men!*[83]

The Japanese study also showed that Vitamin D levels in the sun-exposed group increased by 400%. *As further proof of the efficacy of improving bone mass, the women who had the benefit of sunlight had only one bone fracture in their group. The sunlight-deprived group had six fractures!*

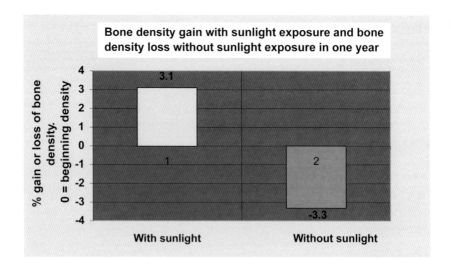

Bone density gain with sunlight exposure and bone density loss without sunlight exposure in one year

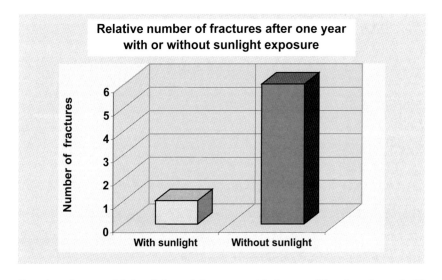

Relative number of fractures after one year with or without sunlight exposure

So what do you think of the advice to avoid the sun like the plague? If regular sunlight exposure cuts the number of fractures by two-thirds or more, shouldn't the medical profession prescribe it?

Several other studies indicate sunlight and vitamin D promote fewer fractures and increased bone mass. One that had elderly Alzheimer's victims as subjects showed similar positive benefits of sunlight.[20] Researchers exposed one group to sunlight for one year, and another was kept in a typical indoor hospital setting. *In the sunlight group a 220% increase in vitamin D levels was found, and bone mass increased by 2.7%. In the indoor group, bone mass decreased by 5.6%. That is a difference of 7.3% in only one year!* The final proof, of course, is with fractures. In the sunlight group, there were three fractures; in the sunlight-deprived group there were eleven or *3.7* times more.

An investigation in Spain concluded that women who actively participated in sun exposure had one-eleventh the chance of a hip fracture as those who did not![109] Another in Switzerland found that only 4% of hip fracture patients had vitamin D blood levels of 30 ng/ml.[110] Imagine what could happen over several years of sunlight exposure along with an appropriate program of exercise. It is also true that smoking and use of certain prescription drugs correlate closely to osteoporosis worldwide. It is entirely possible that a lifestyle involving proper nutrition, exercise and sunlight could prevent this dread disease and improve the quality of life for millions.

UVB from tanning beds also increases bone density.

As we have already seen in previous chapters, it is ultraviolet B light (UVB) that stimulates the skin to produce vitamin D. Since most tanning beds are programmed to produce UVB, could they increase bone mass and strength? An excellent study compared 50 people who used tanning beds regularly with 106 who did not. *The tanning-bed group had 90% higher vitamin D, significantly higher bone density and lower PTH levels.[21]* The users had healthful vitamin D levels of 46 ng/ml compared to only 24 ng/ml for those who did not regularly use tanning beds. You may recall from Chapter 1 that 24 ng/ml lies in the dangerous range and predicts a 100% increased risk for some types of cancers, so it is likely that tanning bed use is an excellent way to prevent both osteoporosis and cancer. Some lament that the UVB from sunlight or tanning beds stimulates the production of endorphins and serotonin (these natural chemicals make people feel happy, relaxed and positive), which leads to an addiction to tanning. They therefore liken tanning to substance abuse.[22,23,] If UVB light is addictive, and thereby causes a profound drop in the incidence of hip fractures, multiple sclerosis, heart disease and the major internal cancers, thank God for the addiction!

These studies beg the questions: Why is the medical community not recommending sunlight exposure as an effective and easy method of preventing death and disability from osteoporosis? Is it recommending tanning bed use in those seasons of the year when UVB is not available? This information is found in the best medical and nutritional journals. Yet, I know of only a few physicians who recommend sunlight to prevent fractures. Those who don't are either guilty of malpractice or ignorant of the facts.

Furthermore, Dr. Marwan Bukhari and colleagues were quoted in the London Times on April 27, 2008 as recommending sunlamps for women due to give birth in winter to use a sun lamp during the final three months of pregnancy to protect their child from osteoporosis in later life. The Times stated, "They made their recommendation as research found that children born to mothers whose final three months of pregnancy included a summer month were 40% less likely to suffer the bone-wasting condition in adult-hood. A mother's exposure to sunlight in that final period ensures the developing baby receives enough vitamin D to form strong bones."[113]

Vitamin D supplementation and osteoporosis

Vitamin D supplements are effective in reducing fracture rates if the dosage is at least 1,000 IU per day.[24] Researchers studied the fracture rates of 48 women who took 1,000 IU per day with 48 who took a placebo. *After two years, four of those taking the placebo had a hip fracture, but not one in the supplemented group. The supplemented group had 59% fewer falls and increased muscle size and strength,* and in another 5-year study, 100,000 IU of vitamin D was administered every four months to a group of elderly people for five years. (That is only a small dose of 833 IU per day). Another group was given a placebo. The supplemented group had a rate for hip, wrist, forearm and spinal column fractures that was only 67% of that of the placebo group.[25] Another investigation showed serum levels of vitamin D to be directly related to the strength of the femur (upper leg bone).[27]

Crohn's disease patients (highly susceptible to osteoporosis) increased bone mass 3-4% per year taking supplements of vitamin D and calcium.[26] All of these studies show clearly that vitamin D supplementation and high serum levels of vitamin D are effective in reducing fractures. The results, I believe, would be impressive with higher daily doses of vitamin D. Remember that sunlight exposure can produce up to 20,000 IU of vitamin D in twenty minutes in light-skinned people,[28] which makes the dosages in these research studies seem quite small. Also be aware that supplementation is not effective for reducing fractures at the typical multivitamin dose of 200-400 IU daily.[29]

Which is most important to prevent osteoporosis, vitamin D or calcium?

Several other investigations have demonstrated that vitamin D/calcium supplementation increases bone mass and decrease fractures.[31-35] However, one study showed that vitamin D taken alone prevented twice as many fractures as calcium taken alone.[33] I reiterate that Vitamin D is far more important than calcium provided there is a minimal amount of calcium available. *A study of postmenopausal women showed that those supplemented with vitamin D and calcium for one year increased bone density by an average of 2.1%. In a group that received calcium only, bone density instead decreased by 2.1%.*[36] When women were assessed for vitamin D, milk and calcium consumption for a period of eighteen years, it was found that those who consumed 1,200 or more milligrams per day of calcium had no fewer fractures than those who consumed 600 milligrams or less.[37] However, those who consumed 500 IU or more of vitamin D per day had a 37% lowered risk of hip fracture compared to those who consumed 140 IU or less. *Neither calcium nor milk consumption showed a protective effect against fractures.*

Calcium is an essential nutrient, but vitamin D is the crucial factor that lets calcium function. The lowest safe level for calcium appears to be about 200 milligrams per day if there is not a heavy acid load due to animal-protein intake. Though calcium *per se* does not prevent osteoporosis, I am certainly not saying that people should not consume more than 200 milligrams (mg) daily. Eating plenty of vegetable foods, especially greens, provides more than 200 mg. For instance, 100 calories of collard greens contains 570 milligrams of calcium; the same quantity of spinach contains 450 milligrams; broccoli, 300 milligrams and arugula (a Mediterranean vegetable) 1,300 milligrams. Skim milk, on the other hand contains only about 355 milligrams per 100 calories. Remember that only vegetable proteins are protective against osteoporosis; animal proteins are one of its causes. Figure 1 showed the relationship between calcium consumption and hip fractures worldwide. The source of the calcium in the countries at the unfavorable part of the chart comes primarily from milk products; calcium in the countries at the favorable end comes primarily from vegetables. There is no protection gained by consuming extreme quantities of calcium.

Dr. Robert Heaney and colleagues showed that when serum levels of vitamin D increase from an average of 20 ng/ml to 34.6 ng/ml, *calcium absorption increases by 65%, and the risk of hip, wrist, forearm or vertebral fracture is reduced by 33%.*[38-40] *Another investigation assessed kidney patients on dialysis who were severely deficient in vitamin D. Treatment with calcitriol dramatically increased the absorption of calcium.*[108]

Perhaps the most conclusive research regarding calcium supplementation *without* sufficient vitamin D was a 2007 meta-analysis by Dr. Heike Bischoff-Ferrari and her colleagues reported in the *American Journal of Clinical Nutrition.*[71] Their analysis excluded studies that combined calcium supplementation with vitamin D, and supplements ranged from 300-1600 milligrams of calcium daily. *They found absolutely no reduction in hip fracture rates among either men or women who took calcium, and they made this statement:* "Pooled results from randomized controlled trials show no reduction in hip fracture risk with calcium supplementation, and *an increased risk is possible.*" There is good reason to suggest that excessive calcium increases the risk of hip fracture: *Women who are in the highest quintile of dairy product consumption at age 20 suffer nearly three times the rate of fracture in old age as those who consume the least.*[111]

A similar meta-analysis performed on studies of calcium supplementation and bone density in children showed that there was little difference in calcium-supplemented children and non-supplemented children.[72]

With sufficient vitamin D (1,400 IU) however, bone density *is* improved.[81] Vitamin D is the key.

Calcium without vitamin D may also be dangerous for the heart. A New Zealand study showed that in those who took 1,000 milligrams of calcium daily, heart-attack rates doubled compared to those who took a placebo.[107]

To summarize: Sunlight exposure, tanning bed use and vitamin D supplementation in sufficient doses can dramatically reduce bone loss and its resultant fractures.

Antidepressants: an emerging factor in osteoporosis

Two research papers in the journal, *Archives of Internal Medicine*, show that taking antidepressants called selective serotonin uptake inhibitors (SSRI's)—the most popular antidepressant drugs—dramatically reduces bone mass in users compared to non-users.[73-74] *The first study demonstrated that elderly women who took SSRI's lost nearly 43% more bone per year than those who did not*. The second established that bone mineral density (BMD) among elderly male SSRI users was about 4% lower at the hip bone and about 6% lower at the spine compared to those reporting no SSRI use. Another investigation reported that SSRI-using adults over the age of 50 were twice as likely to fracture a bone and twice as likely to fall as those who did not use the drugs.[75] These risks were dose-dependent, meaning that as the dosage of the drug increased, there was a accompanying increase in fractures and falling.

The extraordinary story of Dr. Ruth Heidrich

Before leaving the subject of osteoporosis, here is an example of the bone building potential of proper nutrition, sunlight and exercise. Ruth Heidrich, PhD, is a most remarkable woman and a long-time friend who visited our health resort several times and gave electrifying talks on several health issues including cancer, osteoporosis and fitness. Ruth's life was devastated in 1982 when she was diagnosed with breast cancer at age 47. She had been a marathon runner for 14 years and thought her lifestyle of good nutrition would have prevented her cancer. Plus, her genetics were "good," since all four grandparents had lived past 90.

She had a lumpectomy, but physicians said it did not remove all the cancer. They said a mastectomy was needed to prevent the spread of the disease, but later bone scans showed the cancer had already spread. Despite the demoralizing news, Ruth didn't let anything stop her. The morning her surgery was scheduled, she slipped out of the hospital and ran six miles, much to the consternation of the staff. *Three days after, with bandages holding the incisions together, she was out on the beaches and mountains again, training under the Hawaiian sun. That weekend she ran a 10K race and won first place in her age category. Dr. Ruth is not a quitter!*

She was blessed to hear of a clinical research study for breast cancer patients being conducted by Dr. John McDougall, a physician and author of several best-selling books. Dr. McDougall advised Ruth that a condition to participate in the study was to consume a completely vegetarian (vegan), low-fat diet and refuse chemotherapy and radiation, since he wanted to determine if a vegan diet could reverse the cancer. It would be an understatement to say she has followed the counsel. *A year after her surgery, Ruth ran the Great Wall of China; she has run around the pyramids of Egypt; she has gone on to compete several times in the Ironman Triathlons.* She has run 67 marathons, won six gold medals in the Senior Olympics, and has a roomful of first-place trophies from various races—in fact, about 1,000 of them! She was named one of the "ten fittest women in North America" by *Living Fit Magazine* and awarded "The Golden Shoe Award" by *Runner's World Magazine.* Not bad for a former cancer patient, eh?

Ruth has also run and biked in the red mountains of southern Utah, where I accompanied her during her visits to our health institute/resort. Being somewhat of an endurance athlete myself, I twice pedaled a mountain bike from the beach on Maui, Hawaii to the summit of Mt. Haleakala, a climb of 10,000 feet over a distance of thirty-eight miles. I was quite proud of myself, but my male ego was quickly put in its place when I heard that this breast cancer survivor had *run* the same course in a competition called "Run to the Sun," again winning a first place in her age group. Ruth also was invited to Dr. Ken Cooper's Institute for Aerobics Research in Dallas, Texas to challenge the age-group treadmill record held there. She set a new record and returned the next year to break it.

Dr. Cooper, on learning of Ruth's exploits, questioned her about her nutrition program. When he learned that she ate no animal foods—not even dairy products—and took no calcium supplements, he was aghast. He believed her bones were weak, that there was no way she received enough calcium from that diet. He could not have been more wrong. *A bone-density test showed her to have stronger bones than the typical athletic 30-year-old and her bone density has since increased. She is at this writing 73 years old and still has exceptionally high bone density.* That is especially noteworthy, since Ruth's cancer was estrogen-receptor sensitive, which precluded any hormone replacement therapy (HRT). *Her increasing bone mass occurred without HRT, calcium supplementation or dairy foods.*

Although at the time of diagnosis the cancer had spread, since her mastectomy 27 years ago, she has not had any sign of cancer. It is astounding what vegan nutrition, sunlight and exercise can do.

In view of what we have discussed about cancer and osteoporosis, Ruth is doing everything correctly:

1. Although she is a fair-skinned blonde, she uses no sunscreen; the calcium absorbing and anti-cancer benefits of the vitamin D her body produces—under the Solar Power of the Hawaiian sun—are always in full force.

2. Her diet is totally devoid of animal proteins and the accompanying sulphur amino acids that cause decalcification of the bones.

3. That same diet, replete with greens, furnishes ample and easily absorbable calcium. It also furnishes vegetable proteins that are protective against osteoporosis.

4. Her exercise regimen stimulates her bones to keep her bone-mass level high and even increases it.

When Ruth needs protection from over-exposure to the sun, she dons a wide-brimmed hat, long sleeves and pants. She has never had melanoma or common skin cancer in spite of her light skin and regular sun exposure in the tropics.

Dr. Ruth Heidrich has written two inspirational books: *A Race for Life*, and *Senior Fitness* (Lantern Books, NY). These are must-reads, particularly for women who think life is over after a diagnosis of breast cancer.

Solar power, vitamin D and osteomalacia

Osteomalacia is a soft-bone disease known as adult rickets, which results from severe vitamin D deficiency. Deficiency prevents bone from properly mineralizing.[41] *Women who seldom go outdoors, or who are nearly always fully covered with clothing, have an extremely high incidence of osteomalacia at a very young age, even if they live in geographical areas with abundant sunlight.*[42-44] Most victims have vitamin D levels less than 10 ng/ml. Their parathyroid hormones (PTH) are also exceptionally high, which along with the deficiency of vitamin D, which further weakens bones.[45] A French study showed that among women 18 to 49 who wore concealing clothing, 99% were deficient and 82% were severely deficient.[102]

Is fibromyalgia really osteomalacia?

According to Dr Michael Holick, the answer is yes. Fibromyalgia is a condition characterized by chronic pain in the muscles and joint tissues and is usually accompanied by fatigue. Holick says that nearly all of his patients will resolve their discomfort when he prescribes large doses of vitamin D.[46]

The reemergence of rickets

After a century of knowing how to prevent this disastrous children's disease, it is returning, and *cases of rickets are reported as far south as Texas, Georgia and North Carolina,* [63] *Not surprisingly, 83% of cases occur in black children, and 96% are breast-fed, indicating a lack of vitamin D in their mothers' milk.* We must educate expectant mothers to get out in the sun during their pregnancies or at least take a potent vitamin D supplement. Before and after giving birth, these mothers should assure that both they and their babies maintain optimal serum levels of vitamin D. Too many nursing mothers, especially African Americans, are providing vitamin D-deficient milk. Drs. Bruce Hollis and Carol Wagner have shown that *2,000 IU of supplemental vitamin D daily for nursing mothers falls woefully short of achieving healthful serum levels in their babies.*[66] *These researchers then established that 6,400 IU daily is necessary to maintain optimal blood levels in both the nursing mother and her baby.*[114] They also pointed out that infants need vitamin D3, not calcidiol (25(OH)D, since their bodies want to make calcidiol. Thus, nursing mothers should have enough vitamin D intake or production so they have circulating vitamin D3; if they don't have enough intake, then every molecule of D3 will be used to produce calcidiol. When D3 can be measured in the blood, it is a sign that there is sufficient vitamin D intake.

Unfortunately, even women who take prenatal vitamins are often woefully deficient in vitamin D, as are their newborns.[106] Their dosage is simply too small. It is bad enough when unpreventable diseases occur, but when a simple, 100%-effective preventive measure is known, it is inexcusable! If infants do not receive sunlight exposure when it is available, serum vitamin D may be woefully inadequate.[64] Such infants cannot live healthy lives.

Vitamin D and craniotabes

Craniotabes is a skull condition characterized by thin, soft areas, and it has recently been defined as the earliest sign of vitamin D deficiency in newborns.[157] It may signal impending rickets, but until recently, it was considered a physiological anomaly needing no treatment. Obviously, any newborn diagnosed with craniotabes should be immediately checked for vitamin D deficiency to avert full-blown rickets.

Vitamin D, strength and the risk of falling

In the USA, falls account for more unintentional injuries than any other cause and are the leading cause of injury death in the elderly.[88] Yet, there is a simple way to reduce the risk of falling. Elderly patients who took 1,000 IU vitamin D for two years lessened their risk 60%, and muscle size and strength also occurred.[18,30] In some studies, supplemented elderly subjects can go farther and sway less when walking. The tendency to sway among those who have low vitamin D levels is pronounced;[47] those with below-average vitamin D levels sway and stumble 4.4 times more than those with above-average levels.[99,100] Overall physical performance, including strength and endurance, is significantly better in the elderly with high serum levels of vitamin D,[101] and they have fewer falls and fractures.[47]

Other research links vitamin D levels between 16-36 ng/ml with improved lower body strength in those 60 and older, when compared to those with levels less than 16 ng/ml.[48] This relationship persisted regardless of calcium intake, activity level, sex, age, or race. And a three-year study of people over 65 showed that the risk of falling was reduced by 46% in active women and 65% in inactive supplemented women compared to those not supplemented with vitamin D and calcium.[49] In centenarians (individuals at least 100-years old), proper vitamin D levels are critical, yet a study of 104 centenarians (a high fracture group) showed that 99 had undetectable levels.[92]

Fracture risk, however, is not confined to the elderly. Stress fractures caused by physical training among military recruits is 3.6 times higher in those whose vitamin D levels are low,[93,94] and *vitamin D/calcium supplementation reduces the risk of stress fractures by 27% in eight weeks!*[95]

Not only does vitamin D reduce falls by increasing strength, *but balance is also improved by vitamin D combined with calcium, which* is 60% more effective in reducing falls than calcium alone.[50] The elderly fall far more often than younger people, since strength and balance decline in later years. **Nursing home residents who took vitamin D supplements of 800 IU per day were 72% less likely to fall than those who took no vitamin D.**[76] **Another investigation determined that those younger than 75 whose levels were severely deficient—below 10 ng/ml—had five times the risk of falling compared to those whose levels were 30 ng/ml or more.**[77] However, vitamin D alone is not adequate to eliminate falls; exercise is also critical. In one study, t**hose who did not participate in exercise had ten times the rate of falls as those who did.**[78] The exercises included training for strength, coordination, balance and endurance. No doubt all human beings, regardless of age, should exercise daily. The human body is meant to be used. Vitamin D helps to maintain strength and reduce falling, but an unused body still deteriorates. The saying, "Use it or lose it," is never truer than for bone, muscle strength and balance.

Another reason for the increased risk of falling among vitamin D-deficient people is that vitamin D induces the production of nerve growth factor (NGF), which is essential for the proper development and maintenance of nerves. Those with low levels have diminished tactile sense (ability to feel when the skin is touched), which may reduce balance and cause more falls.[115]

In prostate cancer patients treated with vitamin D, 37% improved muscle strength and 25% had a decrease in pain.[51] Another study reported that loss of muscle mass and strength—a condition called sarcopenia—was twice as likely to occur with serum levels of vitamin D lower than 10 ng/ml compared to levels greater than 20 ng/ml [65] High PTH levels, which often accompany low vitamin D levels, correlated even more closely to loss of strength and muscle.

A most impressive result comes from a clinical observation of five vitamin D-deficient patients who suffered from myopathy, a disease of bone and muscle tissue. They were confined to wheelchairs and experienced severe fatigue, weakness, and chronic pain. *After receiving 50,000 IU per week of vitamin D, all regained enough strength and energy within four to six weeks to be mobile and functional, and their aches and pains disappeared.*[52] This study makes me wonder if the pandemic of chronic fatigue is mostly due to vitamin D deficiency.

More on Solar Power and pain

Managing chronic pain accounts for $50 billion in health-care costs yearly in the USA.[53] Of course, the cost in suffering is more significant. Could sunlight and vitamin D help to alleviate chronic pain? The study just mentioned, regarding the debilitated wheelchair patients, is impressive in that all five individuals in the study were able to leave their wheelchairs and live normally without pain. Chronic pain is now a pandemic and has birthed a plethora of advertised products that claim to relieve suffering. Most of them are no better than old-fashioned snake oil. If the real source of the pain is vitamin D deficiency, then no pain pill will be of much benefit other than providing temporary relief. However, a vitamin D capsule or some sunlight exposure might help a great deal. *Five chronic-pain patients at John Hopkins University Medical School were treated with vitamin D, and their pain resolved within a week!*[118] The study was conducted in 1991, and considering the pandemic of chronic pain in the world, it amazes me that no one seems to have paid any attention to this research. Certainly it is a piece of information that the pharmaceutical companies would like to remain well-hidden.

There are many other indications that sunlight and vitamin D reduce pain. Spinal surgery patients with postoperative discomfort were studied for the quantity of pain medication they required.[54] The hospital had a bank of rooms on the sunny side and another on the dark side, referred to respectively as the "bright" and "dim" rooms. Patients in the bright rooms had 46% greater sunlight exposure than those in the dim rooms. *The patients in the bright rooms experienced less pain and took 22% less pain medication than those in the dim rooms, regardless of age. Also impressive was that "bright side" patients reported feeling far less stress.* This important finding will be discussed at length in chapter 15 about the influence of sunlight and vitamin D on mood and mental states.

In a study of 150 chronic pain patients at a Minneapolis care center—most of them young and ambulatory (able to walk)—blood vitamin D levels were measured.[55] *Among dark-skinned subjects, African Americans, black African immigrants and Native Americans, 100% showed deficient levels of vitamin D (less than 20 ng/ml). Eighty-three percent of white patients and 93% of all patients were severely deficient, with average levels below 12 ng/m). Twenty-eight percent had levels below 8 ng/ml (20 nmol/l) and five had undetectable levels.* The authors of this research concluded that "Because osteomalacia is a known cause of persistent, nonspecific musculoskeletal pain, screening all outpatients with such pain for hypovitaminosis D should be standard practice in clinical care." But is such screening being done routinely? Absolutely not.

Millions are being set up for chronic pain with severely low vitamin D levels. A study of teenagers in Boston revealed that 42% had levels of vitamin D lower than 20 ng/ml and that 24% were lower than 15 ng/ml [56] It is likely that if the accurate lower limit for healthful vitamin D levels were used, e.g. 40 ng/ml, the rate of vitamin D deficiency would have reached nearly 100%. *A study of black teenagers in 14 American cities showed an average vitamin D level of about 8 ng/ml and that at least 87% were vitamin D deficient.*[68] One teenage boy was so deficient that he went into hypocalcaemic seizures and broke his leg. A British study showed that immigrants from South Asia suffered 60%-80% more chronic pain than native Englanders, and that many of them had vitamin D levels below 10 ng/ml.[57] However, dark-skinned people in England are not the only ones who suffer from vitamin D deficiency. A study of vitamin D status among white British adults throughout England showed an "alarmingly high" rate of deficiency.[104] Eighty-five percent were at below-adequate levels in winter and spring, and 60% were deficient in summer and fall.

The authors of the research done at the care center in Minneapolis state that "chronic nonspecific musculoskeletal pain is one consequence of hypovitaminosis D [vitamin D deficiency]. For the past 30 years, published reports from Europe have documented persistent, nonspecific musculoskeletal pain in immigrant patients secondary to severe hypovitaminosis D."[55] In one such investigation, vitamin D treatment profoundly reduced the quantity of medication needed among women suffering from acute chronic pain.[91] Their number of hospital visits declined, and nearly two-thirds of them recovered completely.[91] Another study showed that use of morphine was nearly doubled in chronic-pain patients whose vitamin D levels were deficient.[112]

Seventy-five percent of women with early-stage breast cancer are D deficient, and many experience chronic pain. When they are treated with 50,000 IU each week for twelve weeks, chronic pain is reduced by half.[85]

Vitamin D and low-back pain

One of the most common complaints to physicians is low-back pain, and lack of sunlight exposure is closely linked to it.[89] Unfortunately, few doctors are aware.[90] Vitamin D treatment is very effective in dealing with this ailment.[86-87] A 2008 assessment (unpublished at the time of this writing) of 22 studies dealing with back pain showed that those with chronic back pain almost always had inadequate levels of vitamin D, and that in one evaluation of 360 subjects with the condition, 100% had low levels of vitamin D.[116] However, 95% of them improved after vitamin D treatment.

If you know anyone suffering from chronic pain, have them read this section and get their vitamin D blood levels checked. You may save them from a lifetime of suffering.

Vitamin D and chronic pain from diabetic neuropathy

Years ago, a guest at our health resort suffered from painful diabetic neuropathy, a disease of nerve damage associated with diabetes. He stayed for several months, and at the end of that time was pain-free. I felt that this was due to our plant-based diet, and there is little doubt that it was a factor. However, recent research has convinced me that the vitamin D gained from exposure to the Southern Utah sunshine was also important: fifty-one patients with type-two diabetes and neuropathic pain had average serum levels of only 18 ng/ml. After three months of vitamin D3 supplementation, the severity of the pain was reduced by 40-50%.[56] This may be because vitamin D increases production of nerve-growth factor (NGF), a protein that is essential for proper development of nerve cells.[115] Lack of NGF is associated with increased sensitivity to pain.

Solar Power, vitamin D and osteoarthritis

One of the first studies to assess the relationship of vitamin D to arthritis was done in 1996. Seventy-five people with osteoarthritis (the "wear and tear' form) had their vitamin D intake and blood levels assessed. *Those in the highest third had only one-third the progression of the disease as those in the middle and lowest thirds. Low blood levels of vitamin D also predicted greater loss of cartilage in the joints.*[59] Among patients with arthritis of the knee, those with blood levels of vitamin D lower than 20 ng/ml have more disability and more pain and are weaker than those with higher levels.[60] Low vitamin D levels also correlate closely to greater knee pain and walking difficulty.[82]

Solar Power and rheumatoid arthritis (RA)

Both dietary and supplemental vitamin D reduce the risk of RA, which is an autoimmune disease—a disease in which the body's immune system attacks its own tissue (see chapter 11). RA is one of several rheumatic disease that affect bones, muscles, joints and tendons. In a study of 29,000 women, those who ranked in the top third of vitamin D consumption had one-third less risk of RA.[61] In mice studies, vitamin D treatment inhibits the progression of rheumatoid arthritis and minimizes or prevents the symptoms.[62] The same is true in humans. In subjects diagnosed with a form of the disease known as inflammatory arthritis, the lower the

127

vitamin D levels are, the higher is the disease activity.[96] Vitamin D's anti-inflammatory properties and its ability to reduce the autoimmune response are likely responsible for the improvement in RA.[97] Investigations also find that RA is more common in winter, consistent with the idea that vitamin D is a major factor in reducing the risk. [97,98] In a report from researchers in Ireland, it was shown that 70% of patients had low vitamin D levels and that 26% were severely deficient.[117] However, in that report, 21 ng/ml was considered as the deficiency level and 10 as the severe deficiency level. A level of 21 is dangerously deficient. It is likely that all of these patients were under 30 ng/ml.

In our health institute/resort, we observed that guests with arthritis often regained full range of motion in their joints from a week to a month after beginning our program. I assumed that the anti-inflammatory vegetarian nutrition was solely responsible. Now I know that many of the benefits came from sunlight exposure during outdoor exercise.

Vitamin D and athletic performance

Since vitamin D-deficient older people improve balance and muscle strength by improving serum vitamin D levels, it is possible that the same is true for younger people. There is substantial research from Europe that cites improvements in strength, speed and reaction time among athletes exposed to ultraviolet light.[67] This is a subject of another book that Dr. John Cannell and I are currently writing.

What have we learned?

1. When more calcium is lost than is consumed, osteoporosis (brittle bones) results.

2. Populations where calcium consumption is greatest have far more bone fractures than populations with little calcium consumption.

3. Populations where animal-protein consumption is greatest also have far greater rates of bone fractures than populations where there is little animal protein consumption.

4. Sulfur amino acids in animal proteins may be the primary cause of osteoporosis and fractures.

5. Vegetable proteins are protective against osteoporosis.

6. Populations where fractures are most common generally have lower exposure to sunlight than populations where fractures are least common.

7. Sunlight exposure has the ability to build bone mass and profoundly reduce the rate of fractures. This is _reversal_ of osteoporosis.

8. Vitamin D is necessary for the absorption of calcium in the intestine; without it no amount of calcium consumption will halt osteoporosis and subsequent fractures.

9. Vitamin D is also necessary for the absorption of calcium into the bone.

10. Only a small amount of dietary calcium is necessary if serum vitamin D levels are high.

11. Children born to mothers who have low blood levels of vitamin D during late pregnancy have smaller bones than children born to mothers who have adequate levels of vitamin D.

12. UVB exposure from tanning beds increases vitamin D levels and bone strength.

13. Vitamin D supplementation dramatically reduces the rate of bone fractures among osteoporotic women.

14. People suffering from bone loss due to Crohn's disease increase bone mass three to four percent each year with supplements of vitamin D and calcium.

15. Calcium supplements without vitamin D do not prevent osteoporosis and may be dangerous.

16. Osteomalacia (soft bones) is common in women who seldom go outdoors, or who are nearly always fully covered with clothing, even when they live in geographic areas of high sunlight availability.

17. Most cases of what is called fibromyalgia may really be osteomalacia. Dr. Michael Holick has had success in treating fibromyalgia with vitamin D supplements.

18. Strength, balance and reduction of fractures are all positively impacted by vitamin D supplementation.

19. Chronic pain is reduced by vitamin D and sunlight exposure. The same may be true of tanning-bed use.

20. Vitamin D inhibits the progression of various types of arthritis and decreases the loss of joint cartilage.

Chapter 11

Sunlight reduces the risk of multiple sclerosis.

Understanding autoimmune diseases

Multiple Sclerosis (MS) is another devastating autoimmune disease that unnecessarily afflicts millions. It has long been known that dietary habits have a very direct influence on the incidence and prognosis of MS, which is a disease in a similar category to rheumatoid arthritis, lupus erythematosus and type-1 diabetes. *These are diseases in which the immune system attacks the body's own healthy tissue, mistaking that tissue for a foreign invader.* When this happens, a specialized immune-system cell called a T cell, assaults and kills some of the tissue of a targeted organ. Autoimmune diseases, then, are caused by T cells gone awry. In the case of rheumatoid arthritis the immune system attacks the collagen-producing cells of the joints; in the case of type-1 diabetes it attacks and destroys the islet cells that produce insulin; in the case of MS, it attacks the myelin sheath— insulation that surrounds nerve fibers in the brain and spinal cord. When nerve tissue loses its myelin sheath, it is analogous to electric wiring that has lost its rubber insulation; it fails to carry the body's electrical impulses properly and becomes "short circuited." Those who suffer from MS experience numbness, poor coordination and balance, weakness, stiffness and poor vision.

T cells in a person with an autoimmune disease lack the "intelligence" to recognize that they are attacking the wrong tissue. That intelligence, in part, comes from vitamin D, the receptors of which are found in large quantities in mature T cells and even larger concentrations in immature T cells produced in the thymus gland.[1] Without vitamin D stimulation of the receptor sites, these cells will not function properly." When vitamin D is present, however, they have the ability to discern between foreign invaders and the body's own tissue. Animal experiments show that *vitamin D acts as a "selective immunosuppressant,"* meaning that it gives the T cell the ability to distinguish between "good and evil." Vitamin D has shown the ability to "prevent or markedly suppress experimental autoimmune encephalomyelitis, rheumatoid arthritis, systemic lupus erythematosus, type-1 diabetes and inflammatory bowel disease."[1] As will become obvious, vitamin D also has the ability to suppress or prevent MS.

From 85 to 170 people per 100,000 in the USA suffer from MS, and the rate among women from 1991 through 1994 increased by 50% compared to 1982 through 1986.[2] About 2,500,000 people worldwide have MS.[3,4]

The influence of sunlight, latitude and altitude on the incidence of MS

The prevalence of MS is greatest at latitudes that are farthest from the equator, and it is another disease whose incidence has skyrocketed along with increased sunscreen use. Therefore, a lack of UVB/ vitamin D may contribute to increasing MS rates. If this is true, those exposed to the most sunlight would be less likely to develop MS, and indeed, among people living in geographical locations where there are 3,000 hours of available sunlight yearly, rates are quite low.[8]

The geographical distribution of MS confirms the direct correlation between latitude and MS; the further from the equator, where there is less sunlight, the greater the incidence of MS.[9-10,45] *There is more than 100 times the rate of MS in far northern areas as in equatorial areas, where UVB is intense and the rate of MS approaches zero!*

This pattern persists within the USA, where there is far higher MS incidence in northern states.[11] *And in Australia, there is a seven-fold increase in MS incidence between tropical Northern Queensland and Southern Hobart, located in the less sunny part of the country.*[12] Even in small countries like Ireland, MS incidence is far greater in the north than in the south.[13]

Altitude also correlates to MS. In Switzerland MS rates are higher at low altitudes than high altitudes.[15] Areas of high altitude, of course, receive more UVB than areas of low altitude.

Childhood Sunlight exposure and MS

A study on childhood sunlight exposure compared the numbers of daily hours subjects spent in the sunlight when they were six to fifteen years of age.[16] *Those in the lowest sun-exposure category were three times as likely to develop MS as those in the highest.* Those with the *greatest* numbers of actinic keratoses (AK) (precancerous lesions of the skin) and common skin cancers (NMSC) were much less likely to develop MS. People in England with NMSC also have about half the chance of developing MS as those without NMSC.[17] Skin cancer in these studies simply indicates high sunlight exposure—exposure that had occurred incorrectly. Nevertheless, it afforded protection against MS. However, regular sun exposure without burning produces the same benefits without the drawbacks of NMSC, and, a proper diet cuts the chance of NMSC by 94%.

132

An important investigation regarding sunlight exposure in childhood and subsequent risk of MS used identical twins as subjects.[41] Since identical twins have identical genetics, such a study ensures that differences in disease rates are due to environment. The twins were assessed for sun-exposure and the risk of subsequent MS development. Those who had had the highest exposure had reduced MS risks that ranged from 43-75%. For example, a twin who did the most sunbathing had an average 60% reduced risk of MS when compared to the other who did less. Even subjects living above the Arctic Circle in northern Norway, where the "vitamin D winter" is long, had a 45% reduced risk of MS if, as children, they were outdoors consistently during the short summer season.[43]

MS, sunlight and immigration

A study of immigrants born in the sunny West Indies, but who later moved to the United Kingdom (UK), showed they had only one-eighth the rate of MS as their own children born in the UK.[18] Another study assessed MS among people in the West Indies and showed that among people who had immigrated to Europe but returned to the islands after many years, the rate of MS was high. The increase was especially obvious in those who had visited Europe prior to age 15.[19] They developed more than four times more MS than others their age. There are two possible explanations: differences in sunlight or differences in nutrition between the two areas. We will discuss nutrition shortly.

When adults from England (an area of high risk for MS) immigrate to South Africa (a low-risk area), there is little change in their risk of developing MS.[20,21] They develop about six times the incidence of MS as native South Africans. The children who accompany the migrants, however, become highly protected against the disease. This research indicates that to best prevent future development of MS, sun exposure in childhood is important. However, other research shows that there may also be benefits of sun exposure for adults.[22] The researchers state that in Australia, "the prevalence of multiple sclerosis among those migrating before the age of 15 years from the high-risk UKI (England and Ireland) to lower-risk Australia was not significantly different from that among those migrating at or after that age."[22] Obviously, the best advice would be to keep vitamin D levels high regardless of age.

It is not possible for all English children to spend their formative years in South Africa or Australia and then move back to England. They can, however, be encouraged to play outdoors during the summer months and maintain high vitamin D levels by supplementation during winter. It is also important for expectant mothers to keep their vitamin D levels high. Children in northern countries born in May develop significantly more MS as they become adults than those born November.[23] The "vitamin D winter" in the North causes deficiencies in May, and exposure to summer sunlight causes higher levels in November. In the southern hemisphere— in Argentina for example—this relationship to birth month has also been observed, but in reverse order due to the seasonal flip. Most MS patients there are born in September, the last month of winter in that country.[24] *Those mount campaigns against childhood sun exposure are setting children up to become victims of MS.* These people are misinformed and misguided.

Military studies confirm that MS is related to lack of sunlight.

In 1922 Dr. Charles Davenport wrote a paper entitled, "Multiple Sclerosis from the standpoint of geographic distribution and race.[5] He analyzed the MS rate of military draftees and compared it to their states of origin. The highest rates were found in men who grew up in Michigan, Wisconsin, and the extreme northwest—all areas with low UVB availability. There were few cases of MS among those who grew up in southern states. He also noted that those from urban areas had 50% higher MS rates than those from rural areas. Similar studies confirm that relationship. [6,7] In 1979, assessments of the MS rates of USA military personnel were again compared to their states of origin, and the results were nearly identical.[14]

Vitamin D intake and MS

Can vitamin D from food and/or supplements reduce the rate of MS? A study of more than 185,000 women over a period of 10-20 years, divided them into five groups (quintiles), conducted according to the quantity of vitamin D they regularly ingested. Those in the lowest quintile were 50% more likely to contract MS than those in the highest.[25] Interestingly, women who supplemented 400 IU per day or more of vitamin D had a 41% reduced risk of developing MS compared to those who did not supplement. Four hundred IU is miniscule; imagine what might happen with 4,000 IU per day, or with regular sunlight exposure, which produces up to 20,000 IU per day.

Research on EAE

Experimental autoimmune encephalomyelitis (EAE) is a disease that is induced in mice to model and study MS. However, lab procedures that usually induce EAE are ineffective in animals are pre-treated with vitamin D—*the disease is completely prevented.*[26] Vitamin D also prevents the progression when administered at the first symptoms, but withdrawal of the treatment allows the disease to resume. EAE has been reversed by the administration of the "active" form of vitamin D—calcitriol,[27] and UVB irradiation prevents EAE development once it has been induced.[28]

If these same patterns apply to humans, it is critical that everyone's vitamin D levels stay consistently high, preferably over 40 ng/ml. Why take a chance when such a simple habit as regular sunlight exposure and/or taking vitamin D supplements might prevent or halt the progression of this dreaded disease.?

MS and serum levels of vitamin D

When newly diagnosed patients are compared with MS-free subjects, they have significantly lower vitamin D levels, and *when the disease goes into remission, the levels are higher than when the disease is active.*[29] Another investigation found that 77% of all MS patients had vitamin D levels lower than 20 ng/ml—severely deficient.[46] Bone mineral density (BMD) is also significantly lower in MS patients,[30] indicating that vitamin D deficiency plays a part in both MS and osteoporosis. *Another investigation conducted on military personnel found that those with the highest vitamin D levels had a 62% reduced risk compared to those with the lowest.*[40] Other research confirmed that an increasing rate of disability among MS patients directly correlated to decreased vitamin D levels and reduced sunlight exposure,[42] and those with severe disability were three times more likely to be deficient in vitamin D.

An interesting theory on vitamin D, Epstein Barr virus (EVB), infectious mononucleosis (IM) and MS

One researcher from Norway provides evidence that EBV is a precursor for MS, and that low vitamin D levels cannot adequately suppress the virus.[44] Also, IM confers an elevated risk for MS, and EVB is an important risk factor for IM.[48]

The bottom line

Just how much difference could sun exposure and/or vitamin D supplements make in preventing this disease? Dr. William Grant has estimated that "half of the 400,000 people with MS would not have MS if all Americans had the UVB/vitamin D status as those living in the southern states."[31]

The link between nutrition and MS

It is important to understand the relationships of nutrition to MS. Some of the earlier research we cited was looking for factors other than sunlight to explain relationships between MS and latitude.[5-9] Long before the connection between MS and sun was a popular topic, researchers had concluded that fat and animal foods had a close link to the disease. In 1950, Dr. Roy Swank developed a low-fat diet for MS patients.[32] As of this writing he has run a research program for 58 years to study the long-term efficacy of his diet on the longevity, disability level and quality of life of his patients, keeping in contact with them over several decades. He began the experiment with 144 patients who had endured the disease for an average of six years. Their average daily consumption of saturated fat before beginning the program was 125 grams per day, but he instructed them to eat fewer than 20 grams per day in the future. Seventy of the 144 adhered strictly to the diet, consuming an average of 16 grams. Seventy-four patients failed to adhere strictly to the diet though they did lower consumption to 38 grams per day. *After 34 years, 23 of the strict dieters (33%) had died, but only 14 (20%) from MS. Of the less strict subjects, 58 (80%) had died, and 45 (61%) had died from MS.*

The close follow-up of these patients ended after 34 years, but many of them continued to adhere to the dietary program. After 50 years, 15 of the original participants who adhered to the low-fat diet were between 72 and 84 years old. Thirteen were still ambulatory and reported being happy. The other two needed some help to walk but were otherwise well. These results are remarkable. After tenaciously conducting this experiment for over a half century, Dr. Swank concluded that MS patients that followed the diet could expect to survive and be otherwise normal to an advanced age. He then went on to state, "Complete absence of saturated fat in a daily diet might prove beneficial to general health, particularly in relation to cardiac and other circulatory diseases."

Most saturated fats of course, come from animal products—products that also contain proteins that are perhaps even more damaging than saturated fats. It could be that the correlation between saturated fats and MS that Dr. Swank so convincingly discovered is as much a correlation between animal foods and their proteins as it is to saturated fats.

For example, there is a striking relationship between a nation's MS rate and its level of dairy-product consumption. *In fact, the consumption of dairy products is as accurate a predictor of MS as latitude.*[33] With rare exceptions, there is a direct, linear relationship between the quantity of milk products consumed in a country and its MS rate.[34]

As discussed, vitamin D must be converted to "active" D (calcitriol) to have any influence. Animal foods are high in sulphur amino acids that cause an acid blood environment and reduce the body's calcitriol production.[35-36] People who eat more animal foods are more likely to have MS, and it is probable that the combination of low sunlight and high animal-product consumption is largely responsible for the striking geographical distribution of MS. Sunlight and UVB availability decrease at higher latitudes, and the consumption of animal foods increases.

My opinion, however, is that sunlight and vitamin D are the more important factors in preventing MS, with sound nutritional practices following closely. Dr. Grant demonstrates that dietary habits are rather uniform throughout the USA,[37] but MS is 2-3 times more prevalent in the north than in the south.[38] So, when nutrition is a constant, the difference in available sunlight still has a profound affect on the rate of MS. Those who seek the best odds in preventing this dread disease would do well to adopt a program of moderate, frequent sunlight exposure and/or vitamin D supplementation and a diet free of most, if not all, saturated fat and animal proteins.

An interesting personal aside

In 1990 I received a church assignment to look after the welfare of a neighbor family. The wife suffered from crippling MS. I was writing a book at the time and was well-informed of Dr. Swank's research and had also read an excellent book by Dr. John McDougall that thoroughly discussed Swank's work and the relationship of milk and meat to MS. After becoming better acquainted with my neighbor, I visited with copies of Dr. Swank's research in hand and McDougall's ideas in mind. She seemed interested until she heard about saturated fats and dairy product consumption. You see, she worked at a pizza restaurant and dearly loved her product. She was not about to give up pizza simply to reduce her pain and misery and function normally. Pizza was more important than health. Had I recommended a drug, she probably would have willingly swallowed it and waited for the "magic cure."

My wife, Vicki, and I built one of the most popular health resorts in the world, based on low-fat, mostly-vegetarian nutrition. The results our guests obtained were often spectacular in terms of reducing cholesterol, reversing diabetes and arthritis and losing weight. Yet, there were always a few guests who, after being on the program for a day or two, would drive several miles to find a fast-fat restaurant. There are those people who would rather die than change. It is their right, but they amaze me. Fleeting pleasure is more important to them than lasting health and vigor. Hopefully, you will take action. The fact that you have read this far perhaps indicates that you will.

What have we learned?

1. Multiple sclerosis is up to one hundred times more common in northern countries than equatorial countries. This is likely due to the difference in sunlight exposure and vitamin D.

2. Southern Australians are seven times more likely to contract MS than those in sunny northern Australia. The same relationship exists in the USA (sunnier states have a lower incidence).

3. Dr. William Grant has estimated that "half of the 400,000 people with MS would not have MS if all Americans had the UVB/vitamin D status as those living in the southern states."

4. People who as children are in the lowest category of sunlight exposure are more than three times as likely to develop MS as those who are in the highest.

5. A *greater* number of non-melanoma skin cancers (NMSC) and actinic keratoses (precancerous skin lesions) predict a *lesser* risk of MS.

6. Immigrants born in the sunny West Indies who later move to the United Kingdom (UK) have only one-eighth the rate of MS as their own children who are born in the UK.

7. Women in the lowest fifth of vitamin D intake are 50% more likely to contract MS than those in the highest fifth.

8. High serum levels of vitamin D predict low levels of MS.

9. An MS-like laboratory disease induced in animals can be prevented or inhibited by the administration of vitamin D.

10. Milk and saturated fat consumption also correlate very closely to MS risk.

Chapter 12

Solar Power, diabetes and other autoimmune diseases

"Give me the splendid, silent sun, with all his beams full-dazzling!"
Walt Whitman

Solar Power and diabetes

Diabetes is a disease of chronically high blood sugar that can lead to blindness, nerve damage, heart disease and numerous other maladies. There are two types of diabetes: type-1, in which the beta cells of the pancreas do not produce insulin (a hormone that moves sugar from the blood to the cells), and type-2, in which there is generally sufficient insulin, but where blood-sugar levels remain high because the body is resistant to it. Type-1 is generally known as "juvenile" diabetes, and type-2 is generally known as adult-onset diabetes.

In type-1 diabetes, insulin injections are necessary to keep the diabetic alive. In type-2 diabetes, insulin is sometimes necessary, and sometimes "hypoglycemic drugs" are sufficient to control serum sugar levels. Though the result of diabetes–chronically high blood sugar and its associated illnesses–is the same for both types, their causes are completely different. Type-1 is usually an autoimmune disease; the body's immune system attacks the beta cells of the pancreas and the pancreas stops producing insulin. Such attacks are similar to those that cause rheumatoid arthritis and multiple sclerosis. Let's first consider type-2 diabetes, since it accounts for 90% of all diabetes cases.

Type-2 diabetes: its causes and reversal

Type-2 diabetes is the most unnecessary of all degenerative diseases, yet it has increased rapidly as obesity has skyrocketed. These two disorders–obesity and diabetes—march almost in lock step. During the 1990s, obesity increased by 61% and type-2 diabetes increased by 49%.[1] In 2007, the health care and lost productivity of diabetes was $174 billion, an increase of $42 billion over 2006.[44] Diabetes costs are now approaching those of cancer, which in 2006 were $206.3 billion.[45]

Type-2 diabetes is caused by improper nutrition and lack of exercise, the exact causes of obesity. A study in the journal *Diabetes Care* reported research done on 40 type-2 diabetics placed on a low-fat, high-complex-carbohydrate diet and given a walking program.[2] Twenty-three were taking drugs and 17 were on insulin. *At the end of the 26-day program, all but two of those taking the drugs had been able to come off all medication. Of the 17 on insulin, thirteen no longer needed it and two cut their dosages by 50%.* The new diet had roughly 10% of total calories from fat, 70% from complex carbohydrates (whole grains, vegetables, fruits, etc.) and 20% from protein.

In our health resort we used this same plan, but with more exercise, and our guests had astonishing results. Two-thirds of diabetics were free of all medication or insulin in an average of two weeks, and many of the remainder usually needed about two more weeks to be off the meds. Some who were injecting as much as 70-180 units of insulin daily were free from insulin injections in less than a week.

A person usually needs only to stop eating fat, sugar and refined flour and increase whole-food intake—especially vegetables, fruits and whole grains—and walk at least two miles daily to reverse type-2 diabetes. Some "experts" say that diabetes is due to carbohydrates, but they fail to differentiate between refined products (white flour, fruit juices and sugars) and whole brown rice, whole fruits and whole-grain wheat). All carbohydrates are not the same!

Excessive fat consumption was identified as the primary cause of diabetes in 1927, when Dr. E.P. Joslin of Boston wrote in the *Annals of Clinical Medicine*: "With an excess of fat, diabetes begins, and from an excess of fat diabetics die, formerly of coma and recently of atherosclerosis."[3] That same year, Dr. J.S. Sweeney experimented on blood sugar responses to various diets and stated, "in the curves of subjects fed on carbohydrate there is an insignificant rise in blood sugar…those in the carbohydrate group are all strikingly within normal limits…those who were placed on the fat diet and those who were starved manifested a definite decrease of sugar tolerance."[4] In 1930, Dr. I.M. Rabinowich added, "A potential diabetic can be transformed into a completely diabetic individual by the administration of the time-honored carbohydrate-free meal of meat and fat."[5] These researchers knew exactly what caused type-2 diabetes, but few people listened, even though many subsequent studies confirmed their findings.

If this information has been available for decades, why aren't we being told? (1) most physicians have no idea that the information exists, and (2) such information would destroy the market for insulin and hypoglycemic drugs. Pharmaceutical companies will not promote anything that will reduce profits.

Remember that only unrefined complex carbohydrates are healthful, that fats from unrefined nuts, flax and avocados are not nearly as dangerous as other fats, and that some omega-3 fats are absolutely essential for health. Lamentably, nearly all of the fats consumed in Western societies are disease promoting: animal fats and refined, processed polyunsaturated fatty acids (PUFA).

There is a reason for emphasizing the importance of nutrition in diabetes. I have worked with diabetics for thirty years and have seen profound improvements from nutritional changes. Although the book is about sunlight and vitamin D, it is important to understand they are not panaceas. All our ills cannot be cured by a dose of vitamin D.

Sunlight and type-2 diabetes

There are only two studies that indicate an influence of sunlight on type-2 diabetes. One shows that blood-sugar levels are lower during the summer,[6] and the other shows that exposure to UVB increases insulin secretion.[7]

Vitamin D and type-2 diabetes

Research shows that Vitamin D levels correlate closely to insulin sensitivity; the higher the vitamin D levels, the more receptive the body is to the action of insulin, which makes carbohydrates easier to metabolize.[8] This same study shows that the higher the vitamin D levels are, the lower are the blood sugar levels. *Another investigation found that men with the highest vitamin D levels had a 30% reduced risk of type-2 diabetes.*[42] The beta cells of the pancreas (the insulin producing cells) do have vitamin D receptors[9] and function more efficiently when vitamin D levels are higher.[10] Vitamin D stimulates these receptors, and then the beta cells to do a more efficient job of insulin secretion.. Vitamin D supplementation also increases insulin secretion in humans[11] and animals,[12-13] which is likely the reason for the inverse correlation between vitamin D levels and blood-sugar levels.[46]

Another paper reported on a study of adults with impaired sugar tolerance and insulin resistance (both risk factors for diabetes). For three years, half got a placebo and the others vitamin D plus calcium. *The rise in blood-sugar levels was fifteen times higher in the placebo group, and their increase in insulin resistance was eighteen times more.*[48]

Dr. Anastassios Pittas and his colleagues at Tufts University demonstrated that a combination of 800 IU or more of vitamin D, coupled with a high calcium intake over 20 years, produced a 33% reduction in the risk of type-2 diabetes,[14] reduced age-related increases in blood-sugar levels and decreased insulin resistance.[48] *Subjects with high-vitamin D status were about one-third as likely to develop diabetes as those with low levels.[49]*

The incidence of type-2 diabetes varies directly with blood-vitamin D levels among Caucasians and Mexican Americans but not African Americans.[15] Mexican Americans whose vitamin D levels were highest had only 17% of the risk of diabetes as those with the lowest. Among Caucasians, there was a 25% reduced risk when comparing those with high and low levels. *Other research on diabetic women shows that a supplement of 1,332 IU per day for one month correlates with a 21.4% drop in insulin resistance and a 34.3% increase in insulin secretion.[41]* Though type-2 diabetes is a disease caused by poor nutrition and lack of exercise, diabetics can receive considerable benefit from vitamin D. Is the same true for type1?

Vitamin D and diabetic neuropathy

Years ago, one of the guests at our health resort told us that he suffered from very painful diabetic neuropathy, a disease of nerve damage caused by chronically high blood sugar associated with diabetes. He stayed for several months, and at the end of that time, he was pain free. I had felt that his progress was due to our plant-based, low-fat diet, and there is little doubt that the diet was a factor. However, recent research has convinced me that the vitamin D gained from exposure to the Southern Utah sunshine was also exceptionally important in producing his results: fifty-one patients with type-two diabetes and neuropathic pain had average serum levels of only 18 ng/ml. After three months of vitamin D3 supplementation, the severity of the pain was reduced by 40-50%.[56]

Nutrition and type-1 diabetes: Is cow's milk the cause?

Type-1 diabetes is one of the most tragic childhood diseases and requires insulin injections or patches for a lifetime. Even sadder is that proper nutrition during infancy may prevent this illness from occurring. *Even though the underlying mechanisms of type-1 diabetes are different from those of type-2, nutrition plays as strong a part in its cause. The difference is that the offending food is not fat, but milk protein.* Let's analyze the relationship of diet to the occurrence of this disease.

Type-1 diabetes in children correlates closely to the cow's-milk consumption. Cow's milk increases permeability in the intestines of youngsters,[17] which may allow milk proteins to enter the blood before they can be broken down into their constituent amino acids. One theory is that large protein molecules enter the blood, where they are mistaken for foreign invaders.[18] Cow's milk protein has a seventeen amino acid chain that is similar to the protein chains on the beta cells of the pancreas. The immune system creates billions of antibodies against these proteins, and the antibodies attack and destroy the beta cells, which makes the child a type-1 diabetic. It is a case of mistaken identity. The longer a baby is breast-fed before the introduction of cow's milk, the smaller is the chance of type-1 diabetes.[19] My neurosurgeon friend John Clark, MD, who volunteers medical education in Ethiopia, states that 98% of all newborns there die in a year if they are not breast-fed. Mother's milk contains the *correct* antibodies babies need.

The *New England Journal of Medicine* reports that ***all youngsters with type-1 diabetes have vastly increased antibodies to cow's milk protein.[18] Other research shows that children who drink cow's milk before age three were 11 times more likely to develop diabetes than those who consumed none.[20]*** Though the *Journal* article was written in 1992, studies as recent as 2006 indicate that cow's-milk consumption may be a factor in the production of type-1 diabetes.[21] While the National Dairy Council strongly opposes that idea, the theory's validity was further corroborated by an epidemiological study that compared milk consumption rates among children in twelve countries to their rates of type-1 diabetes.[22] The correlation is exceptionally close. As milk consumption increases, type-1 diabetes increases almost in lock-step. In fact, the 96% correlation verges on being prefect. In Figure 1, the lower-left point represents Japan and the upper-right, Finland.[22] Finland's rate of diabetes in this study was 11-times higher than Japan's. In other studies, Finland's rate had thirty-five times the type-1-diabetes rate as Japan.[23]

Animal studies also implicate dairy products as a cause of type-1 diabetes; cow's milk triggers it in rats and mice.[16]

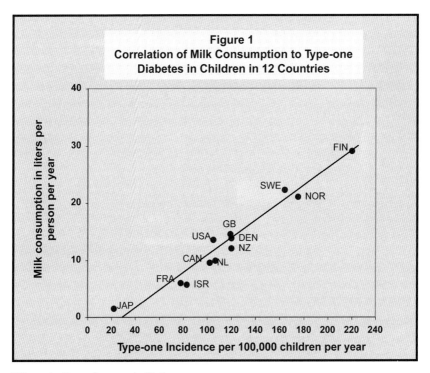

Figure 1
Correlation of Milk Consumption to Type-one Diabetes in Children in 12 Countries

Vitamin D and type-1 diabetes

Vitamin D provides profound protection against type-1 diabetes. Researchers in Norway found that cod liver oil (an oil with a high vitamin D content) taken by expectant mothers substantially reduced the risk.[24] The children of these mothers had only 30% of the diabetes rate of children whose mothers did not take the oil. However, cod-liver oil is not the best supplement. Its vitamin A content is too high, and too much vitamin A intake weakens bones.[50]

Finnish researchers compared diabetes rates of children who were supplemented with those who were less supplemented and found that *the less supplemented children had nearly five times the diabetes rate of those who received 2,000 IU per day.*[25] *The chart below emphasizes the difference between the two groups.*

145

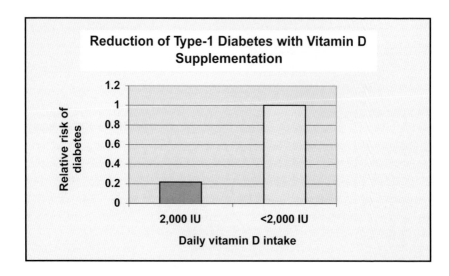

Reduction of Type-1 Diabetes with Vitamin D Supplementation

Relative risk of diabetes

Daily vitamin D intake

Those who received no supplementation had more than eight times the risk of diabetes. The Finns are among the biggest dairy consumers in the world, and their children have the highest rate of type-1 diabetes.[26] If low vitamin D levels contribute to the disease, diabetic children probably have low levels, and that is indeed the case.[27-28] The good news is that vitamin D might be a powerful antidote against cow's milk. The autoantibodies (the autoimmune cells that destroy the beta cells) are detectable long before a child actually manifests any symptoms,[29] and the presence of the antibodies in children inversely correlates to the vitamin D intake of their mothers during pregnancy;[54] the greater the vitamin D intake of the mothers, the lower the risk of diabetes in the children. It is also interesting to note that newly-diagnosed type-1 diabetics have significantly lower serum-vitamin D levels than non-diabetics.[47] *Research on mice reinforces this concept. When the "antidote"– activated Vitamin D–is administered in high doses to mice that otherwise develop the disease, it completely prevents type-1 diabetes from occurring.*[30]

The relationship of sunlight to type-1 diabetes

Australian research shows that the incidence of type-1 correlates closely with latitude; the southernmost part of the country has about three times the rate as the northernmost.[31] And in Newfoundland, Canada, an extremely strong inverse correlation exists between UVB exposure and incidence.[55]

Now let's look at more autoimmune diseases in which vitamin D may play a protective role.

Systemic lupus erythematosus (SLE)

"Lupus" or SLE can attack almost any system of the body, and vitamin D levels are typically quite low in SLE patients.[32-34,123] Since SLE often causes sunlight hypersensitivity, it may be necessary to bring vitamin D to optimal levels by supplementation. Here are some other indications that vitamin D deficiency may predispose to SLE: (1) Hispanics and African Americans are far more likely to develop SLE, and it is more acute and dangerous in these groups than in Caucasians.[51] African Americans have three times the risk, even when the health-care services are equally available to both groups.[51] African Americans are far more likely to suffer from vitamin D deficiency, so the theory that SLE is triggered in part by the deficiency is bolstered by SLE's higher incidence in dark-skinned people. This difference is not due to genetics, since West Africans (the area of origin of most African Americans) do not have high SLE rates.[52] (2) A vitamin D analogue administered to mice with SLE significantly improves longevity.[53]

Inflammatory bowel disease (IBD)

IBD is an autoimmune disease characterized by inflammation of the intestine (colitis) and chronic diarrhea. When IBD is induced in mice, vitamin D and calcium treatments dramatically mitigate the disease.[35] In other research on mice lacking the vitamin D receptor (VDR), IBD and its accompanying colitis became quite severe. All mice without VDR died within eight weeks of IBD; those who had the VDR were all healthy at eight weeks.[36]

Among children who suffer from IBD, vitamin D deficiency is highly prevalent, and the predisposing factors for the disease include dark skin, winter season and lack of vitamin D supplementation.[43]

Crohn's disease

Crohn's, another inflammatory autoimmune bowel disease, causes abdominal pain, inflammation and fibrous tissue buildup. Crohn's is closely correlated to vitamin D deficiency, and moderate sunlight exposure coupled with winter supplementation has been recommended to reduce the severity.[37] Fifty percent of Crohn's patients are vitamin D deficient in winter and 19% in summer. However, "deficient" was defined as vitamin D levels below 20 ng/ml which is critically low. If the goal of 40 ng/ml is used, it is likely that all Crohn's patients are deficient.

Vitamin D and Parkinson's disease

Parkinson's is a progressive disease of the nerves of the brain and/or spinal cord, characterized by weakness, the inability to control some muscular movements, an unusual gait, partial facial paralysis and tremors and is eventually fatal. Parkinson's may or may not be an autoimmune disease, but vitamin D may help to prevent it. Two rat experiments showed that induced Parkinson's could be inhibited by calcitriol.[38-39] Another study showed that abnormal locomotion (movement) in rats with induced Parkinson-like damage could be restored by calcitriol.[39]

Persons with abnormal VDR in the brain and spinal cord also have a much higher risk of Parkinson's.[40] Certainly, sunlight exposure and the higher serum level of Vitamin D that follows would be of value to a Parkinson's patient.

What have we learned?

1. Type-2 diabetes and obesity rates increase together; the more obesity the greater the risk of diabetes.

2. Type-2 diabetes is often reversible with a low-fat, low-refined carbohydrate diet.

3. Serum blood sugar levels are lower in summer than in winter.

4. Exposure to ultraviolet light (UVB) increases insulin secretion in adults.

5. All else being equal, the higher the serum level of vitamin D, the lower the blood sugar level.

6. Vitamin D supplementation increases the secretion of insulin in both humans and animals.

7. Type-1 diabetes is primarily an autoimmune response triggered by milk proteins.

8. D-supplemented children have one-fifth the risk of type-1 diabetes as non-supplemented children.

9. Lupus and inflammatory bowel disease are correlated to low levels of vitamin D.

10. Inflammatory bowel diseases (IBD) correlate to low levels of vitamin D and low sunlight exposure.

11. Laboratory induced IBD in animals is effectively treated with vitamin D.

12. Laboratory induced Parkinson's in animals is inhibited by calcitriol (activated vitamin D) treatment.

Chapter 13

Solar Power, heart disease and high blood pressure

"Open up your heart and let the sunshine in!"
Stuart Hamblen

Heart disease is an arterial (vascular) disease and the number-one killer in the USA. Most heart disease is due to a gradual occlusion (closing) of the heart arteries by calcium and a substance called cholesterol, which forms a deposit called a plaque. ***This occlusion is known as atherosclerosis.*** A plaque may burst, blocking the narrowed area, or fat-laden blood may clot in that area, halting blood flow and preventing oxygen delivery to the tissue. If this happens in heart arteries, a myocardial infarct—a heart attack—occurs. If it happens in the brain, a stroke results. And if the arteries of the limbs are nearly occluded, the disease is called peripheral artery disease (PAD), which can result in a condition known as intermittent claudication and cause terrible pain during walking. Here we will use the general term, "cardiovascular diseases" or (CVD) to cover these conditions.

Poor dietary habits are the primary cause. Populations that consume large quantities of animal-based foods, fried foods and sugar generally have exceptionally high rates; populations who consume few of these foods have low rates.[1] However, sunlight and vitamin D may act to a certain extent as an antidote to such "food poisonings."

Sunlight and heart disease

Serum cholesterol levels in general are good predictors of heart disease. However, when sunlight contacts the skin, cholesterol there is converted to vitamin D, which "uses up" cholesterol in the skin. The used cholesterol is replaced by cholesterol in the blood, thereby lowering serum cholesterol levels, which is important. The Framingham Study, conducted by Dr. William Castelli, followed the health of more than 5,000 residents of Framingham, Massachusetts for over fifty years. ***One of its findings was that no heart attacks occurred in any subjects with cholesterol levels below 150mg%. This finding was true even for those who smoked, had high blood pressure or led inactive lives.***[2] Because his studies convinced him that a diet that pushed cholesterol levels over 150 is the most critical cause of heart disease, Dr. Castelli stated, "When you see the golden arches, you are probably on the way to the pearly gates."[3]

Another study was known as the Multiple Risk Factor Intervention Trial, which studied 360,000 men who were divided into ten groups according to their cholesterol levels and followed for six years to determine heart-disease risk. Death from heart disease increased noticeably in each ascending group. The researchers, stated, ***"In every one of these groups, this relationship held consistently, systematically and without contradiction, and in every one of them it was continuous, strong and graded from the second percent [group] of serum cholesterol on up."[4]***

Sunlight, vitamin D, and CVD

If sunlight exposure helps prevent CVD, then we could expect that disease rates would be lower in summer and higher in winter. A 1996 study indicates that sunlight indeed lowers cholesterol levels and decreases the risk of heart attack.[5] However, the typical winter lack of physical activity could be a factor. In that case sun would have not only a direct influence on cholesterol levels, but also an indirect affect: it is easier to be active outdoors when the weather is warm.

Other research found that "total cholesterol, blood pressure and body mass index [a measure of the degree of fatness of the body] showed pronounced seasonal variations with average levels significantly higher during the winter months in all age groups and both sexes, giving an estimated increase in score risk of 6.8% in men and 3.6% in women."[6] Also, the incidence of stroke is highest in January and lowest in September,[7] and, 77% of stroke patients are vitamin D deficient.[51] CVD peaks in the winter months and is responsible for 20,000 additional deaths per year in England and Wales,[8-9] and in ***Brazil, the heart-attack death rate is 30% higher in winter than summer in those 75 and older[10]***

Dr. Armin Zittermann's review of latitude and rates of CVD demonstrates that CVD occurs much more frequently at higher latitudes.[11] This could be due in part to the fact that those living at lower latitudes have more available sunlight and higher serum levels of vitamin D. Dr. Zittermann points out that in the British Isles, those who live in northern Scotland have twice the rate of CVD as those who live in southern England. Those who live in the more central Midlands, Wales and northern England have intermediate rates. Since there are few differences in nutrition, it is safe to assume that different vitamin D levels make the difference. Altitude may also make a difference. In chapter 1 we established the relationship of UVB availability to altitude and contrasted Phoenix, Arizona (altitude 1,000 feet) with Flagstaff, Arizona (7,000 feet) where 27% more UVB is available due to thinner air at higher altitude.

New Mexico also has considerable altitude differences among the major residential areas. In one study, it was found that as altitude increased, CVD in men decreased.[12] Men who lived at less than 4,000 feet had the most CVD. Those who lived in the 5,000 foot range had 98% of the CVD rate of those living at 4,000 feet or less; for those living in the 6,000 foot range it was 90%; in the 7,000 foot range, 86%, and those living at 8,000 feet had only 72%. The researchers theorized that exercise at higher altitudes is more difficult and therefore strengthens the heart. That theory might have some merit, but it is far more likely that the increased intensity of UVB at higher latitudes caused the drop in CVD.

One might wonder why the benefit increased so dramatically at the highest altitude as compared to the lowest altitude. Dr. Zittermann shows that UVB increases about 4% per 1,000 feet elevation gain near sea level, but increases 8-10% per 1,000 foot elevation gain at altitudes over 8,000 feet, and also states that higher altitude leads to increased UVB availability in late fall and winter.[11] No doubt the same would be true of late winter and early spring. This means that the "vitamin D winter" would be shorter at higher altitudes, and more vitamin D would be produced each year.

Though women did not appear to benefit in the New Mexico study, another showed that both men and women living at high altitudes had a lower risk of CVD, although the influence of altitude was still somewhat greater in men.[13] Furthermore, those at the highest altitudes had about 14% less risk of suffering a stroke.[14]

Vitamin D and peripheral artery disease (PAD)

PAD is a type of CVD which results in occlusion of the arteries of the limbs. It can result in a crippling condition called intermittent claudication, which causes terrible pain when a person tries to walk. Dr. Michal Melamed and colleagues have determined that those with serum-vitamin D levels lower than 17.8 ng/ml have twice the risk of PAD as those with levels over 29.2 ng/ml, and that each 10 ng/ml decrease predicts a 29% increase in PAD.[65]

Serum vitamin D levels, heart attack and stroke

In 1990, a study in New Zealand *found that those below the median level of serum vitamin D suffered 57% more heart attacks than those whose levels were above the median*. They also noted that the greatest number occurred in winter and spring, and that the reduced risk among those with higher levels pertained to all seasons.

Two 2008 studies corroborated those results. Dr. Thomas Wang and colleagues compared the risk of stroke and heart attack with serum-vitamin D levels and found a 62% increased risk in those with lowest levels compared to those with highest levels and also showed that in those with low D levels and high blood pressure had double the risk.[54] Dr. Edward Giovannucci and colleagues reported even more impressive results.[67] *They found that men whose serum levels of vitamin D were less than 15 ng/ml had nearly 2.5 times the rate of heart attack as those whose levels were above 30.* Still other research showed that classic risk factors for cardiovascular disease were higher in those who ranked in the lowest quartile (fourth) of vitamin D levels compared to those whose levels were in the highest quartile.[55] Hypertension was 30% higher, diabetes 98% higher, obesity 129% higher and triglycerides 47% higher.

Sunlight, vitamin D and hypertension (high blood pressure)

Hypertension is a risk factor for CVD, and its incidence is considerably higher in winter than summer. *One study of hypertensive subjects shows that blood pressure levels average 165/90 in winter but 134/74 in the summer, and that both stroke and heart attack rate double in the winter.*[15] Even in children, blood pressure is higher in winter than summer.[63] Supplementation with vitamin D lowers both blood pressure and heart rate in elderly women,[16] which is a desirable because a lower heart rate *generally* indicates a stronger heart. Vitamin D lowers blood pressure by blocking the action of the enzyme called renin, which profoundly raises blood pressure.[64] Renin activates angiotensin which causes vessel constriction. Renin and angiotensin are needed to control blood pressure within healthful levels, but without sufficient vitamin D, the constriction becomes excessive, which may result in hypertension.

Increasing serum vitamin D to 40 ng/ml also reduces hypertension.[17] *In three sessions per week of full-body UVB light treatments, vitamin D levels rose 162% after six weeks and blood pressures dropped six points on both systolic (higher number) and diastolic (lower number) measurements,* and in a study that compared vitamin D levels with the hypertension risk, it was shown *that men who had the lowest D levels also had 6.13 times the risk of developing hypertension. In women, the lowest levels related to a 2.67 times increased risk.*[52] The following graph illustrates the remarkable difference in hypertension risk based on serum vitamin D levels.

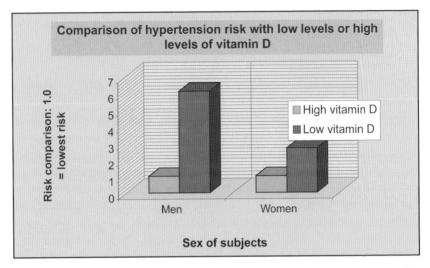

Comparison of hypertension risk with low levels or high levels of vitamin D

Risk comparison: 1.0 = lowest risk

High vitamin D
Low vitamin D

Men   Women

Sex of subjects

The idea that UVB lowers blood pressure is corroborated by studies showing lower rates at higher altitudes.[18]

Blood pressure rises with age almost worldwide, although individuals with optimal D levels have a decreased risk of this age-associated increase.[62] The blood pressure of the Kuna Indians, who live in isolated islands off the coast of Panama, does not rise with age[19] unless they move to Panama City—in which case the rate of hypertension in elderly Kunas is greater than 60%.[20] In their native islands Kunas have absolutely no hypertension whether they were 20, 30 or 60 years old. Urban living takes people indoors and puts them in an area of greater pollution—pollution that filters out UVB.[49] Of course, diet tends to change when people become urbanized, but considering that UVB exposure is proven to maintain healthful blood pressure levels, it is a safe assumption that a significant part of the change for urbanized Kunas is reduced sunlight exposure. Urban vs. rural dwelling has correlated to a rise in both CVD and blood pressure in several other research projects in Africans[21] and Indians,[22] and it has been shown that rural dwellers have higher levels of circulating vitamin D.[23] Also, considerations such as amount of clothing worn, type of work done and amount of time spent indoors all favor the idea that lack of sunlight is a strong risk factor for hypertension.[11]

Sunlight, vitamin D and heart failure

Heart failure is caused by a weakened heart that cannot adequately pump blood, causing fluids back up into the lungs and build up in the feet, ankles, and legs. Sufferers experience extreme fatigue and shortness of breath.

Ultimately the heart gives out and death ensues. *In France, deaths from heart failure are 20% higher than average in January and 15% lower in August—a swing of 35%.[24] A similar study done in Spain found that heart-failure hospital admissions were 25% higher than average in January and 33% lower in August. That is a 58% seasonal swing![26]*

The incidence of heart failure in blacks compared to whites is 40% higher in men and more than 100% higher in women.[48] Remember that dark-skinned people living at high latitudes have lower vitamin D levels—an easily-remedied situation. Not surprisingly, heart failure is related to low vitamin D in all races, and most sufferers have serum levels below 20 ng/ml. Adults with this condition show a history of sedentary, indoor living.[50]

Inflammation is also common with heart failure, and is often caused by proteins called cytokines that are either pro-inflammatory or anti-inflammatory elements of the immune system. *Vitamin D has an amazing ability to inhibit pro-inflammatory cytokine production[45,58] while stimulating the production of anti-inflammatory cytokines[46,58] and is particularly useful in improving the cytokine profiles in patients with congestive heart failure.[58]* Vitamin D has also been shown to prevent the unnatural growth of heart-muscle cells in rats with heart failure.[68] Such cell growth is unnatural and indicates the progressive deterioration of heart muscle characteristic of the disease.

Some have proposed that the surge of winter heart-failure deaths is due to seasonal depression,[27] and a part may be due to that, because sunlight exposure has a profound, positive influence on mood. We will discuss mood in chapter 15.

Heart failure in infants

Tragically, newborns also suffer heart failure, and until lately studies had not considered vitamin D deficiency as a possible cause. However, in a study conducted in southeast England, sixteen infants were identified that had suffered heart failure and hypocalcaemia between 2000 and 2006.[66] Six were of Indian and ten of African ethnicity. Six of them suffered cardiac arrest, three died, eight were placed on lung machines, and two were referred for heart transplants. *The average serum vitamin D level of these children was only 7.4 ng/ml, and some of the infants had undetectable levels.*

Hypocalcaemia is usually caused by insufficient vitamin D in the blood and often results in convulsions and death, but the care givers had not even tried

155

to assure that vitamin D levels were adequate. The researchers concluded with this statement: "Vitamin D deficiency and consequent hypocalcaemia are seen in association with severe and life-threatening infant heart failure. That no infant or mother was receiving the recommended vitamin supplementation highlights the need for adequate provision of vitamin D to ethnic minority populations."

Obviously, a few dollars worth of vitamin D could have prevented this catastrophe. At least the word is getting out.

How does vitamin D reduce plaques in arteries?

Vitamin D may reduce CVD by reducing calcification of the plaques that obstruct arteries. Eighty-three to 90 percent of CVD patients show calcification of their coronary arteries—a far higher percentage than disease-free people.[28-29] Arterial calcium is an excellent measurement to detect severe CVD[30-31] and has been used to predict heart attacks since 1964.[32] If something could reduce calcium deposits in arteries, it would reduce plaques and lower the CVD risk. *Interestingly, there is a strong correlation between calcification of the arteries and decalcification of the bones (osteoporosis).*[33-34] Could there be a lack of something in the blood that might cause plaquing while simultaneously contributing to a loss of bone calcium? In chapter 10, we discussed the strong correlation between osteoporosis and the lack of vitamin D. Could it be the factor that also inhibits the calcification of arteries? Osteoporosis is closely correlated to heart disease.[57] Vitamin D deficiency could certainly be a factor in both, because there is a strong inverse relationship between vitamin D levels and artery calcification; the more D in the blood, the less the calcification.[35] Artery cells have vitamin D receptors (VDR), which when stimulated by vitamin D, inhibit the incursion of calcium.[36] In rats, low levels of calcitriol are associated with massive blood vessel and other soft tissue calcification.[56]

Chapter 10 also showed that serum parathyroid hormone (PTH) levels are much higher when D levels are low, and that high PTH levels trigger bone loss. PTH also is a trigger of arterial calcification and has a part in calcifying both heart muscle and heart valves.[37] PTH levels are also much lower in tanning beds users.[38] According to the most comprehensive studies, blood levels of vitamin D must be at least 32-40 ng/ml to hold PTH levels in check,[39-40] and supplementation with vitamin D has also been shown to lower PTH.[16]

Finally, calcium supplementation of 1,000 milligrams per day is shown to double the risk of heart attacks and increase the risk of stroke by about 50% when compared to those who do not take supplemental calcium, and other studies corroborate the increase in CVD events with calcium supplementation.[60]   Only a small amount of supplemental calcium is needed for those who do not eat correctly, but the vast quantities taken by many postmenopausal women and others may be a detriment to their hearts, especially if not accompanied by a large quantity of vitamin D, which appears to prevent arterial calcification. Remember that too much calcium actually retards the conversion of stored vitamin D (calcidiol) to the potent hormone form, calcitriol, and that large quantities of calcium, without vitamin D (see chapter 10) do not reduce fractures but may actually increase them.[61]

While not all scientists agree on the relationship between vitamin D and calcification of the arteries,[41] there is little disagreement over sunlight and improved CVD health.

Vitamin D and inflammation of the arteries

Inflammation is a response to infection and injury, and arterial inflammation is involved in the development of CVD. Certain chemicals are released into the blood when inflammation is present. These are "markers" of CVD and are useful in predicting its presence.[42-43] One marker is C-reactive protein (CRP) and may not only indicate the presence of CVD, but may be actively involved in the process of atherosclerosis.[42-44] Vitamin D may promote heart and vascular health by its ability to inhibit inflammation. *Vitamin D supplements and injections lower CRP levels by as much as 40%,*[11] and cytokine profiles are improved, which also reduces inflammation.[45,46,58]

If a drug were developed that reduced CVD to the extent that vitamin D does, it would be front page news worldwide. However, since vitamin D therapy sells no expensive, patented drugs, its efficacy in preventing CVD remains generally unknown. That should shortly change with the overwhelming evidence of vitamin D's positive influence.

Beyond vitamin D

In another interesting piece of research of sunlight exposure on CVD, Dr. Peter Hays analyzed the records of first-time heart-attack patients. Amazingly, he found that their chance of survival varied according to whether they were placed on the north (dark) side of the hospital or on the south (sunny) side—survival rate on the sunny side being about 25% better.[47] Dr. Hays assumed that the difference in mortality rates was due to the improved mental health of those patients on the sunny side. It is unlikely that the positive relationship of sunlight to survival of heart disease patients was mediated by vitamin D, since most of the vitamin D-producing UVB is filtered out by window glass. Just being able to see sunlight may have remarkable, positive benefits that are yet to be discovered.

We have now covered the major deadly diseases that are positively influenced by sunlight. We will now turn our attention to other maladies for which "Doctor Sun" should always be consulted.

What have we learned?

1. Heart attacks are uncommon in those with serum cholesterol levels below 150. Sunlight exposure may lower serum cholesterol.

2. High blood pressure (hypertension), high cholesterol levels and stroke incidence are all significantly more prevalent in winter than in summer.

3. People who live at higher altitudes have lower rates of CVD, which includes cerebrovascular disease (which may result in stroke), heart disease, and peripheral artery disease.

4. A few weeks of treatment with ultraviolet light lowers blood pressure substantially.

5. Rural residents, who have higher serum vitamin D levels, have fewer cases of CVD.

6. In Spain, hospital admissions for heart failure are 25% higher than average in January and 33% lower in August—a 58% swing between winter and summer.

7. The risk of heart failure is 40% greater in black men than white men and 100% higher in black women than white women.

8. The lower the level of vitamin D, the greater is the risk of arterial calcification.

9. Vitamin D prevents arterial inflammation.

10. Survival rates for CVD patients in sunny rooms are 25% better than for patients in dark rooms.

11. Higher levels of vitamin D correlate to reduced peripheral artery disease (PAD).

Chapter 14

Solar Power and a potpourri of health concerns

You can make the pathway bright; fill the soul with Heaven's light,
if there's sunshine in your heart."
Church Hymn

Although there has been less research on the positive relationship of sunlight/vitamin D to the diseases discussed in this chapter, there is sufficient indication to include them here.

Periodontal disease (PD)

Periodontal disease (PD) attacks the gum and bone holding the teeth, causing inflammation and bone loss, and it is the number-one cause of tooth loss. Almost 90% of USA citizens have PD.[1] About 51% of teeth are extracted due to PD, compared to 35.4% for caries (cavities).[2] When there is bone loss and inflammation, teeth may become loose and fall out in a process called *attachment loss.*[3]

Since inflammation is involved in cardiovascular disease (CVD) as well, a correlation between CVD and PD is expected. Men with a high rate of PD have a 25% higher risk of CVD than men with minimal PD, and those who are under 50 have a 72% greater risk.[4] Interestingly, both PD and poor oral hygiene are better predictors of death than is CVD.[4] Those with PD also have twice the risk of stroke. Vitamin D decreases the action of inflammatory cytokines—proteins that cause inflammation in tissue and increase the action of anti-inflammatory cytokines.[88-89] These processes are involved in both CVD and PD. Bacteria live in dental plaque and cause an immune cell response that releases pro-inflammatory cytokines in an attempt to destroy the bacteria. Unfortunately, these cytokines cause gum and bone inflammation,[5] but vitamin D dampens the inflammatory response.

In chapter 10 we solidly established vitamin D's impressive bone-building properties; if it dramatically prevents or even reverses osteoporosis, we might expect that it has a role in preventing PD, and indeed research suggests that it is a critical factor in dental health. The bone that holds the teeth is the alveolar ridge. If it degenerates due to lack of density, or is attacked by inflammatory mechanisms, PD is exacerbated, and several studies show that osteoporosis is closely related to alveolar ridge bone loss and loss of teeth.[6-10] Some of the same mechanisms that cause osteoporosis are therefore also a likely cause of PD, so achieving healthful levels of vitamin D should lessen PD's severity. *In one study, subjects who were supplemented with both calcium and vitamin D had a rate of tooth loss 60% lower than those who had taken placebos containing no vitamin D or calcium.[11]* In another, subjects who lacked the vitamin D receptors necessary to stimulate absorption of calcium showed early and severe PD.[12-15]

Attachment loss was shown to be 39 millimeters higher in men and 26 millimeters higher in women whose serum levels of vitamin D were in the lowest fifth compared to those in the highest fifth, [16] and the authors theorize that it is related to low vitamin D levels. The gums of persons who suffer gingivitis (inflammation of the gums) show fewer tendencies to bleed when the gums are probed if their serum vitamin D levels are high, indicating less inflammation.[17]

Dr. John Clark, a neurosurgeon with 45 years experience, read this section and offered suggestions. He told me his observations of conditions that correlated closely to brain and nerve diseases requiring surgery. The three most important factors, in his opinion, are PD, osteoarthritis and calcification of the aorta. All three maladies are related closely to D deficiency. It may not be the primary underlying cause, but it is safe to state that it is a major factor.

Sunlight and dental caries (cavities)

The studies on sunlight and dental cavities that have been reviewed by Dr. Zane Kime[18] are older but of great value. One showed a direct correlation between hours of available sunlight per year and the number of dental caries in Caucasian boys 12 to 14 years of age. In geographic areas with less than 2,200 hours of available sunlight, there were 486 cavities per year per each 100 boys. In areas where there were 3,000 or more hours of sunlight, there were only 290 cavities per year per hundred.[19] The frequency of cavities was also higher in winter than in summer months.[20]

More recently, in 2008, it has been found that pregnant women who are deficient in vitamin D give birth to children whose tooth enamel is weak and who are at much higher risk of dental caries.[173]

Now let's find out if sunlight and vitamin D have an influence on our "largest" pandemic: obesity.

161

Solar Power, vitamin D, overweight and obesity

Overweight is defined as having a body mass index (BMI) higher than 25, and obesity is defined as having a BMI higher than 30.[22] BMI is computed by dividing body weight in kilograms by meters of height squared. BMI is a useful tool for most of the population, although it is inaccurate for people who carry much of their weight as muscle.

Obesity and overweight are increasing rapidly in overfed, undernourished, undersunned, sedentary societies. According to the World Health Organization, 75% of women over 30 are overweight in the USA, Mexico, Turkey, South Africa, Egypt and Malta, and men do not fare much better. Seventy-five percent of men in Britain, Germany, Kuwait, Greece, Argentina, Samoa and New Zealand are overweight.[21]

Obesity is a risk factor for hypertension, high cholesterol, type 2 diabetes, coronary heart disease, stroke, gallbladder disease, osteoarthritis, sleep apnea and other respiratory disorders, and cancers of the endometrium, breast, and colon.[23] The incidence of obesity doubled between 1991 and 1998, and overweight in young people has tripled since 1980.

The primary cause of obesity is a diet high in fats and refined carbohydrates. As such diets become more prevalent in any country, the rate of obesity soars. Witness Japan, China and the countries already mentioned above. They are becoming "westernized" and western rates of obesity are following.

In the USA consider the Pima Indians of Arizona. There was no obesity (and no diabetes) reported among them until about 1920. They were lean and healthy and were known as great distance runners. *During the First World War, many of their young men were inducted into or joined the armed services and returned with a taste for fatty, sugary, nutrient-depleted foods. Today, nearly all adult Pimas are obese, and half of them are type-2 diabetics by the time they are 35!*[24-26] The same happened to the natives of Nauru in Micronesia. When they became wealthy and adopted a Western style of eating, obesity and diabetes skyrocketed.[27] These two ethnic groups are examples of the havoc wrought by the high-fat, low-fiber, high-refined-carbohydrate (flour and sugar) and high-dairy diets that much of the world now consumes. The Pimas' native foods—corn, lima beans, white and yellow teparies, mesquite, and acorns—have very low glycemic responses;[28] since they contain unrefined, complex *carbohydrates*. More recent research shows that the Pima Indians who choose an "Anglo" diet full of fat and refined carbohydrates have 2 ½ times the risk of diabetes as those who choose a somewhat more traditional diet.[29] Of course, diabetes

162

increases nearly in lockstep with obesity.[30] Marked changes are observed when Native Americans who are accustomed to a traditional diet switch to typical American high-fat, high-protein fare. In just five weeks, body weight increases by 7%, and total cholesterol levels increase by 31%, with much of that increase occurring in dangerous LDL cholesterol.[31]

Some contend that obesity has increased while the fat content of the USA diet has decreased; this is *absolutely incorrect*. Both fat and refined carbohydrates have increased. It is just that the ***percentage*** of fat has decreased while the ***total fat*** has increased. It is easy to lower the percentage of fat in the diet without removing any of the fat at all. Let's take the example of a milkshake with 17 grams of fat equaling approximately 150 calories. The entire shake, including the sugar and protein it contains, has about 300 calories. Fifty percent of the calories therefore come from fat. To lower the percentage of fat in the shake, one needs only add three hundred more calories from sugar. Now there are 600 calories in the shake, and 150 fat calories remain. This means that because the fat percentage is now only 25%, it can be labeled a "low-fat" product, without any change in fat content.

Claiming that the "low-fat, high-carb" experiment has been a failure, the high-protein diet hucksters have thrown all carbohydrates into the same category and called them poisons—a mistake that is costing millions of lives by removing fruits and whole grains from the diets of people who succumb to such nutritional propaganda. ***Controlled studies have shown unequivocally that a low-fat, high-unrefined-carbohydrate diet can reverse heart disease and bring about weight loss.***[32] In our health resort, we estimated 110 tons of fat was lost among our guests over twenty years. Our diet was high in unrefined grains and very low in fat. Don't be fooled by high-protein, high-fat nonsense. Sunbathing and vitamin D supplements alone can never reverse the obesity of those who are unwilling to change their eating habits and become active. Nevertheless, sunlight and/or vitamin D may act as adjuncts to weight control.

Vitamin D levels are much lower in obese people,[33-34,145] and ***Norwegian study subjects in the lowest quartile (fourth) of vitamin D consumption had 2.24 times the rate of obesity as those in the highest quartile.***[35] Calcium intake also related to ***greater*** BMI, probably because most calcium consumed came from dairy products, which are extremely high in both fat and sugar. This surprised the researchers, because some studies show that calcium decreases obesity.[35]

Vitamin D may work with calcium to stimulate metabolism in fat cells and thereby reduce obesity.[37,144] A high intake of vitamin D and calcium at breakfast causes a spontaneous and dramatic suppression of appetite and food intake in the following 24-hours.[38] An investigation showed that a high-calcium, high-vitamin D meal increased the burning of calories. However, these last two studies were funded by the Australian Dairy Council.

Women living at 11,000 ft. in Cuzco, Peru are slimmer than women in Lima, near sea level.[39] Their diets are similar, so the high UVB concentration at Cuzco may stimulate more vitamin D production and reduce obesity.

In chapter 13 we noted that heart disease is also lower at higher altitudes, and established that vitamin D and sunlight have positive influences on lessening vascular diseases. As with heart disease, obesity is more prevalent in subjects living further from the equator (where UVB is less available).[40] *As Dr. John Cannell points out, in cultures where women stay covered with clothing and obtain little sunlight, rates of obesity do not vary with altitude,*[41] a strong indication that sunlight exposure and the increase in vitamin D levels are factors in preventing obesity.

Twenty-four hours after exposure to UVB or taking heavy oral doses of vitamin D, obese subjects have only 57% of the rise in serum vitamin D levels as those who were not obese. Vitamin D is stored in fat, and it is likely that the higher the body fat, the less vitamin D is available to be released into the blood.[42-43] *For example, 55% of obese children have vitamin D levels below 20 ng/ml, and 21% have levels below 10.*[93]

Finally, lab experiments show that activated vitamin D inhibits adipogenesis—the production of fat or fat cells.[160, 161] So does vitamin D help control weight? The answer is "probably." Meanwhile, the best advice is to get a reasonable amount of sunlight and vitamin D and eat a low-fat, high fiber diet replete with whole grains and colorful vegetables and fruit. I have had an excellent career helping people lose weight and overcome many maladies by getting lots of sun and optimizing their nutrition. I have seen the results repeatedly and know that it works!

Vitamin D and kidney disease

Vitamin D levels are exceptionally low in adults and children with chronic kidney disease,[126,165] and patients given vitamin D reduce the chance of death by 26%.[164] Whether vitamin D deficiency causes kidney disease, or whether it is a product of kidney disease is not known. Still, it is only common sense to assure that kidney disease sufferers maintain appropriate vitamin D levels, since death rate is reduced.

Vitamin D and Psoriasis

Psoriasis is a skin disease in which cells proliferate rapidly, causing patches of scaly, itching skin. The National Psoriasis Foundation recommends brief, frequent exposures of sunlight as a therapy and report that 80% of those who do it improve or totally clear psoriasis.[44] One of the main commercial therapies is the oral medicine Psoralen, which is taken in combination with sunlight or UV lamp exposure because Psoralen increases the skin's sensitivity to UV. In 1979 in Tucson, Arizona, twelve psoriasis sufferers were given Psoralen and exposed to the abundant sunlight of the southwest. Nine of the twelve experienced significant improvement in the first month, and after three to five months of treatment, all patients experienced complete remission of lesions.[45] The downside of Psoralen is that it is a potent chemical and may produce skin cancer. ***Regular exposure to UVA and Psoralen has been shown to correlate to 83 times the normal incidence of squamous cell carcinoma!***[87] Perhaps the cure is worse than the disease. Other research demonstrates that home UVB lamps are a highly cost-effective method to control psoriasis.[46]

Vitamin D is also used effectively in the treatment of psoriasis. Dr. Michael Holick uses an ointment with activated D—Calcipotriene—which he formulated, and which is 80-90% effective in controlling psoriasis.[47]

Dietary factors may also have a beneficial influence on psoriasis. I once observed the complete disappearance of terrible skin lesions in one of our health resort's massage therapists within two weeks of a dietary change. ***She had been to a dermatologist, a general practitioner and finally to an OBGYN, who she said recommended a complete hysterectomy because he felt her problem might be hormonal.*** She had tried various creams and cortisone, all without any effect. I invited her to try a pure vegetarian nutrition program for two weeks, suspecting that her psoriasis was caused by an allergy to milk, meat or other animal-based foods. She followed the suggestion and her lesions disappeared. A combination of good nutrition and sunlight is probably the best therapy for psoriasis.

Vitamin D and Eczema

Eczema is a skin disorder that occurs primarily in younger people, is characterized by redness and itching, and may produce lesions that discharge pus and become scaly and crusty. Eczema is dramatically improved by UVB treatment[48] and without the use of steroids,[49] which are often recommended for the condition.

Sunlight, vitamin D, sexual performance and fertility

Can sunlight make a difference in sexual behavior or fertility? That is a difficult question to answer with certainty, but there are indications that sunlight exposure and/or vitamin D intake do influence hormones and sexual behavior. Now that I have your undivided attention, let's take a look at the evidence.

In 1939, Dr. Abraham Myerson measured initial levels of circulating testosterone in men and exposed their various body parts to UV.[50] *After five days of chest exposure sufficient to cause reddening, circulating testosterone increased by 120%. After eight days without additional UV exposure, testosterone returned to initial levels. When the genital area was exposed, testosterone levels increased by 200%!* Considering our sex-obsessed society, it is surprising that no studies followed up on Myerson's work.

Other experiments show that rats maintained on vitamin D-deficient diets produce fewer sperm,[51] but sperm production increases when vitamin D is again provided. Vitamin D restores fertility to deficient rats and proper testicular function in deficient chickens.[52] *Female rats mated to deficient males also have 73% fewer successful pregnancies than those mated to vitamin D-sufficient males.*[53] The ovaries and testes of rats that lack vitamin D receptors (VDR) do not function fully and properly,[129] and vitamin D deficiency profoundly reduces sperm production.[130] However, that condition is reversible when vitamin D is restored to optimal levels,[131] which is important since human sperm also contains VDR.[125] Also, most women who are infertile due to polycystic ovary disease, resulting in loss of menstrual cycles, experience restored menstruation and can become pregnant when vitamin D levels are increased.[85]

If vitamin D increases fertility, conception rates should be higher in summer than in winter. In higher latitude countries, where UVB availability varies dramatically during the year, conception rates are indeed at their highest in late summer and birth rates are highest the following spring.[54]

Vitamin D levels are exceptionally low in people with chronic kidney disease,[126] and sufferers generally experience sexual problems,[127,128] including erectile dysfunction in men, decreased libido and fertility in both sexes, and menstrual abnormalities in women. Whether vitamin D is responsible or simply a result of kidney disease is not known.

Considering this information, it might seem that vitamin D deficiency would be an effective method of birth control if one were willing to accept an increased risk of depression, cancer, heart disease, MS, diabetes and osteoporosis! And here is one more point that is somewhat related. Women who consume the largest quantities of vitamin D and calcium have fewer symptoms of PMS.[84]

Sunlight and insomnia

Many elderly individuals have difficulty sleeping long and soundly enough to feel refreshed. A study by Dr. Julie Gammack exposed test subjects to thirty to sixty minutes per day of direct sunlight, [55] and according to the Saint Louis University health web site, "Nursing home patients who were exposed to natural light had improved sleep quality. They had less difficulty falling asleep, fewer episodes of wakefulness during the night and greater satisfaction with the amount of sleep they got." Chalk up another victory for Solar Power!

Vitamin D and hearing loss

Some studies indicated that vitamin D deficiency could contribute to hearing loss in the elderly. Lack of vitamin D reduces microcirculation to the cochlea and impairs calcium metabolism, which may lead to hearing impairment.[82,83] Mice with abnormal vitamin D-receptor genes suffer significant hearing loss, which lends support to the theory.[159]

Low vitamin D intake relates to age-related macular degeneration (AMD)

AMD usually is a gradual loss of central vision due to progressive deterioration of the retina, ultimately resulting in blindness. There is an inverse relationship between AMD and vitamin D intake.[121] Regular fish consumption correlates to a 59% reduced risk, and past vitamin D supplementation correlates to a 33% reduction. Fish and conventional supplements contain little vitamin D. Perhaps 2,000 IU or more per day would more impressively retard macular degeneration.

Sunlight exposure may decrease the risk of myopia (near-sightedness)

Australian researchers demonstrate that myopia in children is directly linked to the number of hours spent indoors, and in Asian societies where children have been decreasing their outdoor activity, the rate of myopia has more than tripled.[122] *Asian children living in Australia spend nearly four times more time outdoors as children of the same genetic background living in Singapore, and those in Singapore are 10 times more likely to be myopic*. The researchers theorize that the difference lies in the production of dopamine by sunlight exposure. Dopamine retards excessive eyeball growth, a condition that leads to myopia.[122] Who is really the most myopic—the youngsters or a medical establishment that promotes the sun-avoidance policies that wreak havoc on both children and adults?

Vitamin D may inhibit parasite growth.

A study of the growth of intracellular parasites shows that calcitriol inhibits parasite growth both in experimental animals and in the lab.[105] Whether that could be replicated in humans is not known. Remember that calcitriol (1,25(OH)D) can be produced in the body only when levels of 25(OH)D are adequate.

Vitamin D and pre-eclampsia

Pre-eclampsia is a disorder in pregnant women that is characterized by edema (fluid accumulation), high blood pressure and excessive urine protein. Pre-eclampsia can progress to eclampsia, which can cause convulsions, coma and death. An investigation found a dose-response relationship—the lower the D levels, the higher the risk of pre-eclampsia.[106] With a decline of 20 ng/ml, there was a doubling of the risk. Additionally, newborn children of women at risk for pre-eclampsia were twice as likely as other children to be vitamin D-deficient. This is important, because vitamin D-deficient newborns are likely to develop rickets and suffer from convulsions.[108]

Sunlight exposure and anaphylaxis

Anaphylaxis, or anaphylactic shock, is an extreme allergic reaction to a protein to which a person has been previously exposed. It is characterized by a profound drop in blood pressure, severe itching and hives, and breathing difficulties. Untreated, it can be lethal. A common cause is bee sting, although many drugs and foods trigger reactions in individuals. When geographical location in the USA is compared to the number of prescriptions for the anti-anaphylaxis drug EpiPen, a strong north-south gradient is apparent, with the highest rates in Massachusetts and the lowest in Hawaii. [107] People living in southern states have about 25-30% of the risk of those living in the New England.

Vitamin D deficiency and epilepsy

There is a much higher rate of vitamin D deficiency in epileptics, but whether there is a cause-effect relationship has not been shown.[109] It would certainly be wise for epileptics, like all others, to maintain high levels of Vitamin D.

Vitamin D and anemia

Anemia is a disorder caused by a reduction of the oxygen-carrying capacity of the blood. It causes pallor, weakness, and breathlessness and fatigue. It has been shown that each 10 ng/mL increase in serum levels of 25 (OH) D is associated with a 29% reduced risk of anemia, whereas each increase of 10 mg/dl of c-reactive protein (CRP) were associated with dramatically increased risk.[167] In chapter 13, we discussed the profound association of vitamin D to lowered levels of CRP, which is an inflammatory chemical that is a strong promoter of heart disease. Vitamin D's ability to control CRP may be the reason for the astounding, positive influence of vitamin D on anemia.

Solar Power, vitamin D and the immune system

We described in chapters 12-13 the beneficial effects of vitamin D for combating inflammatory diseases. Vitamin D also boosts the immune system and enhances the body's ability to kill bacteria or viruses— intercellular invaders—that make their way into body cells. When a mechanism known as a toll-like receptor (TLR) recognizes the invaders, it causes direct antimicrobial (anti-germ) activity by stimulating the action of peptide proteins that bind to and kill viruses (including the AIDS virus— HIV) bacteria and fungi.[73-77,146] The peptides are called cathelicidins, and the human cathelicidin is known as LL-37. The TLR's also activate LL-37 after it is produced.[120] Cathelicidins break down cell walls of viruses and bacteria[78] and may also destroy viruses without cell walls.[120] The gene that turns on cathelicidin is a direct target of vitamin D Receptors (VDR) and is strongly activated by calcitriol. Therefore, Vitamin D triggers LL-37 against all of these "invaders."[79] It also stimulates antimicrobial activity in white blood cells, skin cells and others.[80]

African Americans have lower resistance to tuberculosis, lower levels of vitamin D and reduced ability to stimulate the production and action of cathelicidins, *but when vitamin D is added to the serum of African Americans, there is a dramatically increased production of cathelicidins.*[78]

At the very least, African-American adults should be taking 3,000-5,000 IU of vitamin D every day. Cathelicidins are known to have anti-microbial activity against other bacteria, viruses, fungi and parasites, and also act against leukemia and colon cancer cells.[79]

Vitamin D, sunlight and septicemia

Much of this information comes from two excellent papers, one by Dr. William Grant,[111] unpublished at the time of this writing, and one by Dr. N Mookherjee and colleagues,[112] published in *Expert Opinions on Therapeutic Targets*.

Septicemia is a severe and often deadly blood infection and is a form of sepsis, defined as an infection of tissues by bacteria. Noxious bacteria do damage by attacking tissue or blood, but when they die or when their cell walls rupture, they release a poison (endotoxin), which may do more harm than the bacterial attack itself.

Sepsis accounts for 500,000 emergency-room hospital visits per year in the USA, and the typical stay is nearly five hours.[113] It is one of the most deadly of medical conditions[113] and often results in multiple organ failure and death.[112] There are about 750,000 cases per year, and about 3% of all hospital admissions result in a case of sepsis.[112] Hospitals are not sterile environments, and it is wise to avoid them except in the most dire need!

Sepsis is now one of the top-ten causes of death in the USA and the second leading cause of hospital-associated deaths outside of coronary intensive care units. In North America sepsis and its related disorders kill more people than heart attacks, colon cancer, breast cancer or AIDS. The annual cost for care is about $17 billion, and in the case of severe sepsis, antibiotics have not improved survival. In fact, antibiotics may produce molecules that exacerbate it.[112]

Dr. Grant points out that septicemia incidence is highest in the winter and lowest in the autumn, that rates are also generally highest in the Northeast and lowest in the Southwest, [114] and that African Americans have 1.7 to 4.3 times higher incidence rates than do whites.[115] There is also a rapid increase in risk with age, and several other chronic and infectious diseases are closely associated with that increase.[111] It should be obvious by now that all of these factors indicate vitamin D deficiency; therefore, such a deficiency could play a strong causal role in septicemia, especially since deficiency inhibits the production of cathelicidins, which not only break down the cell walls of noxious germs, but also help to reduce the endotoxins resulting from the breakdown.[117-119]

170

In Australia, melanoma rates have skyrocketed since 1980 when the anti-sun campaign began in earnest in Australia.[116] Sepsis rates jumped simultaneously and coincided with the widespread use of sunscreens.[111] The same is true for viral respiratory infections (see the next section), most cancers, and congestive heart failure,[111] and we have documented throughout this book that several other diseases follow similar patterns. Dr. Grant concludes by stating that the incidence and prevalence features of sepsis are similar to the epidemiological features of vitamin D deficiency based on summertime solar UVB. Certainly, there is no downside to educating the public of the need to keep levels of vitamin D high, as it affords significant protection against this emerging killer.

The influence of sunlight and vitamin D on flu and colds

Some time ago I was addressing a group on the cancer-preventive influences of sunlight and vitamin D, and I mentioned that my wife Vicki and I used a tanning bed during winter. An audience member reported back to me later—with delight—that he had used a tanning bed regularly during the winter and did not experience a cold or flu—extraordinary for him. I was not surprised. Dr. John Cannell and colleagues wrote a remarkable paper[90] showing that cold and flu outbreaks are almost completely seasonal. In the northern hemisphere, they occur in December through March. In the southern hemisphere, outbreaks occur June through September—almost exclusively in winter in both hemispheres. ***The outbreaks in each case occur in times of lowest UVB light and least vitamin D production.*** The paper goes on to explain how Vitamin D stimulates production of cathelicidin, which destroys the cell walls of noxious viruses, including flu viruses. So, when UVB is plentiful, more vitamin D increases the production of cathelicidin.

Shortly after this paper's publication, other researchers, acting on Dr. Cannell's lead, reported results of a three-year study of African-American women.[91] One group was given a placebo and another group received 800 IU per day for two years and 2,000 IU during the third year. The placebo group experienced three times as many cold and flu cases as those who received 800 IU. **The 2,000-IU group had only one cold or flu case the entire year, and none in winter. The placebo group had 24 cases in winter—that is a 24:0 ratio!** So was it just a coincidence that my acquaintance who used the tanning bed stayed unusually free from colds and flu? Here is a graphic representation of the research, formed from data of the study.

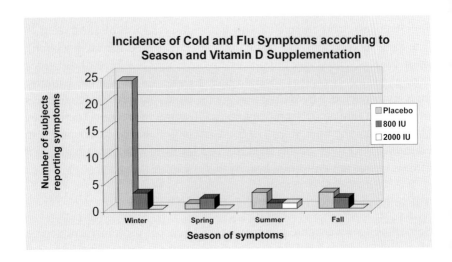

Incidence of Cold and Flu Symptoms according to Season and Vitamin D Supplementation

Number of subjects reporting symptoms

Legend: Placebo, 800 IU, 2000 IU

Season of symptoms: Winter, Spring, Summer, Fall

These findings are especially important because flu shots are not very effective. A review in the *British Medical Journal* came to the following conclusion: *"Evidence from systematic reviews shows that inactivated vaccines [flu shots] have little or no affect on the effects measured."*[101] The review continues, "Reasons for the current gap between policy and evidence are unclear, but given the huge resources involved, a re-evaluation should be urgently undertaken." Some of these flu vaccines also contain mercury, which is highly toxic.[102] A USA evaluation of the influence of vaccination on death from flu stated, "We could not correlate increasing vaccination coverage after 1980 with declining mortality rates in any age group."[103] This was despite the fact that flu shot coverage among the elderly (those most likely to die from flu) increased from 15% to 65% after 1980. [104]

Perhaps flu shots do save some lives, but there is little doubt that vitamin D would do a much better job. *Considering that daily supplementation with 2,000 IU per day of vitamin D can cost as little as $10.00 per year, a tremendous financial burden could be lifted from the health-care system and from the budget of elderly persons!*

Approximately 36,000 people die yearly from flu in the USA, and it is estimated that a pandemic similar to the one in 1918 could kill 1,000,000 or more. The solution: maintain optimal vitamin D levels. This can be done during winter by tanning-bed exposure or with D3 supplementation of at least 2,000 IU per day in the absence of UVB exposure.

Season and pneumonia

Like so many other diseases we have discussed, pneumonia is seasonal, with the lowest rates in summer, an increase in fall and a peak in winter.[171] This indicates that vitamin D may play a part in preventing this serious disease.

Season and "flesh-eating bacteria"

The real name for flesh-eating bacteria is necrotizing fasciitis. It is caused by a type of strep bacteria that is extremely virulent and causes quick infection and death of the tissue it attacks; it does not, however "eat flesh." Necrotizing fasciitis is seasonal, like so many to the diseases we have written about in this book, with the highest incidence in winter.[172] It is likely that sunlight-stimulated vitamin D produces the cathelicidins necessary to keep the disease at bay during the summer.

Season and Low birth weight

Low birth weight is associated with mood, anxiety, depression, high blood pressure and other problems during childhood and afterward. Recent research shows that vitamin D is related to exposure by pregnant women to winter temperatures during a critical developmental time for the fetus.[174,175] This could indicate vitamin D deficiency of the pregnant mother during "vitamin D winter."

Acute lower respiratory infections (ALRI) in newborns and vitamin D deficiency in mother and child

Newborns with ALRI have serum levels of vitamin D that are 79% lower than those of non-infected newborns, and their mothers have levels 70% lower than those of the mothers of non-infected newborns.[153] Among older children who have abnormal VDR, the risk of ALRI was seven times higher than among those whose with normal sites,[158] and children under five were profoundly more likely to suffer ALRI if they had low levels of vitamin D.[154] *Interestingly, children who were placed outside in the sunlight uncovered were less than half as likely to suffer ALRI, and those who had the lowest levels of vitamin D were ten times more likely to contract this terrible infection than those with the highest.*[154] Considering that cathelicidins are present in the lungs and provide the first line of defense against invading organisms,[155] this is not surprising. We have discussed how vitamin D triggers the production of cathelicidins.

Can vitamin D help HIV infected patients?

The answer is not yet definite. However, considering that vitamin D stimulates the production of cathelicidins, it seems reasonable that increasing Vitamin D levels could help HIV infected people. We do know that 82% of HIV infected patients are deficient,[124] and their risk of osteoporosis—another indication of deficiency—is exceptionally high. Giving those with HIV/AIDS vitamin D supplements may also help keep at bay other associated infections.

More on tuberculosis (TB), sunlight and vitamin D

In the early part of the 20th Century, sunlight exposure was used effectively to help TB patients recover (see chapter 1), and sun lamps were used to "cure" a form of TB that was considered incurable. Recently, the interest in Vitamin D to thwart TB is being revisited.[135, 136, 162] Black immigrants to Australia have low vitamin D levels and a much higher risk of TB.[140] Moreover, the effectiveness of vitamin D was demonstrated against the TB bacteria in an experiment in which a single dose of vitamin D (100,000 IU) significantly increased immunity to the TB bacterium.[137] The effectiveness of vitamin D against TB is determined by the production of cathelicidin.[138] Further corroborating vitamin D's essential role is that people who lack vitamin D receptors (VDR) are three times more likely to contract TB as those with normal VDR.[139] Vitamin D also inhibits the body's inflammatory response to TB infection in the lungs.[141,142]

Vitamin D and bacterial meningitis

There is little or no research on the direct affect of sunlight or vitamin D on meningitis, which is an often fatal disease characterized by inflammation of the membranes that cover the brain and spinal cord. However, the disease usually occurs in winter or spring[170], which may be indicative of low vitamin D levels that occur in those seasons.

Sunlight and vitamin D indirectly prevent other diseases by preventing viral infections.

We have discussed at length the ability of vitamin D to destroy viruses and bacteria by stimulating the production of the human cathelicidin, LL-37. Dr. Grant recently wrote a paper linking viral infections to vitamin D deficiency diseases.[147] We have thus far shown the *direct* link between vitamin D and disease risk; Dr. Grant makes the case that D's ability to destroy viruses has a dramatic, positive *indirect* effect in preventing diseases such as cancer, asthma, MS, diabetes and others. Here are some examples from his paper:

1. **The Epstein-Barr virus, in many cases, is associated with the development of multiple sclerosis (MS).[148,149] Therefore, at least part of the reduction of MS risk by vitamin D may be due to the cathelicidins produced in response to vitamin D stimulation. If cathelicidins reduce the Epstein Barr virus, then indirectly vitamin D reduces the risk of MS.**

2. **Similarly, the risk for type-1 diabetes is 4.29 times greater in children who have had viral diseases,[150] and *vitamin D supplements given during lactation reduce the risk by 70%.***

3. **Asthma is also associated with viral infections, which appear to increase risk and exacerbate the disease.[151,152] Vitamin D protects against the asthma development. In part, this may be due to a vitamin D-produced increase in immunity against viruses.**

4. **Viral infections also contribute to the risk for these major cancers: prostate, cervical, Hodgkin's lymphoma, nasopharyngeal, oral, and non-Hodgkin's lymphoma.[147]**

Dr. Grant's findings strongly suggest that through production of LL-37, the risk of many autoimmune diseases and several cancers are reduced. Therefore, maintaining optimal vitamin D levels is critical.

Does Sunlight and vitamin D prevent leprosy?

Leprosy is considered to be a disease that has been eradicated, but in India it still exists. An article in an Indian paper shows that it is much more prevalent in highly urbanized areas that in rural or less polluted areas.[163] From what we have just learned, that should be no surprise.

Other benefits of vitamin D and sunlight

Metabolic syndrome (Met S) and vitamin D

A telling study regarding the relationship of vitamin D to Met S reveals that low vitamin D levels are common in people with the disorder.[92] Met S is a cluster of physiological measurements such as hypertension, abdominal obesity, high triglycerides, low HDL ("good cholesterol") levels, high blood-sugar and insulin resistance, all of which are linked to increased risk of cardiovascular disease and type-2 diabetes. Twenty-five percent of the USA population suffers from Met S. Obviously, people with Met S are at greater risk of degenerative disease and early death.

Could regular doses of vitamin D or summer sun exposure lessen the risk? That is highly likely. Dr. Jose Botella-Carretero, one of the authors of the research just cited,[92] made this statement: *"Our results may be of special interest, given that our patients with and without vitamin D deficiency had similar BMI [body mass index] and waist circumference, so the differences in metabolic syndrome prevalence and lipid levels may indeed reflect a true association between vitamin D status and the metabolic syndrome, irrespective of adiposity."* In other words, low blood levels of vitamin D predicted a higher risk of metabolic syndrome regardless of the degree of obesity.

Sunlight, vitamin D and asthma

The dramatic increase in childhood asthma has paralleled our culture's decline in sunlight exposure, according to Harvard researchers, and they show that the risk is 40% lower in children of women who have the highest vitamin D consumption during pregnancy.[97] Another study shows a more impressive reduction of 52-67%.[100] The researchers believe that inadequate vitamin D levels in the fetus leads to improper development of the lungs and immune system. *Three-year old children whose mothers were in the highest quartile of vitamin D consumption during pregnancy have a 61% reduced risk of a "recurrent wheeze," a symptom of asthma, when compared to those whose mothers were in the lowest quartile.*[97] Each 100-IU increase in vitamin D consumption resulted in a 19% risk reduction. How sad that an inexpensive supplement is not universally recommended for pregnant women who stay indoors.

In another study, asthmatic mice were exposed to ultraviolet light before also being exposed to a common allergen that provokes an asthma attack.[98] Dr. Prue Hart of Australia noted reduced asthma symptoms. Considering the $700 million in yearly costs to treat asthma in Australia alone, a bit of regular sunlight exposure seems a small price to pay.

Asthma is often treated with steroids, but in some individuals, asthma is highly resistant to them. However, when vitamin D3 is added to the steroid treatment, symptoms are greatly reduced.[99] Perhaps sufficient vitamin D supplementation or exposure to UVB light could eliminate the need for any steroids, whose nasty side effects include osteoporosis.

Vitamin D and cystic fibrosis

Cystic fibrosis is a pulmonary disease characterized by excessively viscous (sticky) mucous in the lungs that leads to respiratory infections and impaired pancreatic function. It is considered hereditary, but nearly all sufferers regardless of age, have low levels of vitamin D even when they take supplements.[134,135] Their level of supplementation may not be adequate to raise serum vitamin D to optimal levels, and it is possible that the disease itself suppresses those levels. Physicians would do well to advise higher levels of supplementation and moderate sunbathing in the warm seasons.

Vitamin D and migraines

There is little research on the alleviation of migraines using vitamin D therapy, but Mount Sinai Hospital in New York reports that in two individuals who suffered excruciating headaches, "therapeutic replacement with vitamin D and calcium resulted in a dramatic reduction in the frequency and duration of their migraine headaches."[143] I observed the same in guests who attended our health resort, where sunlight abounded and good nutrition was the rule. Anecdotally, I have heard from people who reduce the frequency and intensity of migraines by using tanning beds.

Sunlight as an antiseptic and antibiotic

In the history section, we mentioned that German microbiologist Robert Koch (who isolated TB bacteria in 1882) showed that sunlight could kill the bacteria. However, even earlier, in 1877, other researchers discovered that sugar water left in the shade became cloudy, indicative of bacterial growth, but if exposed to sunlight, it remained clear.[56]

Sunlight is a potent bactericide. Dr. Zane Kime, in his 1980 book, *Sunlight could Save Your Life*, reviewed the results of research conducted between 1886 and 1909 that showed that all these bacteria were killed by ultraviolet light: anthrax, plague, streptococci, tubercle bacillus, cholera, staphylococcus, colon bacillus and dysentery bacillus. Sunlight was virtually forgotten with the advent of antibiotic drugs, but now the interest has returned. While watching a newscast, I noticed the news ticker along the bottom of the screen announcing, "sunshine is the most effective anti-infection therapy." But is this really news? Dr. Kime cites several early studies on sunlight and infectious diseases that were performed about the same time as the advent of antibiotics. Reports in the scientific literature in the 1940s showed that sunlight killed infectious bacteria or viruses. Kime states …"a number of patients, having such various infections and diseases as blood poisoning, childbirth infections, peritonitis, viral pneumonia, mumps, and bronchial asthma were treated with ultraviolet light therapy to their blood."[57-65] They were, in fact, treated highly successfully.

Dr. Kime also cited research showing that UV therapy killed the flu virus outside the body[66] and destroyed cancer-producing viruses.[67] He reported good results in his own practice in treating fungal infections with sunlight therapy.

Other early research showed that all bacteria within eight feet of low-intensity UV lights were killed in ten minutes.[68]

While visiting in Mexico, a friend invited me to tour a bottled-water plant in a town called Juchipila. It was interesting that the water was exposed to UV as a means of purification. It must work, because I drank it during my visit without ill effects. Sunlight also kills E. coli bacteria in twelve feet of seawater and in waste stabilization ponds.[69-70] I also find it interesting that the Sonicare electric-toothbrush company now sells a sanitizer based on UV. The brush, after use, is placed in the UV sanitizer, and the company claims that it kills millions of germs in 10 minutes.

Nursing pioneer Florence Nightingale insisted that hospitals for wounded troops be constructed for the free entry of light. How many hospitals today follow her brilliant advice? Nosocomial infections (those acquired in a hospital) occur two million times a year and claim the lives of 90,000.[71] Hospital construction returned to the "dark ages" after the advent of antibiotic drugs. *Meanwhile, the solution to most nosocomial infections is right outside the building, and no one will let it in!* At the very least, hospital rooms should be cleansed daily with UV with sufficient strength to kill the surrounding bacteria. Even a hospital's profits would improve; they are businesses, after all. The University of Pennsylvania Center for Health Transformation states, "Nosocomial infections create terrific problems by prolonging hospital stays, occupying scarce bed-days, requiring a greater number of diagnoses, more medication, and a greater burden on doctors and nurses."[72] They estimate, *"If a 300-bed hospital with 10,000 admissions yearly had a 5 percent annual infection rate (500 infections) with costs of $600 to $50,000 depending on the type of infection, the total costs for these infections could be as high as $7.6* *million."*[81] Multiply that by the number of hospitals. Imagine the savings if they let the light in! The patients in such rooms would also be happier and more positive.

Many infectious bacteria are now resistant to antibiotics. Given this reality, it makes sense to return to a sanitation method used successfully for millennia. The antibiotic drug revolution destroyed the promising use of UV and sunlight as an antiseptic, pro-immunity treatment. With the increasing failure of antibiotics, it is time that the interest in UV is renewed. *We have become so obsessed in our pursuit of new antibiotics that we walk in darkness and cannot see the brilliant source of healing right outside the window*.

Vitamin D and longevity

Do those who use vitamin D supplements or receive large quantities from sunlight live longer than those who don't? Research reported in 2007 predicted an increased lifespan of about two years for those who had taken supplements for 5.7 years,[94] and the average supplement was only 528 IU daily. What might 2,000 IU or more per day do? Another study assessed vitamin D levels in colorectal cancer patients and compared them to the risk of patient death over eleven-years. [168] *Those with the highest levels of vitamin D had a 48% reduced risk of dying compared to those with the lowest levels. A similar scientific investigation showed that among those with heart disease, death from any cause over seven years was doubled among those whose vitamin D levels were lowest compared to those whose levels were highest.*[169]

Another investigation showed that vitamin D reduces a major predictor of aging.[95] The sections of DNA found at the ends of chromosomes are known as telomeres, and the shortening of telomeres is considered an indicator of the aging process—the faster the shortening, the faster the aging. The study found that higher D concentrations correlate to longer telomeres and a reduced aging process. Interestingly, osteoporosis, another vitamin D-deficiency disease, also correlates closely to shortened telomeres.[96]

Considering the above information, especially when added to the striking protective effects of vitamin D in reducing the major degenerative and infectious diseases already discussed, it is not surprising that research conducted in August of 2008 showed that people with vitamin D levels below 17.8 ng/ml had four times the chance of death from any cause compared to those who had levels above 32.1 ng/ml.[175] How much more proof must we have to establish the importance of vitamin D to health and quality of life? Will the government act to educate the people?

Vitamin D and nursing-home admissions

The elderly and their children dread the day when being confined to a nursing home is necessary. We have already seen the influence of vitamin D in building bone and muscle strength, reducing sway, enhancing balance and diminishing the risk of falls and arthritis. In the next chapter, the influence of vitamin D in preventing depression and enhancing cognitive ability will be discussed. If vitamin D produces such benefits, those with high levels have an advantage in delaying or preventing their entry into nursing homes. The research supports that idea. *In one investigation, those whose serum vitamin D levels were in the deficient category had three-and-one-half times the risk of being admitted to a nursing home as those whose levels were in the highest category.*[132] Interestingly, even the subjects with "high" levels had nowhere near the optimal level of 50-60 ng/ml. In an aging population, imagine the burden that might be lifted, and the quality of life that might be gained by maintaining optimal levels.

What have we learned?

1. Vitamin D/sunlight reduces oral inflammation, which helps to prevent periodontal disease.

2. Sunlight exposure correlates to reduced risk of dental cavities.

3. Vitamin D and calcium may lower the rate of tooth loss up to 60%.

4. Low vitamin D levels are correlated closely to obesity.

5. Sunlight/UV has been used effectively for many years as a treatment for psoriasis and eczema.

6. There is evidence that UV exposure dramatically enhances fertility.

7. Sleep disorders are markedly improved by morning exposure to natural sunlight.

8. Sunlight is an effective antibiotic and antiseptic and can kill viruses, fungi and bacteria.

9. It is likely that nosocomial (in hospital) infections could be decreased or eliminated by exposing hospital rooms to sunlight and/or full-spectrum UV.

10. Vitamin D and sunlight are powerful immune system enhancers.

11. Tuberculosis may in part be due to vitamin D insufficiency and lack of sunlight exposure.

12. Observational evidence suggests that UV/vitamin D helps reduce migraine headaches.

13. Vitamin D deficiency in pregnant mothers correlates closely to risk of asthma in their children.

14. HIV infected patients usually have very low levels of vitamin D.

15. Most flu and colds may be eliminated by keeping vitamin D levels high.

16. Vitamin D levels in newborns with acute lower

respiratory infection are 79% lower than in non-infected newborns

17. Septicemia (bacterial blood poisoning) correlates to several indications of low vitamin D levels.

18. Sunlight/vitamin D deficiency may cause macular degeneration and myopia.

19. Fertility may be enhanced, and PMS lessened, by high vitamin D levels.

20. The lower the vitamin D levels, the higher is the risk of pre-eclampsia in pregnant women.

21. There is some evidence that vitamin D deficiency contributes to hearing loss.

22. Activated vitamin D (calcitriol) inhibits the growth of parasites in lab animals.

23. Anaphylaxis is several times more common in northern than southern states, indicating that vitamin D may help to prevent this potentially deadly allergic response.

24. Epileptics have a high rate of vitamin D deficiency.

25. Viral infections are closely correlated to many autoimmune diseases and cancers, and vitamin D may reduce these diseases due to its viricidal properties.

26. Metabolic syndrome is closely correlated to vitamin D deficiency.

27. Vitamin D levels are very low in those with cystic fibrosis.

28. Those who take vitamin D supplements live longer than those who do not.

29. Those with the lowest vitamin D levels have 3.5 times the risk of being in a nursing home as those with the highest levels.

Chapter 15

Solar Power fights depression and other mental disorders.

"Sunshine on my shoulders makes me happy."
John Denver

As a child, I lived for the first day of spring. In the cold, high country of the west desert of Utah and east desert of Nevada where I grew up, the winter temperatures often dropped below zero in the winter. My family spent much of the time indoors in that season, and when we did venture forth to feed cattle and do other farm chores, we were well-bundled in clothing. As I mentioned in the introduction, I was often sick and in general, physically and emotionally miserable from November until April. When spring arrived, my physical and mental health dramatically improved. I did not know then that during winter I suffered from a sunlight deficiency. Today, many suffer as I did from the wintertime blues or "seasonal affective disorder (SAD)"

The names of anti-depression drugs are household words in the USA, and the number of people I meet who use them amazes me. Unfortunately, drugs have side effects, one of which, in certain individuals, is violent behavior. We seldom heard of depression as a common disease a generation ago. Has something fundamental changed in the makeup of the brain since then? Or could it be that we have removed some vital factor in our environments that once was in plentiful supply? Could that factor be sunlight? A well-known therapy for depression is bright light therapy, and full-spectrum lighting systems are advised for lifting moods and increasing a sense of well-being.

The typical child watches more than four hours of TV daily.[1] Is it ill-advised to cover them with sunscreen when they finally do leave the house? These are interesting questions, and before we have the answers, more research needs to be done. Nonetheless, there are indications that lack of sunlight may be responsible for the depression pandemic in our modern world—a world in which we have by more time-saving devices and more "toys" than ever before, and a time in which we have leisure than was imaginable in past eras. So why all the gloom and doom in our golden age of gadgets and ease? Do we spend too much time inside and too little where nature intended us to be?

Solar Power and depression

SAD is characterized by depression, irritability, fatigue and inability to concentrate. It is also known as "winter depression." *The symptoms of SAD can be reduced just as effectively with bright-light therapy as with drugs,[2]* and without the side effects. Light therapy also helps non-seasonal depression, although not to the same extent.[3]

So what does sunlight do to relieve "the blues?" The answer lies in a chemical responsible for transmitting impulses in nerves. This "neurotransmitter," serotonin, is a natural "upper" that works in synchronization with the natural "downer," melatonin. When we awake to sunshine, light enters the eye and stimulates serotonin production; we then quickly become awake and invigorated and melatonin is suppressed. At day's end, however, the bright light disappears (or at least that is how nature intended it), melatonin levels rise, and serotonin levels diminish. We begin to feel sleepy, and ideally go to bed for a good night's rest. It is a perfect system for our needs until we stay up far beyond biologically natural hours by using artificial lighting. Lack of serotonin is believed to cause depression, and current antidepressant drugs keep serotonin at high levels. There is bad news about these drugs, however, and good news about sunlight and its influence on depression.

The Food and Drug Administration (FDA), indicates that antidepressant medications known as selective serotonin re-uptake inhibitors (SSRI's) may increase depression in some cases and lead to suicidal thoughts.[4] Some of the brands involved are Paxil, Lexapro, Prozac, Effexor, Zoloft, Wellbutrin, Luvox, Celexa and Serzone, although the FDA listed 34 drugs. The entire list is at fda.gov/cder/drug/antidepressants/. They state the following: "The Food and Drug Administration asks manufacturers of all antidepressant drugs to include in their labeling a boxed warning and expanded warning statements that alert health care providers to an increased risk of suicidality in children and adolescents being treated with these agents, and additional information about the results of pediatric studies."

The FDA lists several additional warnings and instructions about these drugs for children:

- **Antidepressants increase the risk of suicidal thinking and behavior (suicidality) in children and adolescents with MDD (major depressive disorder) and other psychiatric disorders.**
- **Anyone considering the use of an antidepressant in a child or adolescent for any clinical use must balance the risk of increased suicidality with the clinical need.**

184

- Patients who are started on therapy should be observed closely for clinical worsening, suicidality, or unusual changes in behavior.
- Families should be advised to closely observe the patient and to communicate with the prescriber.

Missing are two important facts: first is that SSRI's increase bone loss.[35] *Women who used SSRI's lost nearly 80% more bone per year than non-users.* Secondly, SSRI's don't work very well![64] *A meta-analysis of data on SSRI's submitted to the FDA indicates that placebos (sugar pills) are as effective as SSRI's in reducing depression;* in other words, only drug companies benefit from SSRI's—not depression sufferers.

And now the good news: serotonin levels relate directly to the availability of sunlight. *A study reported in the Lancet in 2002 found that brain serotonin levels were greater during the summer, and higher on sunny days than cloudy ones—the brighter the sunlight, the greater the production of serotonin. The researchers also found that the number of daily hours of bright sunlight was directly related to the production of serotonin by the brain.*[5] But never stare directly into the sun; indirect sunlight, such as that which enters the eye on a sunny day, is sufficient.

Ultraviolet light emitted by tanning beds also enhances mood *apart* from its ability to increase serotonin.[55] A team of r*esearchers (dermatologists) stated that after six tanning bed sessions, their subjects "felt significantly more balanced, less nervous, more strengthened and more satisfied with their appearance."* The researchers, not surprisingly given the anti-tanning bias that currently reigns among dermatologists, then tried to diminish their own findings by saying that the results may have been due to the slight tan that the volunteers gained, since a measurable difference in serotonin and endorphin levels between the subjects and controls was not detected. If mood improves to a significant degree, why should they care if it is due to a tan or serotonin? The fact is that it worked!

Although the brain produces serotonin in response to sunlight entering the eye, there is another class of "feel-good" hormones produced by the skin in response to sunlight or UVB exposure:[6,27] *Endorphins* elevate mood and produce a sense of wellbeing. Dr. Michael Holick also mentions that dopamine, another "upper," is increased with exposure to ultraviolet light,[6] meaning that stimulating the skin with sunlight works its "magic" beyond the production of vitamin D. Considering all of the mood benefits, one might think people could become addicted to ultraviolet light. That is probably the case and at least it is a positive, beneficial addiction when not overdone.

185

As mentioned in chapter 10, at least three articles in professional journals lamented that tanning beds seem addictive,[7,8,28] and other investigations provided evidence that regular sun tanning is addictive.[9, 63] Provided the user is eating low-fat, non-animal foods, replete with antioxidant-rich vegetables and fruits, I can only say, "Hooray for that addiction!"

Vitamin D and depression

Vitamin D, when administered in late winter, produces a positive effect on mood in only five days.[10] One theory for this is that vitamin D stimulates the brain to produce more serotonin. In a wintertime experiment, serum vitamin D levels doubled in six months through supplementation and dramatically increased their scores on a wellbeing assessment when two groups were given either 1,000 IU or 4,000 IU of vitamin D daily.[11] And although both groups improved, the higher dose produced better results. In another investigation, researchers studied the association between vitamin D levels and the risk of mood disorders in the elderly. The results were impressive. *Those whose vitamin D levels were deficient—defined as less than 20 ng/ml—had 11.7 times the incidence of depression when compared to those whose vitamin D levels were higher. Usually an association is considered meaningful when a measured factor correlates to a 50% increase or decrease. In this case, the correlation between vitamin D deficiency and risk of mood disorders was a staggering 1,169 percent![29]* In addition, the researchers measured cognitive ability (mental capabilities). In two of four tests, those with vitamin D deficiency exhibited cognitive performances that were 5.22 times and 3.22 times poorer than those who were not deficient. The graph illustrates the difference in depression between those with higher or lower levels of vitamin D:

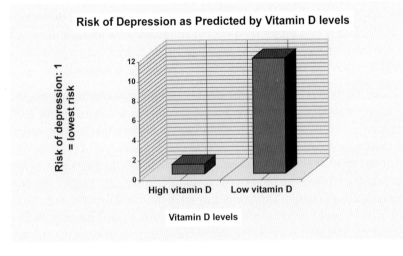

Risk of Depression as Predicted by Vitamin D levels

More on cognitive performance

There are other indications that low levels of vitamin D can lead to "thinking" problems. In chapter 14 we saw that an increased risk of dental diseases correlates to low-vitamin D levels. A recent investigation showed that subjects who had lost the most teeth had more than three-and-and-one-half times the risk of cognitive impairment compared with those who had lost the fewest,[37] an interesting cross-correlation that adds weight to the argument that insufficient vitamin D is a major health crisis. Another study showed that cognitive abilities in people with Alzheimer's disease correlated directly with blood levels of vitamin D, but that levels of vitamins B1, B6 and B12 were not associated with cognitive abilities.[65] Cognitive performance among persons with abnormal vitamin D receptors (VDR) is also dramatically impaired.[38] To think clearly and correctly, proper blood levels of vitamin D are imperative.

Interestingly, children born in the hotter months have an increased risk of learning [69,70] and reading disabilities, including dyslexia.[71] The nervous system's critical time to develop neural connections is in the first months after conception. If the pregnant mother is low in vitamin D during that time, then it could effect the development of the fetus' brain. Conception during fall and winter, when vitamin D levels are low, may predict a greater risk of the birth of a reading-disabled child nine months later. This, of course, is theory, but the idea is intriguing.

Vitamin D and Alzheimer's disease

Vitamin D deficiency is common in Alzheimer's patients,[22] perhaps because they are often hospitalized or house-bound and get little UVB light. *Also, Alzheimer's is 2.8 times more common among those who have the highest quantity of inflammatory cytokines in their blood.*[32] Vitamin D is a potent anti-inflammatory substance,[33] as we have previously discussed,[30,31] so it follows that higher blood levels of vitamin D would reduce the risk of Alzheimer's.

Vitamin D, schizophrenia and influenza

There is a significant association between birth month and schizophrenia in men. In those born in seasons of little sunlight, the rate of schizophrenia is higher. The relationship exists in both the northern and southern hemispheres.[19] Schizophrenia is also more common in dark-skinned migrants to cold climates, and increased rates of schizophrenia is observed in those who are born in urban compared to rural settings.[20] Migrants to colder climates are 4.6 times more likely to develop schizophrenia than are natives.[21] Another observation, brought to my attention by Dr. Grant,[25] cites the possible correlation of influenza during women's pregnancies to increased schizophrenia in their children. Indeed, an investigation conducted in Denmark on the pregnancy histories of women demonstrated *that influenza during pregnancy predicted an 820% increased incidence of schizophrenia in their children.*[59] That result could be at least partially due to brain damage resulting from the high fevers common to flu; it has been shown that there is a very close relationship between fever of the pregnant mother and the risk of later schizophrenia in her children.[67]

But what does this have to do with vitamin D or sunlight? In chapter 14 we established that in summer, when vitamin D production is high, flu is nearly non-existent.[60] Higher vitamin D levels stimulate the production of cathelicidins, which destroy the cell walls of viruses, thereby keeping the flu at bay in summer. It follows that higher levels of vitamin D, by preventing flu, also help reduce the risk of schizophrenia initially provoked during pregnancy. It is possible that vitamin D has a direct affect on the brain that would reduce the risk of schizophrenia and an indirect effect on the brain by reducing the risk of flu. For further dramatic indication that vitamin D is protective against schizophrenia, consider that *infant boys who were not supplemented with vitamin D were 12 times more likely to develop schizophrenia in later life as their cohorts who received supplementation.*[68]

Vitamin D and other disorders of the brain

Other noteworthy research that finds a parallel between insufficient vitamin D and mental disorders:

1. **People born in winter have a greater risk of developing brain tumors both as children[13-14] and as adults[12]**

2. **Prenatal vitamin D deficiency in animals profoundly alters brain development.[15,26] Dr. Darryl Eyles and his colleagues state, "rats born to vitamin D(3)-deficient mothers had profound alterations in the brain at birth. The cortex was longer but not wider, the lateral ventricles were enlarged, the cortex was proportionally thinner and there was more cell proliferation throughout the brain... Our findings would suggest that low maternal vitamin D(3) has important ramifications for the developing brain."[15]**

3. Rats born to vitamin D-deficient mothers also have permanently damaged brains into adulthood[16] and exhibit hyperlocomotion (excessive movement from place to place) at the age of ten weeks.[23] Could this relate to hyperactivity in children? Such rats also show impairment in learning and memory skills.[24]

4. People hospitalized for bipolar disorder and who are exposed to sunlight daily are able to leave the hospital almost four days earlier than those who are not exposed.[17]

5. People hospitalized for SAD have shorter stays when they stay in rooms on the sunny side of the hospital.[18]

6. Anxiety attacks are pandemic in the USA. Two studies of mice with abnormal vitamin D receptors in the brain found an increase in anxiety, aggression, poor grooming, maternal pup neglect and cannibalism.[34,36]

Another vital function of vitamin D is in inducing the production of nerve-growth factor (NGF), a protein that is essential for proper development of nerve cells in the brain and elsewhere.[65]

Is autism a vitamin D-deficiency disorder?

Autism is increasing exponentially and is related to vitamin D deficiency. The Autism Society of America defines autism as "a complex developmental disability that typically appears during the first three years of life and is the result of a neurological disorder that affects the normal functioning of the brain, impacting development in the areas of social interaction and communication skills. Both children and adults with autism typically show difficulties in verbal and non-verbal communication, social interactions, and leisure or play activities."[39]

The cost of autism is about $35 billion annually, and the societal cost for each case is about $3.2 million.[41] The most alarming increase in autism is observed over the past few decades, and its incidence is currently growing at the rate of 10-17% per year.[39] Dr. John Cannell wrote a compelling paper on how autism could be caused, at least in part, by lack of vitamin D during brain development.[40] The rest of this section discusses his primary arguments.

Cannell points out that in 1989, about the time autism began its most rapid increase in incidence, the American Medical Association Council on Scientific Affairs first warned of the perceived dangers of sun exposure and advised keeping infants out of the sun as much as possible.[42] In 1999, when autism risk began to really skyrocket, the American Academy of Pediatrics advised to keep infants out of direct sunlight and to make sure activities minimized sun exposure.[47] In 2002 the Centers for Disease Control reported that the efforts had been quite successful.[47] It is quite possible that the results of all of this "protection" has been an increase in autism. The increase in the incidence of autism has closely paralleled the increase in "sunscare efforts." Both Tourette's syndrome (another nerve disorder) and hyperactivity have also increased with autism.[62] The chart illustrates the frightening autism increase between 1992 and 2003.[48]

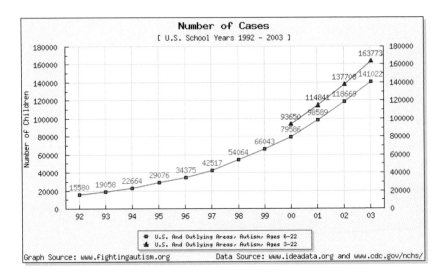

Number of Cases
[U.S. School Years 1992 - 2003]

Graph Source: www.fightingautism.org   Data Source: www.ideadata.org and www.cdc.gov/nchs/

It is obvious that vitamin D is essential for brain development[15,26] and that children are deficient because of sun "protection" measures that lower vitamin D levels. Could this be one of the reasons for the surge in the rate of autism?

Here are more of Dr. Cannell's autism/vitamin D-deficiency links:

1. Both autism and vitamin D deficiency are associated with abnormally high inflammation.[43,44]

2. Low consumption of vitamin D-rich seafood in pregnant women correlates to increased risk of their children's low verbal IQ's, poorer social performance, communication and motor skills.[45]

3. Dark-skinned people are far more likely to be vitamin D deficient because they require more sun exposure to produce it. If the theory is correct, the rate of autism among black children would be higher

than that among white children due to maternal insufficiency and/ or infant insufficiency that would influence brain development. This is exactly the case; children of mothers who have emigrated from Uganda to Sweden, for example, have an autism rate of 15%, which is 200 times that of the general population.[46]

4. There is a close correlation between latitude and autism among countries; the higher the latitude, the higher the rate of autism.[49] High-latitude countries have higher rates of vitamin D deficiency due to a shorter season in which UVB is available to stimulate its production in the skin (see chapter 2). The same relationship of latitude to autism exists within the states of the USA, with northern states having higher rates of autism. [50]

5. In winter, when vitamin D production is low, birth rates of autistic children peak.[51]

6. Rickets and autism show similar urban/rural distribution rates. Rickets is an accepted vitamin D-deficiency disease, and urban children have significantly higher rates of both diseases.[52] Pregnant rural women and their children tend to be outside in the sunshine more their urban counterparts, and in urban settings, more air pollution blocks out UVB light. Poor air quality is directly correlated with autism[53] and with profoundly lower serum levels of vitamin D.[54] For example, the Amish of Pennsylvania—mostly rural farmers—have extremely low rates of autism.[56] *According to Dr. Heng Wang, who treats Amish people in rural Ohio, their rate of autism is 1 in 1,500, compared to 1 in 166 nationally.[57]*

7. Finally, where precipitation rates are high, rates of autism are also high,[56] suggesting a link with sunlight deprivation. Cloudy, rainy weather blocks the UVB light necessary to produce vitamin D.

The theory that autism is a vitamin D-deficiency disorder is reasonable, but until the theory is proven, it would be prudent to assure that pregnant women and young children maintain optimal levels of vitamin D.

What have we learned?

1. Lack of exposure to sunlight may be the primary reason for the increasing incidence of depression in the USA and in other sunlight-deprived countries.

2. A reduction in the symptoms of seasonal affective disorder (SAD) is achieved as effectively with light therapy as with anti-depressant drugs, and without side effects.

3. Antidepressant drugs occasionally cause suicidal thoughts, are expensive, and are a poor substitute for sunlight, exercise and a healthful diet.

4. Serotonin, a natural chemical that makes one feel well, is increased dramatically by sunlight.

5. Vitamin D supplementation or UV exposure may increase feelings of wellbeing by increasing endorphin and dopamine and perhaps other important neurotransmitters.

6. Sunlight is more effective in reducing depression than the commonly used anti-depression drugs.

7. Elderly people with vitamin D levels below 20 ng/ml are almost 12 times as likely to be depressed as those whose levels are above 20.

8. Vitamin D deficiency correlates strongly to poor cognitive performance.

9. Lack of vitamin D in mothers and fetuses may have negative influences on brain development, learning and memory skill. It may also lead to brain tumors.

10. Low vitamin D levels may contribute to Alzheimer's disease, bipolar disorder and anxiety.

11. Vitamin D deficiency increases the risk of flu, and flu increases the risk of schizophrenia.

12. Elderly people who are below 20 ng/ml (50 nmol/L) in blood vitamin D levels have 11.69 times the rate of depression as those who have levels above that value.

13. Autism has increased exponentially as more children avoided the sun and used sunscreens.

Chapter 16
Solar Power and African Americans

There have been several mentions that African Americans suffer a greater degree of degenerative diseases than do Caucasians. But mother nature is not a bigot. When health habits and medical care are the same, disease rates are about equal in the various races; that is, unless another factor is in play. One reason for health differences between blacks and whites in America is that vitamin D deficiency is far more common in blacks—an easily remedied situation.

Here are a few studies that we noted throughout the text:

1. When USA white and black women are compared for vitamin D levels, black women are ten times more likely to be vitamin D deficient.[1]

2. In patients in Minneapolis, Minnesota who were being treated for chronic pain, 100% of African Americans, along with Native Americans, East Africans and Hispanics were vitamin D deficient.[2]

3. Vitamin D is known to be a potent inhibitor of tuberculosis. African Americans have lower resistance to tuberculosis, lower levels of D and lower ability to produce cathelicidin, a natural internal bactericide.[3]

4. A 37-year-old disabled Black woman with myopathy (a muscle disease) was able to leave her wheelchair and function normally after six weeks of vitamin-D therapy.[4]

5. Vitamin D deficiency leads to increased death from the major internal cancers, and a disproportionate number of those cancer deaths occur in African Americans.[5] Dr. William Grant, in summarizing the findings of his study on African Americans and cancer, wrote that "Solar UVB was found significantly inversely correlated with mortality rates for breast, colon, esophageal, gastric and rectal cancers for black Americans."[5] Other research in 2008 corroborated his findings, showing that in the Southeast USA, vitamin D deficiency is about four times more common in African Americans as whites, and suggesting that the greater cancer risks among African Americans is due to that deficiency.[7]

6. Heart disease is twice as prevalent among black men as white men.[6] Although part of the discrepancy may be due to more smoking among black men, it is probable that a significant part is due to vitamin D deficiency. Low sun exposure and low vitamin D levels correlate to increased inflammation, higher cholesterol and hypertension, all risk factors for heart disease. Heart failure is also much more common among blacks—not surprising since we know the efficacy of vitamin D in preventing heart failure.

Now let's discuss what is perhaps the most important study for African Americans. It is often argued that the excessive rates of cancer, diabetes, hypertension, etc. among African Americans are due to lack of access to health care. *If that were the case, black physicians would have approximately the same lower rates of disease as their white counterparts, since black physicians obviously have high access to health care.* However, research shows that even black physicians have a much higher incidence of cancer than their white counterparts.[7] *Nevertheless, black physicians who have habits that provide higher vitamin D levels have approximately the same cancer rates as white physicians.* Had the rates of heart disease, diabetes, hypertension and other diseases also been studied, along with measurements of serum vitamin D levels, I believe the pattern would have been even more clearly established.

Since African Americans have only 50-75% of the serum levels of vitamin D as whites,[5] part—perhaps a large part—of the discrepancy between the health of the races could be rectified by nothing more vitamin D supplementation. That is very good news indeed!

Chapter 17
Tanning beds as health-promoting devices

Sunlight exposure and tanning have been vilified by many (but not all) dermatologists. Tanning beds have been disparaged to an even greater degree and are called "cancer machines" by many in the medical profession and in the popular press. There are movements afoot to make it illegal for those under the age of 18 to even use them. This is woefully misguided and ill-advised. Every beneficial effect of vitamin D that is produced by sunlight exposure is also produced by the use of high-quality tanning beds. What's more, the risks associated with UV overexposure do not appear to be related to regular, non-burning exposure, which tanning beds can provide quite effectively. The following is a list of tanning-bed benefits:

1. Tanning bed use dramatically increases serum-vitamin D levels and bone mass.[1]

2. Whereas a daily 400 IU vitamin D supplement does not maintain healthful levels, tanning bed use increases vitamin D levels by 150% in only seven weeks.[12]

3. Tanning bed use reduces chronic pain.[2]

4. Sun lamps are now being recommended for use by pregnant women who will give birth in a winter month. The recommendation is being made to protect the unborn child from osteoporosis during adulthood.[13]

5. High quality tanning beds, because they provide UVB to both sides of the body simultaneously, stimulate the production of up to 10,000 IU of vitamin D in less than ten minutes. Ten minutes of tanning bed exposure can be done on a lunch break. That means they are more efficient than summer sunlight. Of course, those with darker skin will require a longer time to produce the same amount of vitamin D.

6. It is likely that all benefits of vitamin D can be provided by tanning bed use, including increased resistance to cancer, osteoporosis, heart disease, diabetes, periodontitis, arthritis, infection and other maladies.

7. Tanning beds may be used regardless of outside weather.

8. Tanning beds may be used during "vitamin D winter." This is especially important at higher latitudes that lack sufficient UVB from winter sunlight to stimulate adequate vitamin D production by the skin.

The truth about tanning beds and melanoma

Several studies have investigated the relationship of tanning-bed use to melanoma and a review of 22 investigations done from 1979 through 2002 showed that only four indicated tanning beds increased melanoma risk; eighteen showed no association.[5] One that showed an increased melanoma risk was conducted by Dr. Philippe Autier and colleagues in Belgium in 1991.[6] However, in 2002 Dr. Autier conducted another study in which no association between tanning bed use and melanoma was found.[7] This report stated, *"No result suggested a dose-response curve, and no association was even present for subjects who reported more than 35 hours of cumulated tanning bed use at least 19 yrs before the interview. Our study doesn't support the possibility that tanning bed use could increase melanoma risk."*

I looked for other studies that might have come to contrary conclusions and found one from 2007.[9] It was a meta-analysis of 19 studies that concluded tanning beds do increase the melanoma risk. However, when Dr. William Grant assessed the meta-analysis, he noted that the studies failed to take skin type into consideration.[10] He re-analyzed the data and determined: "These results indicate that when studies largely influenced by inclusion of people with skin phenotype 1 [light-skinned non-tanners] without adjustment for skin phenotype are removed from the meta-analysis, no significant relation is found between tanning bed use and risk of CMM [cutaneous malignant melanoma]."

Several studies between 2003 and 2008 showed mixed results. One of the latest studies showed no significant increase in melanoma with tanning bed use.[8] Another study of five European countries showed that in France, where 20% of the population used tanning beds, their use was associated with a 19% increase in risk of melanoma.[3] In Sweden, where 83% of the population used tanning beds, there was a 38% *decrease* in melanoma. Overall, the risk of melanoma was reduced by 10% in tanning-bed users, although individuals with fair skin and a high number of moles were at increased risk. Clearly, studies that indict tanning beds without taking into consideration skin type are flawed, and if they do not also differentiate between tanning and burning, they are doubly flawed.

Remember that excessive ultraviolet light exposure, whether it comes from sunlight or tanning lamps, causes burning. We have clearly established that burning correlates to an increased risk of melanoma. Unfortunately, most of the studies that associated tanning beds with increased melanoma did not control for burning. Use of either sunlight exposure or tanning beds must be done prudently, so it is best to use professional tanning salons with trained personnel who assess skin type and make recommendations for the maximum time clients should tan.

Dr. Grant also reminds us that UVB is the beneficial wavelength that produces vitamin D. UVA does not produce vitamin D, but does work with UVB to produce a tan. Excessive UVA is harmful in that it penetrates more deeply and generates free radicals that can lead to skin aging and DNA damage, as several studies have shown.[14-17] However, the tan produced by UVA serves as a protection against damage by further UVA. What this means is that it is important to use tanning beds with outputs that mimic the midday, mid-latitude spring-and-summer sunlight, with UVB and UVA in natural balance (the UVB portion of total UV being roughly 3.5-5%, as it is in the spring and summer in much of North America).

Personally, I have no qualms about using tanning beds. Considering the numerous health benefits from high serum vitamin D levels, the slightly increased chance of rarely-fatal common skin cancer does not concern me especially because I am careful to never sunburn.

A very light skin that does not tan, or a skin condition that is sensitive to UV may preclude tanning-bed use by some individuals. Those with freckles and red hair do not generally tan well, and should avoid tanning beds or limit themselves to very short exposures. Others who may have adverse effects to tanning bed exposure are organ transplant recipients, those with many nevi (moles) or those taking photosensitive prescription drugs.[4] If you do not know if your drug is photosensitive, ask a pharmacist. Avoid even the least amount of burning.

Finally, it is a good idea to be checked regularly by a dermatologist to assess any changes that may occur to your skin. *That advice, however, is even more important for those who do not use tanning beds or get regular sunlight, since more melanomas occur among those who receive little or no UVB, or in those irregularly exposed* (see chapter 5).

Chapter 18: Summaries

Summary 1: Important points

I hope you have gleaned much useful information, and that you will use it to enhance the quality of your life. As a final review, here are some of the salient points.

1. Sunlight exposure was used effectively for thousands of years as treatment for numerous diseases. The practice of reasonable sunlight exposure should return to center stage as an essential health measure.

2. Sunlight varies in intensity according to season, latitude, altitude, cloud cover and pollution. Take that into account when planning exposure times and deciding whether to use a tanning bed or vitamin D supplements.

3. In late spring through early fall, a short, whole-body exposure at midday is the best way to receive sunlight. Never, never burn. Cover up after a short time and wear a broad-brimmed hat and light gloves to avoid too much sunlight if you need to stay outside. In early spring and late fall, longer exposure times are needed, and it is not as necessary to cover up exposed body parts during extended periods outdoors.

4. Common skin cancer is easily preventable with a low-fat diet. Processed vegetable oils are dangerous promoters of skin cancer, but a diet based on fresh fruits and vegetables inhibits both common skin cancers (NMSC) and melanoma. NMSC are caused by free-radical attack from the consumption of unhealthful fats combined with sunlight exposure. Eliminate fats, not sunlight. NMSC are easily removed, but major internal cancers, which sunlight helps prevent, are not so easily eliminated and are frequently deadly.

5. Sunlight exposure does not cause melanoma. Sunburning may cause melanoma, but melanomas occur on areas of the body that are seldom exposed to sunlight. Research indicates that regular sunlight exposure helps prevent melanoma, but heavy sunlight exposure while using sunscreens may dramatically *increase* its risk.

6. A greater number of sunburns correlates to a lesser incidence of major internal cancers and other degenerative diseases;

nevertheless, it is never good to burn. Sunburns seem to have a protective effect against these diseases because they are markers for high sunlight exposure and high vitamin D levels and not because sunburn is beneficial. The benefits can be acquired without burning.

7. Vitamin D is one of the chemicals produced by the skin that has such a profound and beneficial influence on health. Sunscreens can prevent 99% of vitamin D production by the skin, and as their use has increased 18-fold since 1972, the incidence of melanoma has tripled. Sunscreens are generally useless and may lead to melanoma by allowing large amounts of unblocked UVA light to penetrate and damage the lower layers of the skin for long periods of time.

8. At least twenty-five major internal cancers are reduced or inhibited by exposure to sunlight and/or high vitamin D levels, including breast, prostate, ovary and colon cancers.

9. Adequate vitamin D, whether from sunlight or supplements, is essential to both bone and muscle strength. Without it, calcium cannot be absorbed either into the blood or into the bone. Rickets, osteomalacia, osteoporosis and bone fractures result from vitamin D deficiency, and from a diet high in animal proteins.

10. Multiple sclerosis (MS) in various countries can be predicted by their latitude. The greater the distance from the equator, the greater is the incidence of MS, because UVB light from sunlight is less available farther from the equator. MS also increases the more a society consumes of milk and other animal foods.

11. Diabetes, both type-1 and type-2, are profoundly linked to low vitamin D levels.

12. Obesity, heart disease, hypertension and stroke are inversely related to sunlight exposure and vitamin D levels.

13. Psoriasis, eczema, and periodontal disease are lessened by sunlight exposure and high serum vitamin D.

14. Fertility is positively influenced by sunlight exposure and high vitamin D levels.

15. Sunlight enhances immune system function by producing vitamin D.

16. Dozens of disorders other than those mentioned in this summary are related to vitamin D deficiency.

17. Sunlight is an excellent antiseptic, and in the first half of the 20th century it was used to kill mumps, diphtheria and pneumonia microorganisms in the blood.

18. Sunlight is an excellent antidepressant, and works at least as well, if not better, than drugs.

19. Lack of sunlight and vitamin D may be responsible for a major part of the excessive disease rates of African Americans and other dark-skinned people. This is a major health concern, and the government should respond with a major education effort.

Summary 2: What you need to know about vitamin D testing and supplementation

1. Have only 25 (OH)D levels assessed; a 1,25(OH)D test is a waste of money.

2. Optimal levels of 25 (OH)D are between 50-70 ng/ml. If they are less than 50 ng/ml, work to increase them by sunlight or tanning-bed exposure or by supplementation. See a doctor first.

3. Vitamin D3 is produced by the skin when it is exposed to UVB light. It is also the only form of vitamin D that should be taken as a supplement. Vitamin D2 is not natural and may form harmful byproducts.

4. To maintain healthful levels of vitamin D in the absence of sunlight or other UVB radiation, 3,000-5,000 IU per day of supplementary vitamin D3 may be necessary; the number will vary according to body size and level of obesity (fatter people will require more).

5. The following chart shows the expected reduction in various disease risk as predicted by serum Vitamin D levels.

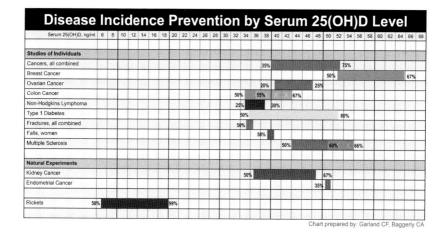

Disease Incidence Prevention by Serum 25(OH)D Level

Serum 25(OH)D, ng/ml	6	8	10	12	14	16	18	20	22	24	26	28	30	32	34	36	38	40	42	44	46	48	50	52	54	56	58	60	62	64	66	68
Studies of Individuals																																
Cancers, all combined																35%								75%								
Breast Cancer																					50%											67%
Ovarian Cancer															20%					25%												
Colon Cancer												50%		55%			67%															
Non-Hodgkins Lymphoma											25%			30%																		
Type 1 Diabetes												50%													80%							
Fractures, all combined												50%																				
Falls, women													50%																			
Multiple Sclerosis															50%								60%		66%							
Natural Experiments																																
Kidney Cancer												50%											67%									
Endometrial Cancer																			35%													
Rickets	50%							99%																								

Chart prepared by: Garland CF, Baggerly CA

References:

All Cancers: Lappe JM, et al. Am J Clin Nutr. 2007;85:1586-91. Breast: Garland CF, et al. J Steroid Biochem Mol Biol. 2007;103:708-11. Colon: Gorham ED, et al. Am J Prev Med. 2007;32:210-6. Diabetes: Hyppönen E, et al. Lancet 2001;358:1500-3. Endometrium: Mohr SB, et al. Prev Med. 2007;45:323-4. Falls: Broe KE, et al. J Am Geriatr Soc. 2007;55:234-9. Fractures: Bischoff-Ferrari HA, et al. JAMA. 2005;293:2257-64. Multiple Sclerosis: Munger KL, et al. JAMA. 2006;296:2832-8. Non-Hodgkin's Lymphoma: Purdue MP, et al. Cancer Causes Control. 2007;18:989-99. Ovary: Tworoger SS, et al. Cancer Epidemiol Biomarkers Prev. 2007;16:783-8. Renal: Mohr SB, et al. Int J Cancer. 2006;119:2705-9. Rickets: Arnaud SB, et al. Pediatrics. 1976 Feb;57(2):221-5.

Epilogue

The future for sunlight looks, shall we say, "bright?" Vicki and I did not take our usual Sun vacation to Cabo San Lucas, Mexico this year due to the need to plan our new health resort and to finish this and another book. Though I do get out in the sun almost daily here in southern Utah, Vicki does not sunbathe often during the winter season. I asked her to have her serum vitamin D levels measured because it concerned me—especially after doing the research for this book. Her tests came back showing a rather anemic 21 ng/ml (52.5 nmol/l). Our physician friend, who is also a believer in alternative medicine, was also concerned and prescribed a single dose of 50,000 IU per week for eight weeks. After seven weeks, her level increased to 56 ng/ml (140 nmol/l)—an impressive change indeed! My own level, using only the sunshine, was 58 ng/ml (145 nmol/l).

Vicki's spectacular increase in vitamin D levels is interesting, but only part of the story. The "normal" range printed on the first test results form was from 8.9 ng/ml to 46.7 ng/ml. The second test form showed a totally different normal range: 32ng/ml to 100 ng/ml. There was a statement as to why the normal ranges had changed: "Recent studies consider the lower limit of 32 ng/ml to be a threshold for optimal health." It referenced a paper by Dr. Bruce Hollis published in the *Journal of Nutrition* in 2005. (Hollis B. *J Nutr.* 2005;135:317-22). In the seven-week period between those two tests, the "safe" lower limit for vitamin D more than tripled! Kudos is due Dr. Hollis and his colleagues who hammer away at the establishment to change conventional thinking on vitamin D.

The tide is turning, and I predict that soon, reasonable sunlight exposure—without sunscreen—will be back in vogue, even among dermatologists. Maybe that's a bit optimistic, but rest assured that most physicians will be extolling the virtues of vitamin D. And you can also bet that pharmaceutical companies will be falling all over each other attempting to be the first to produce the "ultimate vitamin D analogue"—one that will be "better than the real thing." However, it is impossible to fool Mother Nature or to improve on her perfection. Sadly, there is no money to be made from sunlight or dietary vitamin D. Companies will produce a new and inferior molecule, patent it, and then sell it at exorbitant prices. Excuse my cynicism, but when even the *Journal of the American Medical Association* (Lazarou, J. *JAMA* 1998;279:1200-05) admits that **properly prescribed and properly used drugs** are responsible for 106,000 deaths per year, I begin to wonder about the efficacy of drugs and suspect that the drug industry is mainly about money. Properly used prescription drugs as a cause of death places them in fourth place, right behind heart disease, cancer, and iatrogenic (caused by doctors and hospitals) illnesses. There are many fine physicians out there, but you may have to shop to find one. A great test question for a physician is, "What should my serum vitamin D levels be? It he or she doesn't know or gives you the wrong answer, consider finding someone else.

Here's to your health, and may all your days be full of sunshine, love and prosperity!

Suggestions for further reading and other resources

Books on sunlight:

1. *The UV Advantage* by Michael Holick, MD. A must-read book from a scientist who helped make the history of vitamin D.
2. *The Healing Sun* by Richard Hobday.
3. *Sunlight Could Save your Life* by Zane Kime, MD.

Books on nutrition and fitness:

1. *The China Study* **by T.** Colin Campbell, PhD. Of the thousands of books that have been written on health and nutrition, nothing comes close to this magnificent work. Dr. Campbell and colleagues have conducted the largest study of nutrition in history, and the results of that study and others that he reviews leave no doubt in the reader's mind about the best way for human beings to eat for vibrant health. This book is an absolute must read.
2. *Eat to Live* by Joel Fuhrman, MD.
3. *A Race for Life* and *Senior Fitness* by Ruth Heidrich, PhD. These are two of the most inspirational writings available.
4. A Race for Life Cook/rawbook by Dr. Heidrich, available at her web site listed under the next heading.
5. Read anything written by John McDougall, MD, Dean Ornish, MD or Neal Barnard, MD

Web sites dealing with sunlight/vitamin D, health and nutrition:

1. **SUNARC.org**. This is an outstanding web site that is produced by Dr. William Grant. It will keep you informed on the latest research on sunlight, vitamin D and nutrition.
2. **Vitamindcouncil.com**. The site is a treasure trove of information and research on sunlight/vitamin D. It is produced by Dr. John Cannell, who also offers an excellent (and free) newsletter.
3. **Antiaging.com**. An excellent site on anti-aging medicine produced by Philip Lee Miller, MD, the founder of the Los Gatos Longevity Institute.

4. Ruthheidrich.com. An inspirational site where one can learn the health secrets of this amazing breast-cancer survivor and super-fit, world-class athlete.

Other resources:

Dr. Sorenson and his colleagues will soon be building a new health institute/resort and will also be building a web site. Information may be obtained on these and other projects by email: drmarcsorenson@hotmail.com

A few of the beneficial effects of sunlight and/or vitamin D on the human body:

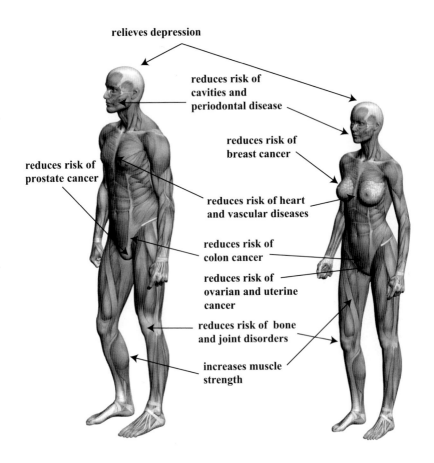

relieves depression

reduces risk of cavities and periodontal disease

reduces risk of breast cancer

reduces risk of prostate cancer

reduces risk of heart and vascular diseases

reduces risk of colon cancer

reduces risk of ovarian and uterine cancer

reduces risk of bone and joint disorders

increases muscle strength

Sunlight and vitamin D have also been correlated to reduced risk of many other major cancers and reduced risk of diabetes, multiple sclerosis, PMS, type-1 diabetes, type-2 diabetes, osteoporosis, depression and numerous other disorders and diseases.

A final word on the importance of Solar Power

By Dr. Gordon Ainsleigh

For those of us involved in advancing the science of sunlight on health, it is frustrating and even maddening to see the critical facts go unreported or misreported for decades, with misinformation out-shouting information most of the time. To date, the only major article for the general public that got all the facts right was in the June 2003 issue of *Reader's Digest*. But that was just five small pages of truth in an ocean of misinformation.

Ignaz Semmelweis, the Austrian physician who realized in 1847 that the childbed fever that was killing 13% of the mothers in his hospital could be prevented by washing and disinfecting the doctors' hands before examining and assisting a birthing mother, had to watch the medical establishment resist his findings and doom millions of women to a death that could easily be prevented. It is thought that the burden of his helpless knowledge led to mental deterioration, and he was committed to an insane asylum in 1865 and died shortly thereafter, some say of an infection and some say by being beaten to death by the staff.

Doctors Peller and Apperley, who found that sun exposure prevents cancer in their 1936-41 studies, had to live out their lives like Semmelweis, watching millions of people suffer and die needlessly because the medical establishment would only acknowledge chemical disease control. Of the doctors who resurrected this science in the late 1970s and early 1980s, Zane Kime is dead, John Eisman is an elder who refuses to retire at a "decent age", and Michael Holick and the Garland brothers, Frank and Cedric, are still under 60 years of age and hope to see the general acceptance of their research before they die.

Throughout these years, at least 150,000 Americans have died needlessly each year because the medical establishment ignores clear evidence that ultraviolet B—the health-giving light that is so abundant in spring and summer sunlight—promotes health and opposes disease. Eisman, Holick and the Garlands have been watching their fellow humans die needlessly for more than 25 years, while I have only been a party to this monumental tragedy for 13 years, although it seems like forever. Like Martin Luther King, we are all asking: "How long, Lord?"

What we who work in the science of sunlight and health have needed for the last ten years of working and waiting—while 150,000 Americans per year suffer and die needlessly from insufficient sun exposure—is a book that tells the whole lifesaving story of frequent moderate sun exposure to the general public, and does it with good logic and scientific accuracy. Scientists are not good at that task, and we gratefully welcome Dr. Marc Sorenson's book, _Solar Power_, to carry toward completion the task to which we have devoted so much of our lives.

H. Gordon Ainsleigh, D.C.

References

Chapter 1: sunlight, vitamin D and health: history and function

1. Whistler, D. *Morbo puerili Anglorum, quem patrio idiomate indigenae vocant The Rickets*. Lugduni Batavorum 1645:1-13.
2. Glisson, F. A treatise of the rickets being a disease common to children. London 1688:1-373.
3. Mellanby, E. Experimental investigation on rickets. *Lancet* 1919;196:407-12.
4. Mellanby, E. Experimental rickets. *Medical Research (G.B.), Special Report Series* 1921;SRS-61:1-78.
5. McCollum, E. Studies on experimental rickets XXI. An experimental demonstration of the existence of a vitamin which promotes calcium deposition. *J. Biol. Chem.* 1922;.53:293-312.
6. Goldblatt, H. et al. A study of rats on a normal diet irradiated daily by the mercury vapor quartz lamp or kept in darkness. *Biochem J.* 1923;17:294-97.
7. Hess, A. Influence of light on the prevention of rickets. *Lancet* 1922;2:1222
8. Steenbock, H. et al. Fat-soluble vitamins. XIX. The induction of calcifying properties in a rickets-producing ration by radiant energy. *Methods Enzymol* 1924;62:209-16.
9. Steenbock, H. et al. The induction of growth promoting and calcifying properties in a ration by exposure to light. *Science* 1924;60:224-25.
10. Beyond Discovery. Unraveling the mystery of vitamin D. National Academy of Sciences Report 2003.
11. Windaus, A. Uber das krystallistierte vitamin D. *Justis. Liebigs. Ann. Chem* 1932;492:226-31.
12. Brockmann, H. Die Isolierung des antirachitischen Vitamins aus Thunfischleberol. *Physiol. Chem* 1936;241:104-15.
13. Cannell, J. Personal communication with author., 2006
14. Garland C. et al. Do sunlight and vitamin D reduce the likelihood of colon cancer? *Int J Epidemiol* 1980;9:227-231.
15. Abe, E. et al. Differentiation of Mouse Myeloid Leukemia Cells Induced by 1 ,25-dihydroxyvitamin D_3 *PNAS* 1981;78:4990-94.
16. Bischoff-Ferrari H. et al. Fracture prevention with vitamin D supplementation: A meta-analysis of randomized controlled trials. *JAMA.* 2005;293(18): 2257-2264.
17. c, A. et al. A prospective study of vitamin D intake and risk of type-2 diabetes in women. Presentation at 65th Annual Scientific Sessions of the American Diabetes Association 2005, abstract # 1772.
18. Sato, Y. et al. Low-dose vitamin D prevents muscular atrophy and reduces falls and hip fractures in women after stroke: a randomized controlled trial. *Cerebrovasc Dis* 2005;20:187-92.
19. Dietrich, T. et al. Association between serum concentrations of 25-hydroxyvitamin D and gingival inflammation. *Am J Clin Nutr* 2005;82:575-580.
20. Dietrich, T. et al. Association between serum concentrations of 25-hydroxyvitamin D3 and periodontal disease in the USA population. *Am J Clin Nutr* 2004;80:108-13.
21. John, E. et al. sun exposure, vitamin D receptor gene polymorphisms, and risk of advanced prostate cancer. *Cancer Res* 2005;65:5470-79.
22. Moan J. et al. Solar radiation, vitamin D and survival rate of colon cancer in Norway. *J Photochem Photobiol B* 2005;78:189-93.
23. Zhou, W. et al. Vitamin D predicts overall survival in early stage non-small cell lung cancer patients. American Association for Cancer Research, 96th Annual Meeting 2005, abstract # LB-231.
24. John, E. et al. Vitamin D and breast cancer risk: The NHANES I Epidemiologic Follow Up Study, 1971-1975 to 1992. *Cancer Epidemiol Biomarkers and Prevention* 1999;8:399-406.
25. Smedby, K. et al. Ultraviolet Radiation Exposure and Risk of Malignant Lymphomas.

JNCI 2005;97:199-209.

26. Vieth, R. et al. Randomized comparison of the effects of the vitamin D$_3$ adequate intake versus 4,000 mcg (4,000 IU) per day on biochemical responses and the wellbeing of patients. *Nutrition Journal* 2004, **3**:8:1475-2891.

27. Bertone-Johnson, E. et al. Calcium and vitamin D intake and risk of incident premenstrual syndrome," *Arch Intern Med* 2005;165:1246-1252.

28. Teng, M. et al. Activated injectable vitamin D and hemodialysis survival: a historical cohort study. *J Am Soc Nephrol* 2005; 16: 1115-1125.

29. Grimes D. et al. sunlight, cholesterol and coronary heart disease. *QJM* 1996;89:579-89.

30. Van der Mei, I. et al. Past Exposure to sun, Skin Phenotype and Risk of Multiple Sclerosis: Case-Control Study. *BMJ* 2003;327:316.

31. Merlino L. et al. Vitamin D intake is inversely associated with rheumatoid arthritis: results from the Iowa Women's Health Study. *Arthritis Rheum.* 2004;50:72-7.

32. Plotnikoff, G. et al. Prevalence of severe hypovitaminosis D in patients with persistent, nonspecific musculoskeletal pain. *Mayo Clinic Proceedings* 2003;78:1463-70.

33. Liel, Y. et al. Low circulating vitamin D in obesity. *Calcif Tissue Int* 1988;43:199-201.

34. Matsuoka, L. et al. sunscreens suppress cutaneous vitamin D3 synthesis. *Journal of Clinical Endocrinology & Metabolism* 1987; 64:1165-68.

35. Fielder, J. Heliotherapy: the principles & practice of sunbathing. Soil and Health Library (online) http://www.soilandhealth.org/index.html.

36. Hobday, R. *The Healing sun.* Findhorn Press 1999:132.

37. Nightingale, F. Notes on Hospitals (third edition) Longman, Roberts and Green 1863.

38. Peller S. Carcinogenesis as a means of reducing cancer mortality. *Lancet* 1936; 2:552-56.

39. Peller S. Skin irritation and cancer in the United States Navy. *Am J Med Sci* 1937;194:326-33.)

40. Apperley, F. The relation of solar radiation to cancer mortality in North America. *Cancer Res* 1941;1:191-95.

41. Moss, R. Another Dissident Dermatologist. Cancerdecisions.com Newsletter. 2005.

42. Bonner, C. Contact Kline Co. http://www.klinegroup.com/

43. Haywood, R. et al. sunscreens inadequately protect against ultraviolet-A-induced free radical damage. *Journal of Investigative Dermatology* 2003;121:862-68.

44. Grant W. et al. Comparisons of estimated economic burdens due to insufficient solar ultraviolet irradiance and vitamin D and excess solar UV irradiance for the United States. *Photochem Photobiol* 2005;81:1276-86.

45. Giovannucci, E. et al. Prospective study of predictors of vitamin D status and cancer incidence and mortality in men. *J Natl Cancer Inst* 2006;98:451.

46. Harris, S. et al. Seasonal changes in plasma 25-hydroxyvitamin D concentrations of young American black and white women. *Am J Clin Nutr* 1998;67:1232-36.

47. Gillie, O. sunlight Robbery: Health benefits of sunlight are being denied by current public health policy in the UK. 2004 Epublication available at http://www.healthresearchforum. org.uk/ sunlight.html.

48. Nesby-O'Dell, S. et al. Hypovitaminosis D prevalence and determinants among African American and white women of reproductive age: third National Health and Nutrition Examination Survey, 1988-1994. *Am J Clin Nutr* 2002;76:187-92.

49. Plotnikoff G. et al. Prevalence of severe hypovitaminosis D in patients with persistent, nonspecific musculoskeletal pain. *Mayo Clin Proc.* 2003;78:1463-70.

50. Grant, W. et al. Benefits and requirements of vitamin D for optimal health. *Alt Med Rev* 2005;10:94-111.

51. Gordon C. et al. Prevalence of vitamin D deficiency among healthy adolescents. *Arch Pediatr Adolesc Med* 2004;158:531-537.

52. Hanley, D. Quoted in Vitamin D. What's enough? Science News Online, Oct 16, 2004.

53. Rucker, D. et al. Vitamin D insufficiency in a population of healthy western Canadians. *Can Med Assn Journal* 2002;166:1517-24.

54. Vieth, R. et al. Age-related changes in the 25-hydroxyvitamin D *versus* parathyroid hormone relationship suggest a different reason why older adults require more vitamin D. *J Clin Endocrinol Metab* 2005;88:185-91.

55. Hollis B. Circulating 25-hydroxyvitamin D levels indicative of vitamin D sufficiency: implications for establishing a new effective dietary intake recommendation for vitamin D. *J Nutr.* 2005;135:317-22.

56. Zadshir A. et al. The prevalence of hypovitaminosis D among USA adults: data from the NHANES III. *Ethn Dis.* 2005;15(4 Suppl 5):S5-97-101.

57. Passeri, G. et al. Low vitamin D status, high bone turnover, and bone fractures in centenarians. *J Clin Endocrinol Metab* 2003;88:5109-5115.

58. Vieth R. Why the optimal requirement for vitamin D3 is probably much higher than what is officially recommended for adults. *J Steroid Biochem Mol Biol* 2004;89-90:575-79.

59. Committee on nutrition; the prophylactic requirement and the toxicity of vitamin D. *Pediatrics* 1963;31:512-30.

60. Lajis, R. Effects of vitamin D overdose. Available at http://www.prn2.usm.my/mainsite/ bulletin/ sun/1996/ sun44.html.

61. An Overview of Cholecalciferol Toxicosis. The American Board of Veterinary Toxicology, 2005.

62. Cannell, J. Toxicity of vitamin D. Paper prepared for the Cholecalciferol Council Sept. 5, 2003. Available at http://www.cholecalciferol-council.com/toxicity.pdf.

63. Tuohimaa P. et al. Both high and low levels of blood vitamin D are associated with a higher prostate cancer risk: a longitudinal, nested case-control study in the Nordic countries. *Int J Cancer* 2004;108:104-08.

64. John, E. et al. sun exposure, Vitamin D receptor gene polymorphisms and risk of advanced prostate cancer. *Cancer Res* 2005;65:5470-79.

65. Tangpricha V. et al. Tanning is associated with optimal vitamin D status (serum 25-hydroxyvitamin D concentration) and higher bone mineral density. *Am J Clin Nutr.* 2004;80:1645-49.

66. Aloia J. et al. A randomized controlled trial of vitamin D3 supplementation in African American women. *Arch Intern Med* 2005;165:1618-23.

67. Martineau A. et al. Effect of vitamin D supplementation on anti-mycobacterial immunity: a double-blind randomized placebo-controlled trial in London tuberculosis contacts. *Int J Tuberculosis Lung Dis* 2005;9: S173.

68. Andiran N. et al. Risk factors for vitamin D deficiency in breast-fed newborns and their mothers. *Nutrition* 2002;18:47-50.

69. American Academy of Pediatrics Press Release, 2003.

70. Hollis B. et al. Vitamin D requirements during lactation: high-dose maternal supplementation as therapy to prevent hypovitaminosis D for both the mother and the nursing infant. *Am J Clin Nutr* 2004;80:1752S-58S.

71. Ala-Houhala, M. et al. Maternal compared with infant vitamin D supplementation. *Arch Dis Child.* 1986;61:1159-63.

72. Javaid, M. et al. Maternal vitamin D status during pregnancy and childhood bone mass at age 9 years: a longitudinal study. *Lancet* 2006;367:36–43.

73. Moon, S. et al. Ultraviolet radiation: effects on risks of prostate cancer and other internal cancers. *Mutat Res* 2005;571: 207–219.

74. Reginster, J. et al. The high prevalence of inadequate serum vitamin D levels and implications for bone health. *Curr Med Res Opin* 2005; 21 (4): 579.

75. Bataille, V. et al. Exposure to tanning beds and risk of cutaneous melanoma in the UK: a case control study. *Euro J Cancer* 2004;40:429-35.

76. Bataille, V. et al. A multicentre epidemiological study on tanning bed use and cutaneous melanoma in Europe. *Euro J Cancer* 2005;41:2141-49.

77. Holick, M. MD. Personal correspondence with the author.

78. Gillie, O. PhD. Personal correspondence with the author.

79. Martineau, A. Effect of vitamin D supplementation on anti-mycobacterial immunity: a double-blind randomized placebo-controlled trial in London tuberculosis contacts. *Int J Tuberculosis Lung Dis* 2005;9:S173.

80. Martineau, A. et al. Vitamin D status of tuberculosis patients and healthy blood donors in Samara City, Russia. *Int J Tuberculosis* Lung Dis 2005;9:S225.

81. Vieth, R. Vitamin D supplementation, 25-hydroxyvitamin D concentrations and safety.

Am J Clin Nutr 1999;69:842-56.

82. Vieth, R. et al. Randomized comparison of the effects of the vitamin D₃ adequate intake versus 100 mcg (4,000 IU) per day on biochemical responses and the wellbeing of patients. *Nutr J* 2004;3:8.

83. Vieth, R. et al. quoted by Cannell, J. Vitamin D newsletter, February 2006. http://www.vitamindcouncil.com.

84. Heaney, R. et al. Human serum 25-hydroxycholecalciferol response to extended oral dosing with cholecalciferol. *Am J Clin Nutr* 2003;77:204-10.

85. Glerup, H. et al. Commonly recommended daily input of vitamin D is not sufficient if sunlight exposure is limited. *J Int Med* 2000;247:260–8.

86. Dawson, Lord. Naked and Unashamed. Lancet March 6, 1932:688.

87. Grant, W. Personal communication with the author, June, 2006.

88. Grant, W. Personal communication with the author, June, 2006.

89. Jablonski, N. et al. The evolution of human skin coloration. *Journal of Evolution* 2000;39:57-106.

90. Cannell, J. Personal communication with the author.

91. Grant, W. An estimate of premature cancer mortality in the USA due to inadequate doses of solar ultraviolet-B radiation. *Cancer* 2002;94:1867-75.

92. Miller, P. Personal communication with author. Dr. Miller's web site can be accessed at www.antiaging.com

93. Stephensen, C. Vitamin D status in adolescents and young adults with HIV infection. *Am J Clin Nutr* 2006;83:1135-41.

94. Cannell, J. et al. Epidemic Influenza and vitamin D. *Epidemiol Infect* 2006;134:1129-40

95. Bodnar, L. et al. Maternal vitamin d deficiency increases the risk of preeclampsia. *J Clin Endocrinol Metab.* 2007;;92:3517-22.

96. Camargo, C. et al. Regional differences in EpiPen prescriptions in the United States: the potential role of vitamin D. *J Allergy Clin Immunol.* 2007;120:131-6.

97. Binkley, N. Low Vitamin D Status despite Abundant sun Exposure. *J Clin Endocrinol Metab 2007;*92: 2130–35.

98. *Harvard Health Letter* July 2007.

99. Harris S. et al. Seasonal changes in plasma 25-hydroxyvitamin D concentrations of young American black and white women. *Am J Clin Nutr.* 1998;67:1232–6.

100. Holick M. et al. Age, vitamin D, and solar ultraviolet. *Lancet.* 1989;2:1104–5.

101. Moore C. et al. Vitamin D intakes by children and adults in the United States differ among ethnic groups. *J Nutr.* 2005;135:2478–85.

102. Belaid, S. et al. Hypovitaminosis D among 18 to 49 years old women wearing concealing clothes, an ignored reality in general practice. *Presse Med* 2007; [Epub ahead of print]

103. Hathcock, A. et al. Risk assessment for vitamin D. *Am J Clin Nutr* 2007;85:6-18.

104. Kirkey, S. Experts prescribe massive increase of vitamin D. Canadian West News Service, September 25, 2007.

105. Dijkstra, S. et al. High prevalence of vitamin D deficiency in newborn infants of high-risk mothers. *Arch Dis childhood* 2007;92:750-53.

106. Vieth, R. et al. The urgent need to recommend an intake of vitamin D that is effective. *Am J Clin Nutr* 2007;85:649-50.

107. Das, G. et al. Hypovitaminosis D among healthy adolescent girls attending an inner city school. *Arch Dis Child* 2006;91:569-72.

108. Talwar, S. et al. Dose response to vitamin d supplementation among postmenopausal African American women. *Am J Clin Nutr* 2007;86:1657-62.

109. Houghton, L. et al. The case against ergocalciferol vitamin D2 as a vitamin D supplement. *Am J Clin Nutr* 2006;84:694-97

110. Armas, L. et al. *J Clin Epidemiol Metab* 2004;89:5387-91.

111. Holick, M. et al. Vitamin D2 is as effective as Vitamin D3 in maintaining circulation concentrations of 25-hydroxyviamin D. *J Clin End0crinol Metab* Dec. 18, 2007. Epub ahead of print.

112. Forsmo, S. et al. Childhood cod liver oil consumption and bone mineral density in a population-based cohort of peri-and postmenopausal women. *Am J Epidemiol*

2008;167:406-11.

113. Ainsleigh, G. Beneficial effects of sun exposure on cancer mortality. *Preventive Medicine* 1993;22:132-140.

114. Grant, W. An estimate of premature cancer mortality in the USA because of inadequate doses of solar ultraviolet-B radiation. *Cancer.* 2002;94:1867-75.

115. Black, H. et al. Role of dietary factors in UV-carcinogenesis. *Cancer Bulletin* 1993;45:232-7.

116. Black, H. et al. Influence of dietary factors on actinically-induced skin cancer. *Mutation Res* 1998;422:185-90.

117. Black, H. et al. Evidence that a low-fat diet reduces the occurrence of non-melanoma skin cancer. *Int J Cancer* 1995;62:165-169.

118. Jacobs, E. et al. Vitamin D insufficiency in Southern Arizona. *Am J Clin Nutr* 2008;87:608-13.

119. Hollis, B. et al. Circulating Vitamin D3 and 25-hydroxyvitamin D in Humans: An Important Tool to Define Adequate Nutritional Vitamin D Status. *J Steroid Biochem Mol Biol.* 2007 March ; 103(3-5): 631–634.

120. Grant, W. Personal communication with author regarding research to be published.

121. Vieth, R. Vitamin D supplementation, 25-hydroxyvitamin D concentrations, and safety. *Am J Clin Nutr* 1999;69:842-56

122. Mark, S. et al Low Vitamin D Status in a Representative Sample of Youth From Quebec, Canada. *Clin Chem.* 2008 Jun 12. [Epub ahead of print]

123. Gordon, C. et al. Prevalence of vitamin D deficiency among healthy infants and toddlers. *Arch Pediatr Adolesc Med.* 2008;162:505-12.

Chapter 2: Seasons and sunlight

1. Webb, A Influence of season and latitude on the cutaneous synthesis of vitamin D3: exposure to winter sunlight in Boston and Edmonton will not promote vitamin D3 in human skin. *J Clin Endocrinol Metab* 1988;67:373-78.

2. EPA website 2005. http://www.epa.gov/ sunwise/doc/uviguide.pdf.

3. National Weather Forecast Service, Flagstaff, AZ 2005.

4. Agarwal, K. The impact of atmospheric pollution on vitamin D status of infants and toddlers in Delhi, India. *Arch Dis Child* 2002;87:111-13.

Chapter 3: Free radicals and antioxidants

1. Karlsson, J. Introduction to nutraology and radical formation. In: *Antioxidants and Exercise*. Illinois: Human Kinetics Press 1997:1-143.

2. Goldfarb, A. et al. Nutritional antioxidants as therapeutic and preventive modalities in exercise-induced muscle damage. *Can. J. Appl. Physiol* 1999;24:249-266.

3. Dekkers, J. et al. The Role of Antioxidant Vitamins and Enzymes in the Prevention of Exercise-Induced Muscle Damage. *Sports Med 1996;* 21: 213.

4. Sjodin, T. Biochemical mechanisms for oxygen free radical formation during exercise. *Sports Med.* 10: 236-254, 1990.

5. Miller, E. et al. Meta-Analysis: High-Dosage Vitamin E Supplementation May Increase All-Cause Mortality. *Ann Intern Med* 2004;142:37-46.

6. Goodman, G. et al. The Beta-Carotene and Retinol Efficacy Trial: incidence of lung cancer and cardiovascular disease mortality during 6-year follow-up after stopping beta-carotene and retinol supplements. *J Natl Cancer Inst* 2004;96:1729-31.

7. Barret, S. Antioxidants and Other Phytochemicals: Current Scientific Perspective. *Quackwatch.org* 2004.

8. Girotti, A. Mechanisms of Lipid Peroxidation. *J Free Rad in Biol and Med* 1985;1:87-95.

9. Brown, K. et al. DNA strand scission by enzymatically generated oxygen radicals. *Arch Biochem Biophys* 1981;206:414-19.

10. Roubai, W. et al. Polymerization of proteins induced by free radical lipid peroxidation. *Arch Biochem Biophys* 1966;113:150-55.

11. Nielsen, H. et al. Covalent binding of peroxidized phospholipid to protein:III Reaction of individual phospholipids with different proteins. *Lipids* 1981;16:215-22.
12. Kime, Z. Methods of refining oil. In: sun*light Could Save Your Life* 1980:126-30.
13. Vieth, W. *Diet and Health*. Quoted on Amazingdiscoveries.org.
14. Liv, J. et al. Vitamin C supplementation restores the impaired vitamin E status of guinea pigs fed oxidized frying oil: *J Nutr* 1998;128:116-22.
15. De Hertog, S. et al. Relation between smoking and skin cancer. *J Clin Oncol* 2001;19:231-238.
16. Rahman, I. et al. Role of antioxidants in smoking- induced lung disease. *Free Rad Biol Med* 1996;21:669-681.

Chapter 4: Solar Power, dietary fat and skin cancer

1. National Cancer Institute 2005. *Cancer Facts and Figures*.
2. Nguyen. T. et al. Nonmelanoma skin cancer. *Current Treatment Options in Oncology* 2002;3:193-203.
3. Watson, A. Tar cancer in mice II. The condition of the skin when modified by external treatment or diet in influencing the cancerous reaction. *BR J Exp Pathol* 1930;11:311-322.
4. Boyd, T. *Ind Med Gaz* 1929;64:564.
5. Baumann, C. et al. Effect of diet on tumors induced by ultraviolet light. *Am J Cancer* 1939;35:213-221.
6. Black, H. et al. Role of dietary factors in UV-carcinogenesis. *Cancer Bulletin* 1993;45:232-7.
7. Black, H. et al. Influence of dietary factors on actinically-induced skin cancer. *Mutation Res* 1998;422:185-90.
8. Black, H. et al. Evidence that a low-fat diet reduces the occurrence of non-melanoma skin cancer. *Int J Cancer* 1995;62:165-169.
9. Liu, G. et al. Omega 3 but not omega 6 fatty acids inhibit AP-1 activity and cell transformation in JB6 cells. Hormel Institute, University of Minnesota, Austin, MN 55912 April 20, 2001.
10. Black, H. et al. Influence of dietary omega-6, -3 fatty acid sources on the initiation and promotion stages of photocarcinogenesis. *Photochem and Photobiol* 1992;2:195-99.
11. Guangming, L. et al. Omega 3 but not omega 6 fatty acids inhibit AP-1 activity and cell transformation in JB6 cells. *Proc Natl Acad Sci* 2001 Jun 19;98(13):7510-5.
12. Simopoulous, A. et al. Omega-6/Omega-3 essential fatty acid ratio: the scientific evidence. *World Review of Nutrition and Dietetics*. Basel, Karger 2003;92:I-XIII.
13. Otley, C. American Cancer Society Statistics 2006.
14. Black, H. et al. Relation of antioxidants and level of dietary lipid to epidermal lipid peroxidation and ultraviolet carcinogenesis. *Cancer Research* 1985;45:6254-6259.
15. Hughes, M. et al. Food intake and risk of squamous cell carcinoma of the skin in a community: The Nambour skin cancer cohort study. *Int J Cancer* 2006; online publication ahead of print.
16. National Cancer Institute. *Cancer Facts and Figures* 2005.

Chapter 5. Solar Power and melanoma: burned by sunscreens?

1. Berwick, M. et al. sun exposure and mortality from melanoma. *JNCI* 2005;97:1-15.
2. Smedby, K. et al. Ultraviolet radiation exposure and risk of malignant lymphomas. *JNCI* 2005;97:199-209.
3. Elwood, J. et al. Melanoma and sun exposure: an overview of published studies. *Int J Cancer* 1997;73:198-203.
4. Kennedy C. et al. The influence of painful sunburns and lifetime sun exposure on the risk of actinic keratoses, seborrheic warts, melanocytic nevi, atypical nevi, and skin cancer. *J Invest Dermatol* 2003;120:1087-93.
5. Garland F. et al. Occupational sunlight exposure and melanoma in the USA Navy. *Arch Environ Health* 1990; 45:261-67.

6. Kaskel, P. et al. Outdoor activities in childhood: a protective factor for cutaneous melanoma? Results of a case-control study in 271 matched pairs. *Br J Dermatol* 2001;145:602-09.

7. Hakansson, N. et al. Occupational sunlight exposure and cancer incidence among Swedish construction workers. *Epidemiology* 2001;12:552-57.

8. Rivers, J. et al. Is there more than one road to melanoma? *Lancet* 2004;363:728-30.

9. Crombie, I. et al. Racial differences in melanoma incidence. *Br J Cancer* 1979;40:185-93.

10. Grant W. et al. Comparisons of estimated economic burdens due to insufficient solar ultraviolet irradiance and vitamin D and excess solar UV irradiance for the United States. *Photochem Photobiol* 2005;81:1276-86.

11. Giovannucci, E. et al. Prospective study of predictors of vitamin D status and cancer incidence and mortality in men. *J Natl Cancer Inst* 2006;98:451.

12. Millen A. et al. Diet and melanoma in a case-control study. *Cancer Epidemiol Biomarkers Prev* 2004;13:1042-51.

13. Ries, L SEER Cancer Statistics Review, 1973-1999 Bethesda, MD: National Cancer Institute, 2002.

14. Matsuoka, L. et al. sunscreens suppress cutaneous vitamin D3 synthesis. *Journal of Clinical Endocrinology & Metabolism* 1987; 64:1165-68.

15. Haywood, R. et al. sunscreens inadequately protect against ultraviolet-A-induced free radical damage. *Journal of Investigative Dermatology* 2003;121:862-68.

16. Garland, C. et al. Could sunscreens increase melanoma risk? American Journal of Public Health, Vol. 82, No. 4, April 1992, pp. 614-15.

17. Reynolds, T. et al. Sun plays havoc with light skin down under. *JNCI* 1992;18:1392-94.

18. Autier, P. et al. sunscreen use, wearing clothes, and number of nevi in 6- to 7- year-old European children. *JNCI* 1998;90:1873-80.

19. Autier, P. et al. sunscreen use and intentional exposure to ultraviolet A and B radiation: a double blind randomized trial using personal dosimeters. *British Journal of Cancer* 2000;83:1243-48.

20. Dennis, L. et al. sunscreen use and the risk for melanoma: a quantitative review. *Ann Intern Med* 2003;139:966-78.

21. Moan, J. et al. The relationship between skin cancers, solar radiation and ozone depletion. *British J Can* 1992;65:916-21.

22. Rivers J. et al. Is there more than one road to melanoma? *Lancet* 2004;28;363(9410):728-30.

23. Maldonado, J. et al. Determinants of BRAF mutations in primary melanomas. *J Natl Cancer Inst* 2003 Dec 17;95(24):1878-90.

24. Beral V. et al. Malignant melanoma and exposure to fluorescent lighting at work. *Lancet* 1982;Aug 7:290-93.

25. Kennedy, A. et al. Fluorescent light induces malignant transformation in mouse embryo cell cultures. *Science* 1980; 207:1209-11

26. Stahl, W. et al. Dietary Tomato Paste Protects against Ultraviolet Light–Induced Erythema in Humans. *J Nutr* 2001;131:1449-51.

27. Aust, O. et al. Supplementation with tomato-based products increases lycopene, phytofluene, and phytoene levels in human serum and protects against UV-light-induced erythema. *Int J Vitam Nutr Res*. 2005;75:54-60.

28. Fazekas Z, et al., Protective effects of lycopene against ultraviolet B-induced photodamage. *Nutr Cancer*. 2003;47(2):181-7.

29. Bain, C. et al. Diet and melanoma. An exploratory case-control study. *Ann Epidemiol* 1993;3:235-38.

30. Brick, W. MD. Emedicine specialties 2004. The article is available at http://www.emedicine.com/med/topic1386.htm.

31. American Melanoma Foundation statistics, 2005.

32. Beasley, D. et al. sunscreen makers sued for misleading health claims. Reuters UK, March 30, 2006.

33. Agredano, Y. et al. Accessibility to air travel correlates strongly with increasing

melanoma incidence. *Melanoma Res* 2006;16:77-81.

34. Westerdahl, J. et al. sunscreen use and malignant melanoma. *Intern J Cancer* 2000;87:145-50.

35. Giovannucci, E. et al. Prospective study of predictors of vitamin D status and cancer incidence and mortality in men. *J Natl Cancer Inst* 2006;98:451.

36. Ainsleigh, G. Beneficial effects of sun exposure on cancer mortality. *Preventive Medicine* 1993;22:132-140.

37. *The chemical sunscreen health disaster.* http://www.skinbiology.com/toxic sunscreens. html. Accessed September 2007.

38. Christophers, A. Melanoma is not caused by sunlight. M*utation Research/Fundamental and Molecular Mechanisms of Mutagenesis* 1998;422:113-17.

39. Reid Sexton and Louise Hall. Sunshine deficiency leads to vitamin D crisis. Sidney, Australia Morning Herald December 9, 2007.

40. van der Mei, I. et al. A high vitamin D insufficiency across Australian populations and latitude. *Environmental Health Perspect* 2007;115:1132-39.

41. Webb, A et al. Calculated ultraviolet exposure for a healthy vitamin D status. *Photochem Photobiol* 2006;82:1697-1703.

42. Turnbull, D. Midday shade boosts vitamin D. University of Southern Queensland press release Friday, December 14, 2007.

43. Grant, W. Roles of solar UV radiation and vitamin D in human health and how to obtain vitamin D. *Expert Rev Dermatol* 2007: pre-publication.

44. Samanek, A, et al. Estimates of beneficial and harmful sun exposure times during for major Australian population centres. *Med J Aust* 2006;184:338-41.

45. Grant, W. An ecologic study of cancer mortality rates in Spain with respect to indices of solar UVB irradiance and smoking. *Int J Cancer* 2007;120:1123-28.

46. Tuohimaa, P. et al. Does solar exposure as indicated by the non-melanoma skin cancers protect from solid cancers? Vitamin D as a possible explanation. *Eur J Cancer* 2007;43:1701-12.

47. Devesa, S. et al. *Atlas of Cancer Mortality in the United States,* 1950-1994. NIH publication 99-4564, 1999.

48. Grant, W. *Solar ultraviolet irradiance and cancer incidence and mortality.* Chapter 2. Edited by Jorg Reichrath, Landes Bioscience 2007.

49. Rhodes, A. Melanoma's public message. Guest editorial 2003;34.

50. Proposed Rules. *Federal Register* # 165. 2007;72: 49070.

51. Calafat, A. et al. Concentrations of the Sunscreen Agent, Benzophenone-3, in Residents of the United States: National Health and Nutrition Examination Survey 2003ñ2004. (available at http://dx.doi.org/).

52. Wolff, M. et al. Prenatal Phenol and Phthalate Exposures and Birth Outcomes. National Institutes of Health USA Department of Health and Human Services. doi:10.1289/ ehp.11007 (available at http://dx.doi.org/)

53. Environmental Working Group: Americans Carry Body Burden of Toxic Sunscreen Chemical. March 25, 2008. (available at http://www.ewg.org/node/26212).

54. Lau, C. et al. Lau C, Rogers JM. 2004. Embryonic and fetal programming of physiological disorders in adulthood. *Birth Defects Res C Embryo Today* 2004;72:300-12.

55. Bryden A. et al. 2006. Photopatch testing of 1155 patients: results of the U.K. multicentre photopatch group. *The British journal of dermatology* 155:737-47.

56. Rodriguez E, Valbuena MC, Rey M, Porras de Quintana L. 2006. Causal agents of photoallergic contact dermatitis diagnosed in the national institute of dermatology of Colombia. *Photodermatol Photoimmunol Photomed* 2006;22:189-92.

57. Hayden C. et al.. Systemic absorption of sunscreen after topical application. *Lancet* 1997:350:863-64.

58. Kunz P. et al. Comparison of in vitro and in vivo estrogenic activity of UV filters in fish. *Toxicol Sci* 2006:90:349-61.

59. Risheng, M. et al. UV Filters with Antagonistic Action at Androgen Receptors in the MDA-kb2 Cell Transcriptional-Activation Assay. *Toxicological Sciences* 2003;74:43-50.

60. Pickart, L. The Chemical Sunscreen Health Disaster. 2000-2008. (available at http://

www.skinbiology.com/toxicsunscreens.html)

61. Grant, W. Personal communication with author regarding pre-publication research.
62. Gorham, E. et al. Do sunscreens increase risk of melanoma in populations residing at higher latitudes? *Ann Epidemiol* 2007 ;17:956-63.
63. Garland, C. et al. Rising trends in melanoma. An hypothesis concerning sunscreen effectiveness. *Ann Epidemiol.* 1993 3:451.
64. Moan, J. et al. [Is UV-A a cause of malignant melanoma?]. Tidsskr Nor Laegeforen 1994; 114: 935-38
65. Setlow, R. Spectral regions contributing to melanoma: a personal view. *J Investig Dermatol Symp Proc.* 1999;4:46-9.
66. Brand, R. et al. Sunscreens containing physical UV blockers can increase transdermal absorption of pesticides. *Toxicol Ind Health.* 2003;19:9-16.
67. Pont, A. et al. Active ingredients in sunscreens act as topical penetration enhancers for the herbicide 2,4 dichlorophenoxyacetic acid. *Toxicol Appl Pharmacol.* 2004;195:348-54.
68. Osborne, J. Et al. Vitamin D and systemic cancer: is this relevant to malignant melanoma? *Br J Dermatol* 2002;147:197-213.

Chapter 6 Solar power and cancer-prevention mechanisms

1. Giovannucci, E. The epidemiology of vitamin D and colorectal cancer: Recent findings. *Curr Opin Gastroenterol* 2006;22:24-9.
2. Mathiasen, I. et al. Apoptosis induced by vitamin D compounds in breast cancer cells is inhibited by Bcl-2 but does not involve known caspases or p53. *Cancer Res.* 1999;59:4848-56.
3. Diaz, G. et al. Apoptosis is induced by the active metabolite of vitamin D_3 and its analogue EB1089 in colorectal adenoma and carcinoma cells: possible implications for prevention and therapy. *Cancer Res* 2000;60:2304-12.
4. Swamy, N. et al. Inhibition of proliferation and induction of apoptosis by 25-hydroxyvitamin D3-3beta-(2)-Bromoacetate, a nontoxic and vitamin D receptor-alkylating analog of 25-hydroxyvitamin D3 in prostate cancer cells. *Clin Cancer Res.* 2004;10:8018-27.
5. Miller, E. et l. Calcium, vitamin D, and apoptosis in the rectal epithelium. *Cancer Epidemiology Biomarkers & Prevention* 2005;14: 525-28.
6. Miyaura, C. et al. 1,25-dihydroxyvitamin D_3 induces differentiation of human myeloid leukemia cells. *Biochem Biophys Res Comm* 1981;102:937.
7. Suda, T. et al. Modulation of cell differentiation, immune responses and tumor promotion by vitamin D compounds. *Bone Min Res* 1986;4:1.
8. Tokar E, et al. Chemoprevention of prostate cancer by cholecalciferol (vitamin D3): 25-hydroxylase (CYP27A1) in human prostate epithelial cells. *Clin Exp Metastasis* 2005;22:265-73.
9. Niendorf A, et al. Effect of 1,25-dihydroxyvitamin D_3 on human colon cancer in vitro. *J Steroid Biochem* 1987;27: 825.
10. Lointier, P. et al. The role of vitamin D_3 in the proliferation of a human colon cancer cell line in vitro. *Anticancer Res* 1987;7:817.
11. Holt, P. et al. Colonic epithelial cell proliferation decreases with increasing levels of serum 25-hydroxy vitamin D. *Cancer Epidemiol Biomarkers Prev* 2002;11:113-9.
12. Chen, T. et al. The in vitro evaluation of 25-hydroxyvitamin D3 and 19-nor-1alpha,25-dihydroxyvitamin D2 as therapeutic agents for prostate cancer. *Clin Cancer Res* 2000;6:901-08 (invasiveness and proliferation).
13. Shokravi, M. et al. Vitamin D inhibits angiogenesis in transgenic murine retinoblastoma. *Inv Oph* 1995;36:83-7.
14. Mantell, D. et al. 1,25-Dihydroxyvitamin D_3 inhibits angiogenesis in vitro and in vivo. *Circulation Research.* 2000;87:214.
15. Nakagawa, K. et al. 22-Oxa-1{alpha},25-dihydroxyvitamin D3 inhibits metastasis and angiogenesis in lung cancer. *Carcinogenesis* 2005;26:1044-54.
16. Bao, B. et al. 1{alpha},25-dihydroxyvitamin D3 inhibits prostate cancer cell invasion via modulation of selective proteases. *Carcinogenesis* 2006;27:32-42.
17. Nakagawa, K. et al. 22-Oxa-1{alpha},25-dihydroxyvitamin D3 inhibits metastasis and

angiogenesis in lung cancer. *Carcinogenesis* 2005;26:1044-54.

18. Nakagawa K. et al. 1alpha,25-Dihydroxyvitamin D(3) is a preventive factor in the metastasis of lung cancer. *Carcinogenesis* 2005;26:429-40.

19. El Abdaimi, K. et al. The vitamin D analogue EB 1089 prevents skeletal metastasis and prolongs survival time in nude mice transplanted with human breast cancer cells. *Cancer Research* 2000;60:4412-4418.

20. Lokeshwar B. et al. Inhibition of prostate cancer metastasis in vivo: a comparison of 1,23-dihydroxyvitamin D (calcitriol) and EB1089. *Cancer Epidemiol Biomarkers Rev.* 1999;8:241-48.

21. Kremer, R. et al. Prevention of skeletal metastasis with the vitamin D analog EB1089: comparison with palmidronate therapy. Paper presented at the International Symposium on Predictive Oncology and Intervention Strategies; Paris, France; February 9 - 12, 2002. Available at http://www.cancerprev.org/Journal/Issues/26/101/1093/4556.

22. Weitsman, G. et al. Vitamin D sensitizes breast cancer cells to the action of H2O2: mitochondria as a convergence point in the death pathway. *Free Radic Biol Med* 2005 Jul 15;39(2):266-78.

23. Ravid, A. et al. The role of reactive oxygen species in the anticancer activity of vitamin D. *Recent Results Cancer Res* 2003;164:357-67.

24. Lappe, J. et al. Vitamin D and calcium supplementation reduces cancer risk: results of a randomized trial. *Am J Clin Nutr* 2007;85:1586ñ91.

25. Pilz S. et al. Low serum levels of 25-hydroxyviamin D predict fatal cancer in patients referred to coronary angiography. *Cancer Epidemiol Biomarkers Prev* May 2008; [Epub ahead of print].

26. Bao, B. et al. Protective role of 1a, 25-dihydroxyvitamin D3 against oxidative stress in nonmalignant human prostate epithelial cells. *The International Journal of Cancer* 2008;122, 2699-2706.

Chapter 7. Solar Power, breast Cancer and other women's cancers

1. Cancer Facts and Figures 2005. American Cancer Society.

2. Gorham, E. et al. Acid haze air pollution and breast and colon cancer mortality in 20 Canadian cities. *Can J Pub Health* 1989;80:96-100.

3. Garland, C et al. Geographic variation in breast cancer mortality in the United States: a hypothesis involving exposure to solar radiation. *Prev Med* 1990;19:614-22.

4. Gorham, E. et al. sunlight and breast cancer incidence in the USASR. *Int J Epidemiol* 1990;19:820-824.

5. Morabia, A. et al. Geographic variation in cancer incidence in the USASR: estimating the proportion of avoidable cancer. *Prev Med* 1992;21:151-161.

6. Grant W. An estimate of premature cancer mortality in the United States due to inadequate doses of solar ultraviolet-B radiation. *Cancer.* 2002;94,1867-75.

7. John, E. et al. Vitamin D and breast cancer risk: The HANES 1 epidemiologic follow-up study, 1971-1975 to 1992. *Cancer Epidemiology Biomarkers and Prevention* 1999;8:399-406.

8. Lowe L. et al. Plasma 25-hydroxy vitamin D concentrations, vitamin D receptor genotype and breast cancer risk in a UK Caucasian population. *Eur J Cancer* 2005;41:1164-699.

9. Bertone-Johnson E. et al. Plasma 25-hydroxyvitamin D and 1,25-dihydroxyvitamin D and risk of breast cancer. *Cancer Epidemiol Biomarkers Prev* 2005:8:1991-97.

10. Zinser G. et al. 1,24(S)-dihydroxyvitamin D2, an endogenous vitamin D2 metabolite, inhibits growth of breast cancer cells and tumors. *Anticancer Res* 2005;25:235-41.

11. Milliken E. et al. EB1089, a vitamin D receptor agonist, reduces proliferation and decreases tumor growth rate in a mouse model of hormone-induced mammary cancer. *Cancer Lett* 2005;229:205-15.

12. Wigington D. et al. Pamidronate and 1,24(S)-dihydroxyvitamin D2 synergistically inhibit the growth of myeloma, breast and prostate cancer cells. *Anticancer Res* 2005;3B:1909-17.

13. Grant, W. et al. Breast cancer—risk and reduction factors. SUNARC website, March 22, 2004.

14. Hoyer-Hansen M. et al. Vitamin D analog EB1089 triggers dramatic lysosomal changes and Beclin 1-mediated autophagic cell death. *Cell Death Differ* 2005;10:1297-1309.

15. Berube S. et al. Vitamin D and calcium intakes from food or supplements and mammographic breast density. *Cancer Epidemiol Biomarkers Prev* 2005;14:1653-59.

16. Weitsman G. et al. Vitamin D sensitizes breast cancer cells to the action of H2O2: mitochondria as a convergence point in the death pathway. *Free Radic Biol Med.* 2005;39:266-78.

17. Lipkin, M. et al. Vitamin D, Calcium and Prevention of Breast Cancer: A Review. *J American Coll Nutr* 1999;18: 392S-397S.

18. Robsahm, T. et al. Vitamin D3 from sunlight may improve the prognosis of breast, colon-and prostate cancer. *Cancer Causes Control.* 2004;15:149-58.

19. Blask, D. et al. Growth and fatty acid metabolism of human breast cancer (MCF-7) xenografts in nude rats: impact of constant light-induced nocturnal melatonin suppression. *Breast Cancer Res Treat* 2003;79:313-20.

20. Lefkowitz, F. et al. sunlight, vitamin D and ovarian cancer mortality rates in USA women. *Int J Epidemiol* 1994;23:1133-36.

21. Grant, W. An estimate of premature cancer mortality in the USA because of inadequate doses of solar ultraviolet-B radiation. *Cancer.* 2002;94:1867-75.

22. Freedman, D. et al. sunlight and mortality from breast, ovarian, colon, prostate, and nonmelanoma skin cancer: a composite death certificate based case-control study. *Occup Environ Med* 2002;59:257-62.

23. Grant, W. Ecologic studies of solar UVB radiation and cancer mortality rates. *Recent Results Cancer Res* 2003:164:371-77.

24. Salazar-Martinez E. et al. Nutritional determinants of epithelial ovarian cancer risk: a case-control study in Mexico. *Oncology.* 2002;63:151-57.

25. Salazar-Martinez E. et al. Dietary factors and endometrial cancer risk. Results of a case-control study in Mexico. *Int J Gynecol Cancer* 2005;15:938-45.

26. Megdal, S. et al. Night work and breast cancer risk: a systematic review and meta-analysis. *Eur J Cancer* 2005;41:2023-32.

27. Schernhammer, E. et al. Night work and risk of breast cancer. *Epidemiology* 2006;17:108-11.

28. Garland, C. et al. Geographic variation in breast cancer mortality in the United States: a hypothesis involving exposure to solar radiation. *Prev Med* 1990;19:614-22.

29. Garland, C. Paper presented to the 97th Annual Meeting of the American Association for Cancer Research, April 4, 2006, abstract # 4008.

30. Knight, J. Paper presented at the 97th Annual Meeting of the American Association for Cancer Research, April 4, 2006, abstract # 4009.

31. Lim, H. et al. Cancer survival is dependent on season of diagnosis and sunlight exposure. *Int J Cancer* 2006 May 2. Epublication ahead of print.

32. Mohr, S. et al. Is ultraviolet B irradiance inversely associated with incidence rates of endometrial cancer? An ecological study of 107 countries. *Preventive Medicine* article in press, November 2007.

33. Lappe, J. et al. Vitamin D and calcium supplementation reduces cancer risk: results of a randomized trial. *Am J Clin Nutr* 2007;85:1586–91.

34. Garland, C et al. What is the dose-response relationship between vitamin D and cancer risk? *Nutrition Reviews* 2007;65:S91-5.

35. Knight J. et al. Vitamin D and reduced risk of breast cancer: a population-based case-control study.

36. Abbas, S. et al. Serum 25 hydroxyvitamin D and risk of postmenopausal breast cancer—results of a large case-control study. *Carcinogenesis* 2007. Oct. 31 [Epub ahead of print].

37. Garland, C. et al. Vitamin D and prevention of breast cancer: pooled analysis. *J steroid Biocem & Molecular Biology* 2006 Pre-publication.

38. Brisson, J. et al. Synchronized seasonal variations of mammographic breast density and

plasma 25-hydroxyvitamin D . *Cancer Epidemiol Biomarkers Prev 2007;16:929-33.*

39. Goodwin, P. et al. Pre-publication announcement by American Society of Oncology, May 15, 2008

40. Sharif B. Mohr, MPH, Cedric F. Garland, Dr. PH, Edward D. Gorham, MPH, PhD, William B. Grant, PhD, and Frank C. Garland, PhD, . Relationship between Low Ultraviolet B Irradiance and Higher Breast Cancer Risk in 107 Countries. *The Breast Journal*, 2008;14:255–60.

41. Ferlay J, et al. GLOBOCAN 2002: cancer incidence, mortality and prevalence worldwide: IARC Cancer-Base No. 5.

Chapter 8. sunlight, vitamin D and prostate cancer

1. John, E. et al. sun exposure, vitamin D receptor polymorphisms and risk of advanced prostate cancer. *Cancer Res* 2005;65:5479.

2. Schwartz, G. et al. Prostate Cancer and skin pigmentation: a case-control study. *J Urol* 1993;149:396A.

3. Weinrich, S. et al. Low sun exposure and elevated serum prostate specific antigen in African American and Caucasian men. *AM J Health Stud* 2001;17:148-55.

4. Freedman, D. et al. sunlight and mortality from breast, ovarian, colon, prostate and non-melanoma skin cancer: a composite death certificate based case-control study. *Occup environ Med* 2002;59:257-62.

5. Hanchette, C. et al. Geographic patterns of prostate cancer mortality: Evidence for a protective effect of ultraviolet radiation. *Cancer* 1992;70:2861-69

6. Schwartz, G. et al. Is vitamin D deficiency a risk factor for prostate cancer? [hypothesis] *Anticancer Res* 1990;10:1307-11.

7. John, E. et al. Residential sunlight exposure is associated with a decreased risk of prostate cancer. *J Steroid Biochem Mol Biol* 2004;89:-90.

8. Luscombe, C. et al. Exposure to ultraviolet radiation: association with susceptibility and age at presentation with prostate cancer. *Lancet* 2001;358:641–42.

9. Moon, S. et al. Ultraviolet radiation: effects on risks of prostate and other internal cancers. *Mutat Res* 2005; 571:207–219.

10. Bodiwala, D. et al. Prostate cancer risk and exposure to ultraviolet radiation: further support for the protective effect of sunlight. *Cancer Lett* 2003;192:145-49.

11. Robsahm, T. et al. Vitamin D3 from sunlight may improve the prognosis of breast-, colon- and prostate cancer (Norway). *Cancer Causes Control* 2004;15:149-58.

12. Schwartz, G. et al. Is vitamin D deficiency a risk factor for prostate cancer? [hypothesis]. *Anticancer Res* 1990;10:1307-11.

13. Tuohimaa P. et al. Both high and low levels of blood vitamin D are associated with a higher prostate cancer risk: a longitudinal, nested case-control study in the Nordic countries. *Int J Cancer.* 2004;108:104-8.

14. Feskanich, D. et al. Vitamin A intake and hip fractures among postmenopausal women. *JAMA.* 2002;287:47-54.

15. Ikezoe T. et al. CCAAT/enhancer-binding protein delta: a molecular target of 1,25-dihydroxyvitamin D3 in androgen-responsive prostate cancer LNCaP cells. *Cancer Res.* 2005;65:4762-68.

16. Wigington D. et al. Pamidronate and 1,24(S)-dihydroxyvitamin D2 synergistically inhibit the growth of myeloma, breast and prostate cancer cells. *Anticancer Res.* 2005;25:1909-17.

17. Lokeshwar, B. et al. Inhibition of prostate cancer metastasis in vivo: a comparison of 1,25-Dihydroxyvitamin D (Calcitriol) and EB1089. *Cancer Epidemiol Biomarkers Prev.* 1999;8:241–48

18. Schwartz, G. et al. 1a25-Dihydroxyvitamin D (calcitriol) inhibits the invasiveness of human prostate cancer cells. *Cancer Epidemiol. Biomarkers Prev.* 1997;6:727–32.

19. Bao, B. et al. 1alpha,25-dihydroxyvitamin D3 inhibits prostate cancer cell invasion via modulation of selective proteases. *Carcinogenesis.* 2006;27:32.

20. Majeski, S. et al. Vitamin D is a potent inhibitor of tumor cell induced angiogenesis. *J*

Investig Dermatol Symp Proc 1996;1, 97–101.

21. Miller, G. et al. The human prostatic carcinoma cell line LNCaP expresses biologically active specific receptors for 1 alpha, 25-dihydroxyvitamin D3. *Cancer Res.* 1992;52:515–20.

22. Blutt, S. et al. Calcitriol-induced apoptosis in LNCaP cells is blocked by overexpression of Bcl-2. *Endocrinology* 2000;141:10–17.

23. Woo, T. et al. Pilot study: potential role of nutrient vitamin D (cholecalciferol) in patients with isolated PSA relapse after definitive therapy. *Nutr Cancer* 2005;51:32-36.

24. Beer, T. et al. High-dose weekly oral calcitriol in patients with a rising PSA after prostatectomy or radiation for prostate carcinoma. *Cancer.* 2003;97:1217-24.

25. Schwartz, G. Vitamin D and the epidemiology of prostate cancer. *Semin Dial* 2005;18:276-89.

26. Sakr, W. et al. The frequency of carcinoma and intraepithelial neoplasia of the prostate in young adult patients. *J Urol* 1993;150:379-85.

27. Breslow, N. et al. Latent carcinoma of the prostate at autopsy in seven areas. The International Agency for Research on Cancer, Lyons, France. *Int J Cancer* 1977;20:680-88.

28. Yatani, R. et al. Geographic pathology of latent prostate carcinoma. *Int J Cancer* 1884;29:611-16.

29. Bell, N. et al. Evidence for alteration of the vitamin D-endocrine system in Blacks. *J Clin Invest* 1985;76:470-73.

30. Nakamura, K. et al. Fish as a major source of vitamin D in the Japanese diet. *Nutrition* 18;2002:415-16.

31. Takeuchi, A. et al. High-performance liquid chromatographic determination of vitamin D3 in fish liver oils and eel body oils. *J Nutr Sci Vitaminol* (Tokyo) 1984;30:421-30.

32. Nakamura, K. et al. Serum 25-hydroxyvitamin D levels in active women of middle and advanced age in a rural community in Japan. *Nutrition* 1999;15:870-73.

33. Nakamura, K. et al. Serum 25-hydroxyvitamin D concentration and related dietary factors in peri- and postmenopausal Japanese women. *Am J Clin Nutr* 2000;71:1161-65.

34. Ewings, P. et al. A case-control study of cancer of the prostate in Somerset and East Devon. *Br J Cancer* 1996;74:661-66.

35. Engeset, D. et al. Fish consumption and breast cancer risk. The European Prospective Investigation into Cancer and Nutrition (EPIC). *Int J Cancer* 2006. E publication ahead of print.

36. American Cancer Society Statistics, 2005.

37. Grant, W. et al. Comparisons of estimated economic burdens due to insufficient solar ultraviolet irradiance and vitamin D and excess solar UV irradiance for the United States. *Photochem Photobiol* 2005;81:1276-86.

38. Grant, W. et al. Benefits and requirements of vitamin D for optimal health: a review. *Altern Med Rev* 2005;10:94-111.

39. Grant, W. Lower vitamin-D production from solar ultraviolet-B irradiance may explain some differences in cancer survival rates. *JNMA* 2006;98:364.

40. Giovannucci, E. et al. Prospective study of predictors of vitamin D status and cancer incidence and mortality in men. *J Natl Cancer Inst* 2006;98:451.

41. Lagunova, Z. et al. Prostate cancer survival is dependent on season of diagnosis. *The Prostate* 2007;9999:1-9.

42. Schwartz, G. et al. UV, latitude, and spatial trends in prostate-cancer mortality: all sunlight is not the same. *Cancer Causes Control* 2006;8:1092-1101.

43. Skinner, H et al. Vitamin D intake and the risk for pancreatic cancer in two cohort studies. *Cancer Epidemiol Biomarkers Prev* 2006;15:1688-95.

44. Touhimma, P. et al. Interactions of factors related to the metabolic syndrome and vitamin D on risk of Prostate Cancer. *Cancer Epidemiol Biomarkers Prev* 2007;16:302-7.

45. Li, H. et al. A Prospective Study of Plasma vitamin D metabolites, vitamin D receptor polymorphisms and prostate cancer. *PLoS Med.* 2007;4:e103.

46. Beer, T. Double –Blinded randomized study of high-dose calcitriol plus docetaxel vompared with placebo plus docetaxel in androgen-independent prostate cancer: a report

from the ASCENT investigators. *J Clin Oncol* 2007;20:669-74.

47. Bao, B. et al. 1alpha, 25 hydroxyvitamin D3 inhibits prostate cancer cell invasion via modulation of selective proteases. *Carcinogenesis* 2006;27:32.

48. Forsmo, S. et al. Childhood cod liver oil consumption and bone mineral density in a population-based cohort of peri-and postmenopausal women. *Am* J *Epidemiol* 2008;167:406-11.

49. Bao, B. et al. Protective role of 1a, 25-dihydroxyvitamin D3 against oxidative stress in nonmalignant human prostate epithelial cells. *The International Journal of Cancer* 2008;122, 2699-2706.

Chapter 9. Solar Power, colon cancer and other internal cancers

1.   Platz, E. et al. Plasma 1,25-dihydroxy- and 25-hydroxyvitamin D and adenomatous polyps of the distal colorectum. *Cancer Epidemiol Biomarkers Prev* 2000; 9:1059-65.

2.   Peters, U. et al. Vitamin D, calcium, and vitamin D receptor polymorphism in colorectal adenomas. *Cancer Epidemiol Biomarkers Prev* 2001;10:1267.

3.   Peters, U. et al. Circulating vitamin D metabolites, polymorphism in vitamin D receptor, and colorectal adenoma risk. *Cancer Epidemiol Biomarkers Prev* 2004;13:546-52.

4.   McCullough, M. et al. Calcium, vitamin D, dairy products, and risk of colorectal cancer in the Cancer Prevention Study II Nutrition Cohort (United States). *Cancer Causes Control* 2003;14:1-12.

5.   Grau, M. et al. Vitamin D, calcium supplementation, and colorectal adenomas: results of a randomized trial. *J Natl Cancer Inst.* 2003;95:1765-71.

6.   Tangrea, J. et al. Serum levels of vitamin D metabolites and the subsequent risk of colon and rectal cancer in Finnish men. *Cancer Causes Control* 1997;8:615-25.

7.   Feskanich D. et al. Plasma vitamin D metabolites and risk of colorectal cancer in women. *Cancer Epidemiol Biomarkers Prev* 2004;13:1502-08.

8.   Garland, C. et al. Serum 25-hydroxyvitamin D and colon cancer: eight-year prospective study. *Lancet* 1989;2:1176-78.

9.   Garland, C. et al. The role of vitamin D in cancer prevention9. *Am J Pub Health* 2006;96:252-61.

10. Feskanich, D. et al. Plasma vitamin D metabolites and risk of colorectal cancer in women. *Cancer Epidemiol Biomarkers Prev* 2004;13:1502-08.

11. Spina, C. et al. Colon cancer and solar ultraviolet B radiation and prevention and treatment of colon cancer in mice with vitamin D and its Gemini analogs. *J Steroid Biochem Mol Biol.* 2005;97:111-20.

12. Tangpricha, V. et al. Vitamin D deficiency enhances the growth of MC-26 colon cancer xenografts in Balb/c mice. *J Nutr* 2005 Oct;135(10):2350-4.

13. Huerta, S. et al. 1alpha,25-(OH)(2)-D(3) and its synthetic analogue decrease tumor load in the Apc(min) Mouse. *Cancer Res* 2002;62:741-46.

14. Gorham, E. et al. Vitamin D and prevention of colorectal cancer. *J Steroid Biochem Molecular Biol* 2005;97:179–94.

15. Garland, C. et al. Do sunlight and vitamin D reduce the likelihood of colon cancer? *Int. J. Epidemiol* 1980;9:227–31.

16. Mizoue, T. et al. Ecological study of solar radiation and cancer mortality in Japan. *Health Phys* 2004;87:532-38.

17. Moan, J. et al. Solar radiation, vitamin D and survival rate of colon cancer in Norway. *J Photochem Photobiol B* 2005;78:189-93.

18. Chao, A. Meat consumption and risk of colorectal cancer. *JAMA* 2005;293:172-82.

19. Larsson, S. et al. Red meat consumption and risk of cancers of the proximal colon, distal colon and rectum: the Swedish Mammography Cohort. *Int J Cancer* 2005;113:829-34.

20. Norat, T. et al. Meat, fish, and colorectal cancer risk: the European Prospective Investigation into cancer and nutrition. *J Natl Cancer Inst* 2005;97:906.

21. English, D. et al. Red meat, chicken, and fish consumption and risk of colorectal cancer. *Cancer Epidemiol Biomarkers Prev* 2004;13:1509-14.

22. Luchtenborg, M. et al. Meat and fish consumption, APC gene mutations and hMLH1

expression in colon and rectal cancer: a prospective cohort study (The Netherlands). *Cancer Causes Control* 2005;16:1041-54.

23. Grant, W. Risk and risk reduction factors for colon cancer. UVB/vitamin D and colorectal cancer essay. Available at http://www. SUNARC.org./colorectalcan402.htm.

24. Appleton, B. et al. Inhibition of aflatoxin-initiated preneoplastic liver lesions by low dietary proteins. *Nutr Cancer* 1982;3:200-06.

25. Dunaif, G. et al. Relative contribution of dietary protein level and aflatoxin B$_1$ dose in generation of presumptive preneoplastic foci in rat liver. *J Natl Cancer Inst* 1987;78:365-69.

26. Youngman, L. et al. High-protein intake promotes the growth of preneoplastic foci in Fischer #344 rats: evidence that early remodeled foci retain the potential for future growth. *J Nutr* 1991;121:1454-61.

27. Youngman, L. et al. Inhibition of aflatoxin B$_1$-induced gamma-glutamyl transpeptidase positive (GGT+) hepatic preneoplastic foci and tumors by low protein diets: evidence that altered GGT+ foci indicate neoplastic potential. *Carcinogenesis* 1992;13:1607-13.

28. Dunaif, G. et al. Dietary protein level and aflatoxin B1-induced preneoplastic hepatic lesions in the rat. *J Nutr.* 1987;117:1298-302.

29. Horio, F. et al. Thermogenesis, low-protein diets, and decreased development of AFB1-induced preneoplastic foci in rat liver. *Nutr Cancer.* 1991;16:31-41.

30. Campbell, T. The China Study. Benbella Books 2005.

31. Singh, P. et al. Dietary risk factors for colon cancer in a low-risk population. *Am J Epidemiol* 1998;148:761-74.

32. Grant, W. Risk and risk reduction factors for colon cancer. *UVB/vitamin D and colorectal cancer essay.* Available at http://www. SUNARC.org./colorectalcan402.htm.

33. Grant, W. An estimate of premature cancer mortality in the USA due to inadequate doses of solar ultraviolet-B radiation. *Cancer* 2002;94:1867-75.

34. Kawa, S. et al. Inhibitory effect of 22-oxa-1,25-dihydroxyvitamin D3, maxacalcitol, on the proliferation of pancreatic cancer cell lines. *J Steroid Biochem Mol Biol* 2005;97:173-77.

35. Schwartz, G. et al. Pancreatic cancer cells express 25-hydroxyvitamin D-1 alpha-hydroxylase and their proliferation is inhibited by the prohormone 25-hydroxyvitamin D3. *Carcinogenesis* 2004;25:1015-26.

36. Kawa, S. et al. Inhibitory effect of 220-oxa-1,25-dihydroxyvitamin D3 on the proliferation of pancreatic cancer cell lines. *Gastroenterology* 1996;110:1605-13.

37. Albrechtsson, E. et al. Vitamin D receptor is expressed in pancreatic cancer cells and a vitamin D3 analogue decreases cell number. *Pancreatology* 2003;3:41-6.

38. Kaewsakhorn, T. et al. Effects of calcitriol, seocalcitol, and medium-chain triglyceride on a canine transitional cell carcinoma cell line. *Anticancer Res* 2005;25:2689-96.

39. Konety, B. et al. Effects of vitamin D (calcitriol) on transitional cell carcinoma of the bladder in vitro and in vivo. *J Urol* 2001;165:253-8.

40. Heuch, J. et al. Risk of primary childhood brain tumors related to birth characteristics: a Norwegian prospective study. *Int J Cancer* 1998;77:498-503.

41. McNally, R. et al. An infectious aetiology for childhood brain tumors? Evidence from space-time clustering and seasonality analyses. *Br J Cancer* 2002;86:1070-77.

42. Brenner, A. et al. Season of birth and risk of brain tumors in adults. *Neurology* 2004;63:276-81.

43. Eyles, D. et al. Vitamin D3 and brain development. *Neuroscience* 2003;118:641-53.

44. Ko, P. et al. Maternal vitamin D3 deprivation and the regulation of apoptosis and cell cycle during rat brain development. *Brain Res Dev Brain Res* 2004;153:61-8.

45. Naveilhan, P. et al. Induction of glioma cell death by 1,25(OH)2 vitamin D3: towards an endocrine therapy of brain tumors? *J Neurosci Res* 1994;37:271-77.

46. Fujioka, T. et al. Prevention of renal cell carcinoma by active vitamin D3. *World J Surg* 2000;24:1205-10.

47. Suzuki, T, et al. 1,25-Dihydroxyvitamin D3 suppresses gene expression of eukaryotic translation initiation factor 2 in human promyelocytic leukemia HL-60 cells. *Cell Struct Funct* 2005;30:1-6.

48. Luong QT, et al. Vitamin D compounds in leukemia. *J Steroid Biochem Mol Biol.* 2005;97:195-202.

49. Sharabani, H. et al. Cooperative antitumor effects of vitamin D(3) derivatives and rosemary preparations in a mouse model of myeloid leukemia. Int J Cancer. 2006;118:3012-21.

50. Ikezoe T. et al. HIV-1 protease inhibitor ritonavir potentiates the effect of 1,25-dihydroxyvitamin D(3) to induce growth arrest and differentiation of human myeloid leukemia cells via down-regulation of CYP24. *Leuk Res* 2006 Jan 30 [Epub ahead of print].

51. Bastie J. et al. Cooperative action of 1alpha,25-dihydroxyvitamin D3 and retinoic acid in NB4 acute promyelocytic leukemia cell differentiation is transcriptionally controlled. *Exp Cell Res* 2005;310:319-30.

52. Jung, S. et al. 1,25(OH)2-16ene-vitamin D3 is a potent antileukemic agent with low potential to cause hypercalcemia. *Leuk. Res.* 1994;18:453-63.

53. Zhou, W. et al. Vitamin D is associated with improved survival in early-stage non-small cell lung cancer patients. *Cancer Epidemiol Biomarkers Prev* 2005;14(10):2303-09.

54. Nakagawa, K. et al. 22-Oxa-1alpha,25-dihydroxyvitamin D3 inhibits metastasis and angiogenesis in lung cancer. *Carcinogenesis* 2005;26:1044-54.

55. Nakagawa, K. et al. 1 alpha,25-Dihydroxyvitamin D(3) is a preventive factor in the metastasis of lung cancer. *Carcinogenesis* 2005;26:429-40.

56. Smedby, K. et al. Ultraviolet Radiation Exposure and Risk of Malignant Lymphomas. *JNCI* 2005;97:199-209.

57. Porojnicu, A. et al. Season of diagnosis is a prognostic factor in Hodgkin's lymphoma: a possible role of sun-induced vitamin D. *Br J Cancer* 2005;5;93:571-74.

58. Grant, W. Ecological Study of Dietary and Smoking Links to Lymphoma. *Altern Med Rev* 2000;5:563-562.

59. Wigington, D. et al. Pamidronate and 1,24(S)-dihydroxyvitamin D2 synergistically inhibit the growth of myeloma, breast and prostate cancer cells. *Anticancer Res* 2005;25:1909-17.

60. Grant, W. Lower vitamin-D production from solar ultraviolet-B irradiance may explain some differences in cancer survival rates. *J Natl Med Assoc* 2006;98:357-64.

61. Giovannucci, E. et al. Prospective study of predictors of vitamin D status and cancer incidence and mortality in men. *J Natl Cancer Inst* 2006;98:451.

62. Cancer Facts and Figures 2005, American Cancer Society.

63. Grant, W. Ecologic studies of solar UVB radiation and cancer mortality rates. *Recent Results Cancer Res* 2003;164:371-77.

64. Ainsleigh, G. Beneficial effects of sun exposure on cancer mortality. *Preventive medicine* 1993;22:132-140.

65. Adami, H. et al Primary and secondary prevention in the reduction of cancer morbidity and mortality. *Eur J Cancer* 2001;37:S118-127.

66. Vieth, R. Personal communication with author.

67. Garland, C et al. What is the dose-response relationship between vitamin D and cancer risk? *Nutrition Reviews* 2007;65:S91-5.

68. Otani, T. et al. Plasma vitamin D and risk of colorectal cancer: the Japan Public Health Center Based Prospective Study. *Br J Cancer* 2007;6:446-51.

69. Mohr, S. et al. Could Ultraviolet B irradiance and vitamin D be associated with lower incidence of lung cancer? *J Epidemiol community Health* 2008;62:69-74.

70. Porojnicu, A. et al. Seasonal and geographical variations in lung cancer prognosis in Norway. *Lung Cancer* Nov 2006 pre-publication document.

71. Zhou, W. et al. Circulating 25-hydroxyvitamin D levels predict survival in early-stage non-small-cell lung cancer patients. *J Clin Oncology* 2007;25:479-85.

72. Mohr, S. et al. Are low ultraviolet B and high-animal-protein intake associated with risk of renal cancer? *Int J Cancer* 2006.Pre-publicattion paper.

73. Gorham, E. et al. Optimal vitamin D status for colorectal cancer prevention: a quantitative meta analysis. *Am J Prev Med* 2007;32:210-16.

74. Emory University (2008, April 14). Vitamin D And Calcium Influence Cell Death In

The Colon, Researchers Find. *Science Daily*. Retrieved May 2, 2008, from http://www. sciencedaily.com /releases/2008/04/080413161052.htm.

75. Grant, W. Personal communication with author, June 2, 2008.
76. Regulska, M. et al. Inhibitory effects of 1,25-dihydroxyvitamin D3 and its low-calcemic analogues on staurosporine-induced apoptosis. *Pharmacol Rep* 2007;59:393-401.
77. van Ginkel, P. et al. 1 alpha-Hydroxyvitamin D2 inhibits growth of human neuroblastoma. *J Neurooncol* 2007;85:255-62.
78. Shokravi, M. et al. Vitamin D inhibits angiogenesis in transgenic murine retinoblastoma. *Inv Oph* 1995;36:83-7.
79. Albert, D. et al. Vitamin D analogs, a new treatment for retinoblastoma: The first Ellsworth Lecture. *Ophthalmic Genet* 2002;23:137-56.

Chapter 10. Boning up: Solar Power, osteoporosis, arthritis and pain.

1. Lips, P. et al. Vitamin D physiology. *Prog Biophys Mol Biol* 2006; Feb 28: Epub ahead of print.
2. McGowan, J. National Institutes of Health 2003.
3. National Alliance for Nutrition and Activity 2005 statistics.
4. Abelow, B. et al. Cross-cultural association between dietary animal protein and hip fracture: a hypothesis. *Calcif Tissue Int* 1992;50:14-18.
5. Frassetto, L. et al. Worldwide incidence of hip fracture in elderly women: Relation to consumption of animal and vegetable foods. *J Gerontol* 2000;55A:M583-92.
6. Fourteen studies cited in Sorenson, M. *Megahealth*. Evans Publishing, NY 1995 pp 177-79.
7. Zemel, M. et al. Calcium utilization: effect of varying level and source of dietary protein. *Am J Clin Nutr* 1988;48:880-83.
8. Sherman, H. Calcium requirements of maintenance in man. *J Biol Chem* 1920;4:21-27.
9. Breslau, N. et al. Relationship of animal protein-rich diet to kidney stone formation and calcium metabolism. *J Clin Endocrinol Metab* 1988;66:140.
10. Langman, C. et al. Calcitriol Metabolism during chronic metabolic acidosis. *Semin Nephrol* 1989;9:65-71.
11. Javaid, M. et al. Maternal vitamin D status during pregnancy and childhood bone mass at age 9 years: a longitudinal study. *Lancet* 2006;367:36–43.
12. Hosking, D. Calcium homeostasis in pregnancy. *Clin Endocrinol (Oxf)* 1996;45:1–6.
13. Zamora, S. et al. Long-term effect of early vitamin-D supplementation on bone mineral status in prematurely born infants. *J Pediatr Gastroenterol Nutr* 2000;31:94.
14. Zamora, S. et al. Vitamin D supplementation during infancy is associated with higher bone mineral mass in prepubertal girls. *J Clin Endocrinol Metab* 1999;84:4541-44.
15. Sowers, M. et al. Lower peak bone mass and its decline. *Baillieres Best Pract Res Clin Endocrinol Metab* 2000;14:317–29.
16. Vieth, R. et al. Age-related changes in the 25-hydroxyvitamin D *versus* parathyroid hormone relationship suggest a different reason why older adults require more vitamin D. *J Clin Endocrinol Metab* 2005;88;185-91.
17. Hollis, B. Circulating 25-hydroxyvitamin D levels indicative of vitamin D sufficiency: implications for establishing a new effective dietary intake recommendation for vitamin D. *J Nutr.* 2005;135:317-22.
18. Sato, Y. et al. Amelioration of osteoporosis and hypovitaminosis D by sunlight exposure in stroke patients. *Neurology* 2003;61:338-42.
19. Nguyen, T. et al. Prediction of osteoporotic fractures by postural instability and bone density. *BMJ* 1993;307:1111-15.
20. Sato, Y. et al. Amelioration of osteoporosis and hypovitaminosis d by sunlight exposure in hospitalized, elderly women with Alzheimer's disease: a randomized controlled trial. *J Bone Miner Res.* 2005;20:1327-33.
21. Tangpricha, V. et al. Tanning is associated with optimal vitamin D status (serum 25-hydroxyvitamin D concentration) and higher bone mineral density. *Am J Clin Nutr* 2004;80:1645-49.

22. Warthan, M. et al UV light tanning as a type of substance-related disorder. *Arch Dermatol* 2005;141:963-96.

23. Feldman, S. et al. Ultraviolet exposure is a reinforcing stimulus in frequent indoor tanners. *J Am Acad Dermatol* 2004;51:45-51.

24. Sato, Y. et al. Low-dose vitamin D prevents muscular atrophy and reduces falls and hip fractures in women after stroke: a randomized controlled trial. *Cerebrovasc Dis* 2005;20:187-92.

25. Trivedi, D. et al. Effect of four monthly oral vitamin D3 (cholecalciferol) supplementations on fractures and mortality in men and women living in the community: randomized double blind controlled trial. *BMJ* 2003;326:469.

26. Siffledeen, J. et al. Randomized trial of etidronate plus calcium and vitamin D for treatment of low bone mineral density in Crohn's disease. *Clin Gastroenterol Hepatol* 2005;3:122-32.

27. Bischoff-Ferrari, H. et al. Positive association between 25-hydroxy vitamin D levels and bone mineral density: A population-based study of younger and older adults. *Am J Med* 2004;116:634-39.

28. Hollis B. Circulating 25-hydroxyvitamin D levels indicative of vitamin D sufficiency: implications for establishing a new effective dietary intake recommendation for vitamin D. *J Nutr* 2005;135:317-22.

29. Bischoff-Ferrari, H. et al. Fracture prevention with vitamin D supplementation: a meta-analysis of randomized controlled trials. *JAMA* 2005;293:2257.

30. Bischoff-Ferrari, H. et al. Higher 25-hydroxyvitamin D concentrations are associated with better lower-extremity function in both active and inactive persons aged 60 y. *Am J Clin Nutr* 2004;80:752-58.

31. Gallagher, J. et al. Treatment of postmenopausal osteoporosis with high doses of synthetic calcitriol: A randomized, controlled study. *Ann Intern Med* 1990;113:649-55.

32. Chapuy, M. et al. Combined calcium and vitamin D3 supplementation in elderly women: confirmation of reversal of secondary hyperparathyroidism and hip fracture risk: The Decalyos II Study. *Osteoporosis Int* 2002;13:257-64.

33. Tilyard, M. et al. Treatment of postmenopausal osteoporosis with calcitriol or calcium. *N Engl J Med* 1992;326:357-62.

34. Chapuy, M. et al. Vitamin D3 and calcium to prevent hip fractures in elderly women. *N Engl J Med* 1992;327:1637-42.

35. Dawson-Hughes, B. et al. Effect of calcium and vitamin D supplementation in bone density of men and women 65 years of age or older. *N Engl J Med* 1997;337:670-76.

36. Chen, J. et al. 1-alpha- Vitamin Hydroxyvitamin D3 treatment decreases bone turnover and modulates calcium-regulating hormones in early postmenopausal women. *Bone* 1997;20:557-62.

37. Feskanich, D. et al. Calcium, vitamin D, milk consumption, and hip fractures: a prospective study among postmenopausal women. *Am J Clin Nutr* 2003;77:504-11.

38. Heaney, R. et al. Calcium Absorption Varies within the Reference Range for Serum 25-Hydroxyvitamin D. *J Am Coll Nutr* 2003;22:142-46.

39. Trivedi, D. et al. Effect of four monthly oral vitamin D_3 (cholecalciferol) supplementation on fractures and mortality in men and women living in the community: randomized double blind controlled trial. *BMJ* 2003;326:469.

40. Heaney, R. et al. Long-latency deficiency disease: Insights from calcium and vitamin D. *Am J Clin Nutr* 2003;78:912-19.

41. Holick, M. et al. The vitamin D epidemic and its health consequences. *J Nutr* 2005;135:2739S-48S.

42. Sahibzada, A. et al. Presentation of osteomalacia in Kohistani women. *J Ayub Med Coll Abbottabad* 2004;16:63-5.

43. Rajeswari, J. et al. Aetiology and clinical profile of osteomalacia in adolescent girls in northern India. *Natl Med J India* 2003;16:139-42.

44. Al-Jurayyan, N. et al. Nutritional rickets and osteomalacia in school children and adolescents. *Saudi Med J* 2002;23:182-85.

45. Narchi, H. et al. Case-control study of diet and sun exposure in adolescents with

symptomatic rickets. *Ann Trop Pediatr* 2000;20:217-21.

46. Holick, M. The UV advantage. Ibooks Inc. New York, 2003. p 87.

47. Janssen, H. et al. Vitamin D deficiency, muscle function, and falls in elderly people. *Am J Clin Nutr* 2002;75:611–15.

48. Bischoff-Ferrari, H. et al. Higher 25-hydroxyvitamin D concentrations are associated with better lower-extremity function in both active and inactive persons aged >60 y. *Am J Clin Nutr* 2004;80:752-58.

49. Bischoff-Ferrari, H. et al. Effect of cholecalciferol plus calcium on falling in ambulatory older men and women. *Arch Intern Med* 2006;166:424-430.

50. Bischoff-Ferrari, H. et al. Is fall prevention by vitamin D mediated by a change in postural or dynamic balance? *Osteoporosis Int.* 2006;17:656-63.

51. Van Veldhuiszen, P. et al. Treatment of vitamin D deficiency in patients with metastatic prostate cancer may improve bone pain and muscle strength. *J Urol* 2000;163:187-90.

52. Prabhala, A. et al. Severe myopathy associated with vitamin D deficiency in western New York. Arch Intern Med 2000;160:1199-1203.

53. Katz, W. et al. Musculoskeletal pain and its socioeconomic implications. *Clin Rheumatol* 2002;21 Suppl 1:S2-4.

54. Walch, J. et al. The effect of sunlight on postoperative analgesic medication use: a prospective study of patients undergoing spinal surgery. *Psychosom Med* 2005;67:156-63.

55. Plotnikoff, G. et al. Prevalence of severe hypovitaminosis D in patients with persistent, nonspecific musculoskeletal pain. *Mayo Clin Proc* 2003;78:1463-70.

56. Gordon, C. et al. Prevalence of vitamin D deficiency among healthy adolescents. *Arch Pediatr Adolesc Med.* 2004;158:531-37.

57. Macfarlane, G. et al. An excess of widespread pain among South Asians: are low levels of vitamin D implicated? *Ann Rheum Dis* 2005;64:1217-19.

58. Kaur, M. et al. Indoor tanning relieves pain. *Photodermatol Photoimmunol Photomed* 2005;21:278.

59. McAlindon, T. et al. Relation of dietary intake and serum levels of vitamin D to progression of osteoarthritis of the knee among participants in the Framingham Study. *Ann Intern Med* 19961;125:353-9.

60. Baker, K. et al. Hypovitaminosis D and its Association with Muscle Strength, Pain and Physical Function in Knee Osteoarthritis (OA): A 30-month Longitudinal, Observational Study. American College of Rheumatology Presentation Number: 1755 Oct. 17, 2004.

61. Merlino, L. et al. Vitamin D intake is inversely associated with rheumatoid arthritis: Results from the Iowa Women's Health Study. *Arthritis & Rheumatism* 2004;50:72-77.

62. Cantorna, M. et al. 1,25-Dihydroxycholecalciferol inhibits the progression of arthritis in murine models of human arthritis. *J Nutr*1998;128:68-72.

63. Weisberg, P. et al. Nutritional rickets among children in the United States: review of cases reported between 1986 and 2003. *Am J Clin Nutr* 2004;80(6 Suppl):1697S-705S.

64. Alouf, B. et al. Incidental finding of vitamin-D deficient rickets in an otherwise healthy infant—a reappraisal of current vitamin-D supplementation guidelines. *J Natl Med Assoc* 2005;97:1170-73.

65. Visser, M. et al. Low vitamin D and high parathyroid hormone levels as determinants of loss of muscle strength and muscle mass (sarcopenia): the Longitudinal Aging Study Amsterdam. *J Clin Endocrinol Metab* 2003;88:5766-72.

66. Hollis B. et al. Vitamin D requirements during lactation: high-dose maternal supplementation as therapy to prevent hypovitaminosis D for both the mother and the nursing infant. *Am J Clin Nutr* 2004;80:1752S-58S.

67. Cannell, J. Personal communication with author.

68. Stephensen, C. Vitamin D status in adolescents and young adults with HIV infection. *Am J Clin Nutr* 2006;83:1135-41.

69. Reid Sexton and Louise Hall. sunshine deficiency leads to vitamin D crisis. *Sidney, Australia Morning Herald* December 9, 2007.

70. Schnadower, D. et al. Hypocalcemic seizures and secondary femoral fractures in an adolescent with primary vitamin D deficiency. *Pediatrics* 2006;118:2226-30.

71. Bischoff-Ferrari, H. et al. Calcium intake and hip fracture in men and women: a meta-analysis of prospective cohort studies and randomized, controlled trials. *Am J Clin Nutr* 2007;86:1780-90.

72. Winzenberg, T. et al. Effects of calcium supplementation on bone density in healthy children: a meta-analysis of randomized controlled trials. *BMJ* 2006;333:763-64.

73. Diem, S. et al. Use of antidepressants and rates of hip bone loss in older women: the study of osteoporotic fractures. *Arch Intern Med* 2007;167:1240.

74. Haney, E. et al. Association of low bone mineral density with selective serotonin uptake inhibitor use by older men. *Arch Intern Med* 2007167:1246-51.

75. Richards, J. et al. Effect of selective serotonin reuptake inhibitors on the risk of fracture. *Arch Intern Med* 2007;167:188-94.

76. Broe, K. et al. A higher dose of vitamin D reduces the risk of falls in nursing home residents: a randomized, multiple-dose study. *J Am Geriatric Soc* 2007;55:234-49.

77. Snijder, M. et al. Vitamin D status in relation to one-year risk of recurrent falling in older men and women. *J Clin Endocrinol Metab* 2006;91:2890-95.

78. Swanenburg, J. et al. Effects of exercise and nutrition on postural balance and risk of falling in elderly people with decreased bone mineral density: randomized controlled trial pilot study. *Clin Rehabil* 2007;21:523-34.

79. Takasu, H. et al. c-Fos protein as a target of anti-osteoclastogenic action of vitamin D, and synthesis of new analogs. *J Clin Invest* 2006;116::528-35.

80. Hauschka, P. Hauschka Laboratory entry regarding bone-cell biology online 2004. Accessed January 2, 2008. http://www.childrenshospital.org/cfapps/research/data_admin/Site31/mainpageS31P13.html.

81. Hitz, M. et al. Bone mineral density and bone markers in patients with a recent low-energy fracture; effect of 1 y of treatment with calcium and vitamin D. *Am J Clin Nutr* 2007;86:251-59.

82. Wang, J. et al. Low Vitamin D Levels are Associated with Greater Pain and Slow Walking Speed in Patients with Knee Osteoarthritis. Presentation 199: American College of Rheumatology Annual Scientific Meeting, Boston, Mass. Oct. 2007.

83. Nguyen, N. Identification of high-risk individuals for hip fracture: a 14-year prospective study. *J bone Miner Res* 2005;20:1921-28.

84. Fisher, A. et al. Relationships between myocardial injury, all -cause mortality, vitamin D, PTH, and biochemical Bone turnover markers in older patients with hip fractures. *Ann Clin Lab Science* 2007;37:222-232.

85. Khan, Q. vitamin D supplementation reduces fatigue and muscle pain in women with early-stage breast cancer: Presented at 30th San Antonio Breast Cancer Symposium, December, 2007.

86. Al Faraj S, et al. Vitamin D deficiency and chronic low back pain in Saudi Arabia. *Spine* 2003;28:177-79.

87. Plehwe WE, Carey RPL. Spinal surgery and severe vitamin D deficiency. *Med J Aust* 2002;176: 438-39.

88. Hoskin, A. Fatal falls: trends and characteristics. *Stat Bull Metrop Insur Co.* 1998;79:10-15.

89. Lofti, A. Hypovitaminosis D in female patients with chronic low-back pain. *Clin Rheumatol* 2007;26:1895-1901.

90. Lewis, P. vitamin D deficiency may have role in chronic low back pain. *BMJ* 2005;330:1220-21.

91. de Torrente de la Jara, G. et al. Female asylum seekers with musculoskeletal pain: the importance of diagnosis and treatment of hypovitaminosis D. *BMC Fam. Pract.* 2006;23:7-14.

92. Passeri, G, et al. Low vitamin D status high bone turnover and bone fractures in centenarians. *J Clin Endocrinol Metab* 2003;88:5109-5115.

93. Ruohola, J. et al. Association between serum 25(OH0d concentrations and bone stress fractures in Finnish young men. *J Bone Miner Res* 2006;21:1483-88.

94. Givon, U. et al. Stress fractures in the Israeli defense forces from 1995-1996. *Clin Orthop Relat Res* 2000;373:227-32.

95. Lappe, J. et al. Stress fracture reduced by vitamin D and calcium. 53rd annual Orthopedic Research Society meeting, San Diego, California, Feb. 2007.

96. Patel, S. et al. Serum vitamin D metabolite levels may be inversely associated with current disease activity in patients with early inflammatory polyarthritis. *Arthritis Rheum* 2007;56;2143-49.

97. Cutolo, M. et al. Vitamin D in rheumatoid arthritis. *Autoimmune Rev* 2007;7:59-64.

98. Cutolo, M. et al. Circannual vitamin D serum levels and disease activity in rheumatoid arthritis: Northern versus Southern Europe. *Clin Exp Rheumatol* 2006;24:702-4.

99. Okuno, J. et al. Correlation between vitamin D and functional capacity, physical function among Japanese frail elderly living in the community. *Nippon Ronen Igakkai Zasshi* 2007;44:634-40.

100. Kwon, J. et al. Concomitant lower serum albumin and vitamin D levels a re associated with deceased objective physical performance among Japanese community-dwelling elderly. *Gerontology* 2007;53:322-38.

101. Houston, D. et al. Association between vitamin D status and physical performance: the INCHANTI study. *J Gerontol A Biol Sci Med Sci* 2007;62:440.

102. Belaid, S. et al. Hypovitaminosis D among 18 to 49 years old women wearing concealing clothes, an ignored reality in general practice. *Presse Med* 2007; [Epub ahead of print]

103. Parra, E. et al. Unpublished report in *Toronto Globe and Mail*, December 19, 2007. Written by Martin Mittelstaedt.

104. Hypponen, e. et al. Hypovitaminosis D in British adults at age 45 y: nationwide cohort study of dietary and lifestyle predictors. *Am J Clin Nutr* 2007;85:860-68.

105. Hooten, M. et al. Presentation to American Society of Anesthesiologists, October 2007.

106. Bodnar, L. et al. High prevalence of vitamin D insufficiency in black and white pregnant women residing in the northern United Sates and their neonates. *J Nutr* 2007;137:305-6.

107. Bolland, M. et al. Vascular events in healthy older women receiving calcium supplementation: randomized controlled trial. *BMJ* January 16, 2008, Epub prior to publication.

108. Sheikh, M. Role of vitamin D-dependent and vitamin D independent mechanisms in absorption of food calcium. *J Clin Investig* 1988:81:126-132.

109. Larrosa, M. vitamin D deficiency and related factors in patients with osteoporotic hip fracture. *Med Clin* (BARC) 2008;130:6-9.

110. Bischoff-Ferrari, H. et al. Severe vitamin D deficiency in Swiss hip-fracture patients. Bone 2007 Nov 28 [Epub ahead of print]

111. Cumming, R. et al. Case-control study of risk factors for hip fractures in the elderly. *Am J Epidemiol.* 1994 ;139:493-503.

112. Turner, M. et al. Prevalence and Clinical Correlates of Vitamin D Inadequacy among Patients with Chronic Pain. *Pain Med.* 2008 Mar 11 [Epub]

113. Sun Lamps help Unborn Babies Beat Osteoporosis. *London Times* April 27, 2008.

114. Wagner C. et al. High-dose vitamin D3 supplementation in a cohort of breastfeeding mothers and their infants: a 6-month follow-up pilot study. *Breastfeed Med.* 2006;1:59-70.

115. Carlson, A. et al. Is vitamin D deficiency associated with peripheral neuropathy? *The Endocrinologist* 2007;17:319-25.

116. Leavitt, S. Quoted online in Newind Press: Vitamin D may help alleviate chronic back pain. http://www.newindpress.com/NewsItems.asp?ID=IE320080626061955&Page=3&Title=Features+-+Health+%26+Science&Topic=-162

117. Haroon, M. Report to European Union League Against Rheumatism , June 13, 2008.

118. Gloth, F. et al. Can vitamin D deficiency produce an unusual pain syndrome? *Arch Intern Med* 1991;152:1662-4.

Chapter 11. sunlight reduces risk of multiple sclerosis

1. Deluca, H. et al. Vitamin D: its role and uses in immunology. *FASEB J* 2001;15:2579-85.

2. Noonan, C. et al. Prevalence estimates for MS in the United States and evidence of an

increasing trend for women. *Neurology* 2002;58:136-38.

3. MS Society Statistics accessed March 16, 2006.
4. National Institutes of Health, MS Foundation 2006.
5. Davenport, C. et al. Multiple Sclerosis from the standpoint of geographic distribution and race. *Arch Neurol Psychiatry* 1922;8:51-58.
6. Acheson, E. et al. Some comments on the relationship of the distribution of multiple sclerosis to altitude, solar radiation and other variables. *Acta Psychiat* (Scand) 1960;35 (suppl 147):132-47.
7. Norman, J. et al. Epidemiology of multiple sclerosis in USA veterans: 2. Latitude, climate, and risk of multiple sclerosis. *J Chron Dis* 1983;36:551-59.
8. Goldberg, P. et al. Multiple sclerosis: vitamin D and calcium as environmental determinants of prevalence (a viewpoint). Part I: sunlight, dietary factors and epidemiology. *Int J Environ Studies* 1974;6:19–27.
9. Alter, M. et al. Multiple sclerosis and nutrition. *Arch Neurol* 1974;31:267-72.
10. Kurtkze, J. et al. Geography in multiple sclerosis. *J Neurol* 1977;215:1-26.
11. Hernan, M. et al. Geographic variation of MS incidence in two prospective studies of USA women. *Neurology* 1999;53:1711-18.
12. McLeod, J. et al. Epidemiology of multiple sclerosis in Australia. With NSW and SA survey results. *Med J Aust* 1994;160:117-22.
13. McGuigan, C. et al. Latitudinal variation in the prevalence of multiple sclerosis in Ireland, an effect of genetic diversity. *J Neurol Neurosurg Psychiatry* 2004;75:572-76.
14. Kurtzke, J. et al. Epidemiology of multiple sclerosis in USA veterans: 1. Race, sex, and geographic distribution. *Neurology* 1979;29:1228-35.
15. Kurtzke, J. et al. On the fine structure of the distribution of multiple sclerosis. *Acta Neurol Scand* 1967;43:257-82.
16. van der Mei, I. et al. Past exposure to sun, skin phenotype, and risk of multiple sclerosis: case-control study. *BMJ* 2003;327:316-321.
17. Goldacre, M. et al. Skin cancer in people with multiple sclerosis: a record linkage study. *J Epidemiol Community Health* 2004;58:142-44.
18. Elian, M. et al. Multiple sclerosis among the United Kingdom-born children of immigrants from the West Indies. *J Neurol Neurosurg and Psychiatry* 1987;50:327-32.
19. Cabre, P. et al. Role of return migration in the emergence of multiple sclerosis in the French West Indies. *Brain* 2005;128:2899-2910.
20. Dean, G. et al. Annual incidence, prevalence and mortality of multiple sclerosis in white South African-born and in white immigrants to South Africa. *BMJ* 1967;2:724-730.
21. Kurtzke, J. et al. A method for estimating the age at immigration of white immigrants to South Africa with an example of its importance. *S Afr Med J* 1970;44:663-669.
22. Hammond, S. et al. The age-range of risk of developing multiple sclerosis: evidence from a migrant population in Australia. *Brain* 2000;123:968-74.
23. Willer, C. et al. Timing of birth and risk of multiple sclerosis: population based study. *BMJ* 2005;330;120-24.
24. Leutic, G. et al. Response to Willer *BMJ* Jan. 13 2005. *BMJ* online http://bmj. bmjjournals.com/cgi/eletters/330/7483/120#92412.
25. Munger, K. et al. Vitamin D intake and the incidence of multiple sclerosis. *Neurology* 2004;62:60-65.
26. Cantorna, M. et al. 1,25-Dihydroxyvitamin D3 reversibly blocks the progression of relapsing encephalomyelitis, a model of multiple sclerosis. *Proc Natl Acad Sci U S A* 1996;93:7861-64.
27. Spach, K. et al. Gene expression analysis suggests that 1,25-dihydroxyvitamin D3 reverses experimental autoimmune encephalomyelitis by stimulating inflammatory cell apoptosis. *Physiol Genomics*. 2004;18:141-51.
28. Hauser, S. et al. Prevention of experimental allergic encephalomyelitis (EAE) in the SJL/J mouse by whole body ultraviolet irradiation. *J Immunol* 1984;132:1276-81.
29. Soilu-Hanninen, M. et al. 25-Hydroxyvitamin D levels in serum at the onset of multiple sclerosis. *Mult Scler* 2005;11:266-71.
30. Ozgocmen, S. et al. Vitamin D deficiency and reduced bone mineral density in multiple

sclerosis: effect of ambulatory status and functional capacity. *J Bone Miner Metab* 2005;23:309-13.

31. Grant, W. Ultraviolet B (UVB) radiation and vitamin D are important risk reduction factors for multiple sclerosis; viral infections are an important risk factor; dietary fat is a minor risk factor. SUNARC.org. accessed March 16, 2006.

32. Swank, R. et al. Review of MS patient survival on a Swank low saturated fat diet. *Nutrition* 2003;19:161–62.

33. Agranoff, B. et al. Diet and the geographical distribution of multiple sclerosis. *Lancet* 1974;2:1061-68.

34. Malosse, D. et al. Correlation between milk and dairy product consumption and multiple sclerosis prevalence: a worldwide study. *Neuroepidemiology* 1992;11:304-12.

35. Breslau, N. et al. Relationship of animal protein-rich diet to kidney stone formation and calcium metabolism. *J Clin Endocrinol Metab* 1988;66:140.

36. Langman, C. et al. Calcitriol Metabolism during chronic metabolic acidosis. *Semin Nephrol* 1989;9:65-71.

37. Grant W. An estimate of premature cancer mortality in the United States due to inadequate doses of solar ultraviolet-B radiation. *Cancer.* 2002;94,1867-75.

38. Hernan, N. et al. Geographic variation of MS incidence in two prospective studies of USA women. *Neurology* 1999;53:1711-18.

39. Agarwal. K. et al. The impact of atmospheric pollution on vitamin D status of infants and toddlers in Delhi, India. *Arch Dis Child* 2002;87:111-13.

40. Kassandra, L. et el. Serum 25 Hydroxyvitamin D Levels and Risk of Multiple Sclerosis. *JAMA* 2006;296:2832-38.

41. Islam, T. Childhood sun exposure influences risk of multiple sclerosis in monozygotic twins. *Neurology* 2007;69:381-88.

42. van der Mei, I. et al. Vitamin D levels in people with multiple sclerosis and community controls in Tasmania, Australia. *J Neurol* 2007;254:581-90.

43. Kampman, M. Outdoor activities and diet in childhood and adolescence relate to MS risk above the Arctic Circle. *J Neurol* 2007;254:471-77.

44. Holmey, T. vitamin D status modulates the immune response to Epstein Barr Virus: synergistic effect of risk factors in multiple sclerosis. *Med Hypothesis* 2008;70:66-69.

45. Hayes, C. et al. Vitamin D and multiple sclerosis. *Proc Soc Exp Biol Med* 1997;216:21-27.

46. Nieves, J. et al. High prevalence of vitamin D deficiency and reduced bone mass in multiple sclerosis. *Neurology* 1994;44:1687-92.

47. MacNeal, R. et al. Update on sun protection and tanning in children. *Curr Opin Pediatr* 2007;19:425-29.

48. Grant, W. Personal communication with author June2, 2008.

Chapter 12. Solar Power, diabetes and autoimmune diseases

1. Mokad, A. et al. The continuing epidemics of obesity and diabetes in the United States. *JAMA*, 2001; 286:1195-1200.

2. Barnard, J. et al. Response of non-insulin-dependent diabetic patients to an intensive program of diet and exercise. *Diabetes* Care 1982;5:370-74.

3. Joslin, E. et al. Atherosclerosis and Diabetes. *Ann Clin Med* 1927;5:1061-80.

4. Sweeney, J. et al. Dietary factors that influence the dextrose-tolerance test: a preliminary study. *Arch Intern Med* 1927;40:818-830.

5. Rabinowich, I. et al. Experiences with a high-carbohydrate, low-calorie diet for the treatment of diabetes mellitus. *Can Med Assn J* 1930;23:489.

6. Ishii, H. et al. Seasonal variation of glycemic control in type 2 diabetic patients. *Diabetes* Care 2001;24;1503.

7. Colas, C. et al. Insulin secretion and plasma 1,25(OH)$_2$D after UV-B irradiation in healthy adults. *Hormone and Metabolic Research* 1988;21:154-155.

8. Chiu K. et al. Hypovitaminosis D is associated with insulin resistance and beta cell dysfunction. *Am J Clin Nutr* 2004;79:820-25.

9. Brown, A. et al. Vitamin D. *American J of Physiol* 1999;277(2 Pt 2):F157-75.

10. Norman, A. et al. Vitamin D deficiency inhibits pancreatic secretion of insulin. *Science* 1980;209, 823-25.

11. Gedik, O. et al. Effects of vitamin D deficiency and repletion on insulin and glucagons secretion in man. *Diabetologia* 1986;29:142-45.

12. Nyomba, B. et al. Influence of vitamin D status on insulin secretion and glucose tolerance in the rabbit. *Endocrinology*, 1984;115:191-97.

13. Cade, C. et al. Vitamin D₃ improves impaired glucose tolerance and insulin secretion in the vitamin D-deficient rat in vivo. *Endocrinology* 1986;119:84-90.

14. Pittas, A. et al. Vitamin D and calcium intake in relation to type 2 diabetes in women. *Diabetes Care* 2006;29:650-66.

15. Scragg, R. et al. Serum 25-hydroxyvitamin D, diabetes, and ethnicity in the Third National Health and Nutrition Examination Survey. *Diabetes Care* 2004;27:2813-18.

16. Scott, F. et al. Cow milk and insulin-dependent diabetes mellitus: Is there a relationship? *Am J Clin Nutr* 1990;51:489-91.

17. Troncone, R. et al. Increased intestinal sugar permeability after challenge in children with cow's milk allergy or intolerance. *Allergy* 1994;49:142-46.

18. Karjalainen, J. et al. A bovine albumin peptide as a possible trigger of insulin-dependent diabetes mellitus. *N Engl J Med* 1992;317:302-07.

19. Virtanen, S. et al. Diet, cow's milk protein antibodies and the risk of IDDM in Finnish children. Childhood diabetes in Finland study group. *Diabetologia* 1994;37:381-87.

20. Kostraba, J. et al. Early exposure to cow's milk and solid foods in infancy: Genetic predisposition and risk of IDDM. Diabetes 1993;42:288-95.

21. Birgisdottir B. et al. Lower consumption of cow milk protein A1 beta-Casein at 2 years of age, rather than consumption among 11- to 14-year-old adolescents, may explain the lower incidence of type 1 diabetes in Iceland than in Scandinavia. *Ann Nutr Metab* 2006;50:177-83.

22. Dahl-Jorgensen, K et al. Relationship between cow's milk consumption and incidence of IDDM in childhood. *Diabetes Care* 1991;14:1081-83.

23. LaPorte, R. et al. Geographic differences in the risk of insulin-dependent diabetes mellitus: the importance of registries. *Diabetes Care.* 1985;8 Suppl1:01-07.

24. Stene, L. et al. Use of cod liver oil in pregnancy associated with lower risk of type-1 diabetes in the offspring. *Diabetologia* 2000;43:1093-98.

25. Hypponen, E. et al. Intake of vitamin D and risk of type 1 diabetes: a birth-cohort study. *Lancet* 2001;358:1500-03.

26. Dahl-Jorgensen, K. et al. Relationship between cows' milk consumption and incidence of IDDM in childhood. *Diabetes Care* 1991;14:1081-83.

27. Arreola, F. et al. Bone mineral content, 25-hydroxycalciferol and zinc serum levels in insulin-dependent (type I) diabetic patients. *Arch Invest Med (Mex)* 1990;21:195-99.

28. Pozzilli, P. et al. Low levels of 25-hydroxyvitamin D3 and 1,25-dihydroxyvitamin D3 in patients with newly diagnosed type 1 diabetes. *Horm Metab Res.* 2005;37:680-83.

29. Kukreja, A. et al. Autoimmunity and diabetes. *J Clin Endocrinol Metab* 1999;84: 4371–78.

30. Mathieu, C. et al. Prevention of autoimmune diabetes in NOD mice by 1,25 dihydroxyvitamin D3. *Diabetologia* 1994;37:552–58.

31. Staples, J. et al. Ecologic analysis of some immune-related disorders, including type-1 diabetes, in Australia: latitude, regional ultraviolet radiation, and disease prevalence. *Environmental Health Perspectives* 2003;111:518-523.

32. Kamen, D. et al. Vitamin D deficiency in systemic lupus erythematosus. *Autoimmun Rev* 2006;5:114-7.

33. Huisman, A. et al. Vitamin D levels in women with systemic lupus erythematosus and fibromyalgia. *J Rheumatol* 2001;28:2535-39.

34. Becker, A. et al. Bone density and 25-OH vitamin D serum level in patients with systemic lupus erythematosus. *Z Rheumatol* 2001 Oct;60(5):352-8.

35. Zhu, Y. et al. Calcium and 1 alpha,25-dihydroxyvitamin D3 target the TNF-alpha pathway to suppress experimental inflammatory bowel disease. *Eur J Immunol*

2005;35:217-24.

36. Froicu, M. et al. A crucial role for the vitamin D receptor in experimental inflammatory bowel diseases. *Mol Endocrinol* 2003;17:2386-92.

37. Gilman, J. et al. Determinants of vitamin D status in adult Crohn's disease patients, with particular emphasis on supplemental vitamin D use. *Eur J Clin Nutr*. 2006 Feb 22; [Epub ahead of print].

38. Sanchez, B. et al. 1,25-Dihydroxyvitamin D(3) increases striatal GDNF mRNA and protein expression in adult rats. *Brain Res Mol Brain Res* 2002;108:143-46.

39. Wang, J. et al. Vitamin D(3) attenuates 6-hydroxydopamine-induced neurotoxicity in rats. *Brain Res* 2001;904:67-75.

40. Kim, J. et al. Association of vitamin D receptor gene polymorphism and Parkinson's Disease in Koreans. *Korean Med Sci 2005; 20: 495-98.*

41. Borissova, A. et al. The effect of vitamin D3 on insulin secretion and peripheral insulin sensitivity in type 2 diabetic patients. *Int J Clin Pract* 2003;57(4):258-61.

42. Mattila, C. Serum 25-hydroxyvitamin D concentration and subsequent risk of type-2 diabetes. *Diabetes Care* 2007;30:2569-70.

43. Pappa, H. et al. Vitamin D status in children and young adults with inflammatory bowel disease. *Pediatrics* 2006;118:1950-61.

44. American Diabetes Association news release, January 2008.

45. American Cancer Society, Cancer Facts and Figures 2007.

46. Need, A. et al. Relationship between fasting serum glucose, age, body mass index and serum 25 hydroxyvitamin D in postmenopausal women. *Clin Endocrinol* 2005;62:738-41.

47. Littorin, B. et al. Lower levels of plasma 25 –hydroxyvitamin D among young adults at diagnosis of autoimmune type-1 diabetes compared with control subjects: results from the nationwide Diabetes Incidence Study in Sweden (DISS). *Diabetologia* 2006;49:2847-52.

48. Pittas, A. et al. The effects of calcium and vitamin D supplementation on blood glucose and markers of inflammation in nondiabetic adults. *Diabetes Care* 2007;30:980-86.

49. Pittas, A. Review: the role of vitamin D and calcium in type-2 diabetes. A systematic review and meta-analysis. *J Clin Endocrinol Metab* 2007.

50. Forsmo, S. et al. Childhood cod liver oil consumption and bone mineral density in a population-based cohort of peri-and postmenopausal women. *Am J Epidemiol* 2008;167:406-11.

51. Alarcon, G. et al. Systemic lupus erythematosus in three ethnic groups: III. A comparison of characteristics early in the natural history of the LUMINA cohort. Lupus in minority populations: Nature vs. Nurture. *Lupus* 1999;8:197-209.

52. Arnson, Y. et al. Vitamin D and autoimmunity: New aetiological considerations. *Ann Rheum Dis* 2007;66:1137-42.

53. Abe, J. et al. Prevention of immunological disorders in MRL/1 mice by a new synthetic analogue of vitamin D3. *J Nutr Sci Vitaminol* 1990;36:21-31.

54. Fronzac, C. et al. In utero dietary exposures and risk of islet autoimmunity in children. *Diabetes Care* 2003;26:3237-42.

55. Sloka, S et al. Time series analysis of ultraviolet B radiation and type-1 diabetes in Newfoundland. *Pediatr Diabetes* 2008, Jan 24 [Epub].

56. Lee, P. et al. Vitamin D as an analgesic for patients with type 2 diabetes and neuropathic pain. *Arch Intern Med*. 2008;168:771-2.

Chapter 13. Solar Power, heart disease and high blood pressure

1. Review of the literature found in Sorenson, M. *Megahealth*. Evans Publishing, NY, 1995. Also see Campbell, T. *The China Study*. Benbella 2005.

2. Castelli, W. Epidemiology of coronary heart disease: The Framingham Study. *Am J Med* 1984;76:4-12.

3. Castelli, W. Quoted in Barnard, N. *The Power of Your Plate* Book Publishing Company, Summertown, TN 1990, p. 20.

4. Stamler, J. et al. Is the relationship between serum cholesterol and risk of premature

death from coronary heart disease continuous and graded? *JAMA* 1986;256:2823-28.

5. Grimes, D. et al. sunlight, cholesterol and coronary heart disease. *QJM* 1996;89:579-89.

6. Ulmer, H. et al. Estimation of seasonal variations in risk factor profiles and mortality from coronary heart disease. *Wien Klin Wochenschr* 2004 Oct 30;116(19-20):662-8.

7. Sheth, T. et al. Increased winter mortality from acute myocardial infarction and stroke: the effect of age. *J Am Coll Cardiol* 1999;33:1916-19.

8. Pell, J. et al. Seasonal variations in coronary heart disease. *QJM* 1999;92:689-96.

9. Weerasinghe, D. et al. Seasonality of coronary artery deaths in New South Wales, Australia. *Heart* 2002;88:30-34.

10. Sharovsky, R. et al. Increase in mortality due to myocardial infarction in the Brazilian city of Sao Paulo during winter. *Arq Bras Cardiol* 2002;78:106.

11. Zittermann, A. et al. Putting cardiovascular disease and vitamin D insufficiency into perspective. *Br J Nutr* 2005;94:483-92.

12. Mortimer, E. et al. Reduction in mortality from coronary heart disease in men residing at high altitude. *N Engl J Med*;1977;17;296:581-85.

13. Gordon, R. et al. Coronary heart disease at high altitudes. *N Engl J Med* 1977;297:60-62.

14. Gordon, R. et al. Altitude and CBVD death rates show apparent relationship. *Stroke* 1977;8:274.

15. Charach, G. et al. Seasonal changes in blood pressure and frequency of related complications in elderly Israeli patients with essential hypertension. *Gerontology*. 2004 Sep-Oct;50(5):315-21.

16. Pfeifer, M. et al. Effects of a short-term vitamin D(3) and calcium supplementation on blood pressure and parathyroid hormone levels in elderly women. *J Clin Endocrinol Metab* 2001;86:1633-37.

17. Krause, R. et al. Ultraviolet B and blood pressure. *Lancet* 1998;352:709-10.

18. Hultgren H. et al. Reduction of systemic arterial blood pressure at high altitude. *Adv Cardiol* 1970;5:49-55.

19. Hollenberg, N. et al. Age, renal perfusion and function in island-dwelling indigenous Kuna Amerinds of Panama. *Nephron*. 1999;82:131-38.

20. Hollenberg, N. et al. Aging, acculturation, salt intake, and hypertension in the Kuna of Panama. *Hypertension* 1997;29:171-76.

21. Muna, W. et al. Cardiovascular Disorders in Africa. *World Health Stat Q* 1993;46:125-33.

22. Gutpa, R. et al. Cholesterol lipoproteins, triglycerides, rural-urban differences and prevalence of dyslipidaemia among males in Rajasthan. *J Assoc Physicians India* 1997;45:275-79.

23. Chapuy, M. et al. Healthy elderly French women living at home have secondary hyperparathyroidism and high bone turnover in winter. EPIDOS Study Group. *J Clin Endocrinol Metab*1996;81:1129-33.

24. Boulay, F. et al. Seasonal variation in chronic heart failure hospitalizations and mortality in France. *Circulation*. 1999;100:280-86.

25. Stewart, S. et al. Heart failure in a cold climate. Seasonal variation in heart failure-related morbidity and mortality. *J Am Coll Cardiol* 2002;39:760-76.

26. Martinez-Selles, M. et al. Annual rates of admission and seasonal variations in hospitalizations for heart failure. *Eur J Heart Fail* 2002;:779-86.

27. Sher, L. et al. Effects of seasonal mood changes on seasonal variations in coronary heart disease: role of immune system, infection, and inflammation. *Med Hypotheses* 2001;56:104-06.

28. Agatston, A. et al. Quantification of coronary artery calcium using ultrafast computed tomography. *J Am Coll Cardiol* 1990;15:827-32.

29. Honye, J. et al. Morphological effects of coronary balloon angioplasty in vivo assessed by intravascular ultrasound imaging. *Circulation* 1992;85:1012.

30. Feldman, C. et al. Detection of coronary artery disease based on the calcification index obtained by helical computed tomography. *Arq Bras Cardiol* 2000;75:471-80.

31. Kitamura, A. et al. Evaluation of coronary artery calcification by multi-detector row

computed tomography for the detection of coronary artery stenosis in Japanese patients. *J Epidemiol* 2005;15:187-93.

32. Baedenkopf, W. et al. Calcification in the coronary arteries and its relationship to arteriosclerosis and myocardial infarction. *Am J Roentgenol* 1964;92:865-71.

33. Banks, L. et al. Effect of degenerative spinal and aortic calcification on bone density measurements in post-menopausal women: links between osteoporosis and cardiovascular disease? *Eur J Clin Invest* 1994;24:813-17.

34. Barengolts, E. et al. Osteoporosis and coronary atherosclerosis in asymptomatic postmenopausal women. *Calcif Tissue Int* 1998;62:209-13.

35. Watson, K. et al. Active serum vitamin D levels are inversely correlated with coronary calcification. *Circulation* 1997;96:1755-60.

36. Davies, M. et al. Pathophysiological mechanisms of vascular calcification in end-stage renal disease. *Kidney Int* 2001;60:472-79.

37. Rostand, S. et al. Parathyroid hormone, vitamin D, and cardiovascular disease in chronic renal failure. *Kidney Int* 1999;56:383-92.

38. Tangpricha, V. et al. Tanning is associated with optimal vitamin D status (serum 25-hydroxyvitamin D concentration) and higher bone mineral density. *Am J Clin Nutr* 2004;80:1645-49.

39. Hollis, B. et al. Circulating 25-hydroxyvitamin D levels indicative of vitamin D sufficiency: implications for establishing a new effective dietary intake recommendation for vitamin D. *J Nutr.* 2005;135:317-22.

40. Vieth, R. et al. Age-related changes in the 25-hydroxyvitamin D *versus* parathyroid hormone relationship suggest a different reason why older adults require more vitamin D. *J Clin Endocrinol Metab* 2005;88;185-91.

41. Norman, P. et al. Vitamin D, Shedding Light on the Development of Disease in Peripheral Arteries. *Arterioscler Thromb Vasc Biol* 2005;25:39-46.

42. Van Lente, F. et al. Markers of inflammation as predictors in cardiovascular disease. *Clin Chim Acta* 2000;293:31-52.

43. Shishehbor, M. et al. Inflammation and atherosclerosis. *Curr Atheroscler Rep* 2004 Mar;6(2):131-39.

44. Li, J. et al. C-reactive protein is not only an inflammatory marker but also a direct cause of cardiovascular diseases. *Med Hypotheses* 2004;62:499-506.

45. Muller, K. et al. 1,25-Dihydroxyvitamin D3 inhibits cytokine production by human blood monocytes at the post-transcriptional level. *Cytokine* 1992;4:506-12.

46. Canning, M. et al. I-alpha,25-Dihydroxyvitamin D3 (l,25(OH)(2)D(3)) hampers the maturation of fully active immature dendritic cells from monocytes. *Eur J Endocrinol* 2001;145:351-57.

47. Beauchemin, K. et al. Dying in the dark: sunshine, gender and outcomes in myocardial infarction. *J R Soc Med* 1998;91:352-54.

48. American Heart Association. Heart and stroke statistics – 2004 update.

49. Agarwal, K. The impact of atmospheric pollution on vitamin D status of infants and toddlers in Delhi, India. *Arch Dis Child* 2002;87:111-13.

50. Zitterman, A. et al. Vitamin D insufficiency in congestive heart failure: Why and what to do about it? *Heart Fail Rev.* 2006;11:25-33.

51. Poole, K. et al. Reduced vitamin D in acute stroke. *Stroke* 2006;37:243-45.

52. Forman, J. et al. Plasma Hydroxyvitamin D and risk of Incident Hypertension. (*Hypertension.* 2007;49:1-7.)

53. Scragg, R. et al. Myocardial infarction is inversely associated with plasma 25-hydroxyvitamin D3 levels: a community-based study. *Int J Epidemiol* 1990;19:559-63.

54. Wang, T. et al. Vitamin D deficiency and risk of cardiovascular disease. *Circulation* 2008;117 pre-publication copy.

55. Martins, D. et al. Prevalence of cardiovascular risk factors and the serum levels of 25-Hydroxyvitamin D in the United States. *Arch Intern Med* 2007;167:1159-65.

56. Zittermann, A. et al. Vitamin D and vascular calcification. *Curr Opin Lipidol* 2007;18:41-46.

57. Wannamethee, S. et al. Height loss in older men: associations with total mortality and incidence of cardiovascular disease. Arch Intern Med 2006;166:2546-52.
58. Schleithoff, S. et al. Vitamin d supplementation improves cytokine profiles in patients with congestive heart failure: a double-blind, randomized, placebo-controlled trial. *Am J Clin Nutr* 2006;83:731-2.
59. Serum 25-hydroxyvitamin D3 concentrations and carotid artery intima-media thickness among type-2 diabetics. *Clin Endocrinol (Oxf)* 2006;65:593-97.
60. Bolland, M. et al. Vascular events in healthy older women receiving calcium supplementation: randomized controlled trial. *BMJ* January 16, 2008, Epub prior to publication.
61. Bischoff-Ferrari, H. et al. Calcium intake and hip fracture in men and women: a meta-analysis of prospective cohort studies and randomized, controlled trials. *Am J Clin Nutr* 2007;86:1780-90.
62. Judd, S. Et al. Optimal vitamin D status attenuates the age-associated increase in systolic blood pressure in white Americans: results from the third National Health and Nutrition Examination Survey. *Am J Clin Nutr* 2008;87:136-41.
63. Polat, M. et al. the Effect of seasonal changes on blood pressure and urine specific gravity in children living in Mediterranean climate. *Med Sci Monit* 2006;12:CR186-90.
64. Sigmund, C. Regulation of rennin expression and blood pressure by vitamin D3. *J Clin Invest* 2002;110:155-56.
65. Melamed, M. et al "Vitamin D May Protect Against Peripheral Artery Disease." *Science Daily* 20 April 2008. [Available at <http://www.sciencedaily.com / releases/2008/04/080416140954.htm].
66. Maiya, S. et al. Hypocalcaemia and vitamin D deficiency: an important, but preventable cause of life-threatening heart failure. *Heart* 2008;94:581-84.
67. Giovannucci, E. et al. 25-hydroxy-vitamin D and risk of myocardial infarction in men. *Ann Intern Med* 2008;168:1174-80.
68. Mancuso, P. et al. 1,25-Dihydroxyvitamin-D3 Treatment Reduces Cardiac Hypertrophy and Left Ventricular Diameter in Spontaneously Hypertensive Heart Failure-prone (cp/+) Rats Independent of Changes in Serum Leptin. *J Cardiovasc Pharmacol.* 2008;51:559-64.

Chapter 14. Solar Power and a potpourri of health concerns.

1. Dentalinsurance.com 2006.
2. Phipps, K. et al. Relative contribution of caries and periodontal disease in adult tooth loss for an HMO dental population. *J Pub Health Dent* 1995;55:250-52.
3. Hideout, C. et al. Effect of vitamin D and calcium on Periodontitis. *J Periodontal* 2005;76:1576-87.
4. Destrehan, F. et al. Dental disease and risk of coronary heart disease and mortality. *BMJ.* 1993;306:688-91.
5. Page, R. et al. The etiology and pathogenesis of periodontitis. *Commend Contain Educe Dent* 2002;23:11-14.
6. Teal, M. et al. The relationship between bone mineral density and periodontitis in postmenopausal women. *J Periodontal* 2000;71:1492–8.
7. Payne J. et al. Longitudinal alveolar bone loss in postmenopausal osteoporotic/osteopenic women. *Osteoporos Int* 1999;10:34–40.
8. Bando, K. et al. Bone mineral density in periodontally healthy and edentulous postmenopausal women. *Ann Periodontol* 1998;3:322–6.
9. Krall, E. et al. Increased risk of tooth loss is related to bone loss at the whole body, hip, and spine. *Calcif Tissue Int* 1996;59:433–47.
10. Payne, J. et al. The association of cigarette smoking with alveolar bone loss in postmenopausal females. *J Clin Periodontol* 2000;27:658–64.
11. Krall, E. et al. Calcium and vitamin D supplements reduce tooth loss in the elderly. *Am J Med* 2001;111:452-56.
12. Hennig, B. et al. Association of a vitamin D receptor gene polymorphism with localized

early-onset periodontal diseases. *J Periodontol* 1999;70:1032.

13. Inagaki, K. et al. Vitamin D receptor alleles, periodontal disease progression, and tooth loss in the VA dental longitudinal study. *J Periodontol.* 2003;74:161-67.
14. de Brito Junior, R. et al. Polymorphisms in the vitamin D receptor gene are associated with periodontal disease. *J Periodontol* 2004;75:1090-95.
15. Tachi, Y. et al. Association of vitamin D receptor gene polymorphism with periodontal diseases in Japanese and Chinese. *Nucleic Acids Res Suppl* 2001;1:111-12.
16. Dietrich, T. et al. Association between serum concentrations of 25-hydroxyvitamin D$_3$ and periodontal disease in the USA population. *Am J Clin Nutr* 2004;80:108-13.
17. Dietrich, T. et al. Association between serum concentrations of 25-hydroxyvitamin D and gingival inflammation. *Am J Clin Nutr* 2005;82:575-80.
18. Kime, Z. sun*light Could Save Your Life*. World Health Publications, Penryn, CA 1980 pp 180-81.
19. East, B. et al. Mean annual hours of sunshine and the incidence of dental caries. *Am J Pub Health* 1939;29:77.
20. McBeath, E. et al. The role of vitamin D in control of dental caries in children. *J Nutr* 1938;15:547.
21. World Health Organization, Sept 22, 2005.
22. Medicinenet.com 2003.
23. Department of Health and Human Services, Centers for Disease Control and Prevention, March, 2006.
24. Nabhan, G. Native Seed Search information packet, Tucson, A. 1990.
25. Nabhan, G. Personal communication, 1990.
26. Nabhan, G. Food, health and native American agriculture. *J Gastronomy* 1989;12:68-81.
27. Ringrose, H. et al. Nutrient intakes in an urbanized Micronesian population with a high diabetes prevalence. *Am J Clin Nutr* 1979;32:1334-41.
28. Brand, J. et al. Plasma glucose and insulin responses to traditional Pima Indian meals. *Am J Clin Nutr* 1990;51:416-20.
29. Williams, D. et al. The effect of Indian or Anglo dietary preference on the incidence of diabetes in Pima Indians. *Diabetes Care.* 2001;24:811-16.
30. Knowler, W. et al. Obesity in the Pima Indians: its magnitude and relationship with diabetes. *Am J Clin Nutr* 1991;53:1543S-51S.
31. McMurry, M. et al. Changes in lipid and lipoprotein levels and body weight in Tarahumara Indians after consumption of an affluent diet. *NEJM* 1991;325:1704-08.
32. Ornish, D. Can lifestyle changes reverse coronary heart disease? The lifestyle heart trial. *Lancet* 1990;336:129-33.
33. Liel, Y. et al. Low circulating vitamin D in obesity. *Calcif Tissue Int* 1988;43:199-201.
34. Parikh, S. et al. The Relationship between Obesity and Serum 1,25-Dihydroxy Vitamin D Concentrations in Healthy Adults. *J Clin Endocrinol Metab* 2004;89(3):1196-99.
35. Kamycheva, E. et al. Intakes of Calcium and Vitamin D Predict Body Mass Index in the Population of Northern Norway. *J Nutr* 2002;132:102–06.
36. Ellinger, F. et al. The influence of ultraviolet rays on body weight. *Radiology* 1939;32:157.
37. Shi, H. et al. 1a,25-Dihydroxyvitamin D3 modulates human adipocyte metabolism via nongenomic action. *FASEB J* 2001;15:2751-53.
38. Ping-Delfos, W. et al. Acute suppression of spontaneous food intake following dairy calcium and vitamin D. *Asia Pac J Clin Nutr* 2004;13(Suppl):S82.
39. Lindgarde, F. et al. Body adiposity, insulin, and leptin in subgroups of Peruvian Amerindians. *High Alt Med Biol.* 2004;5:27-31.
40. Schmitt, L. et al. Patterns in the within-population variability of stature and weight. *Ann Hum Biol* 1988;15:353-64.
41. Cannell, J. *The Vitamin D Newsletter*, Sept. 2004. http://www.vitamindcouncil.com.
42. Wortsman, J. et al. Decreased bioavailability of vitamin D in obesity. *Am J Clin Nutr* 2003;72:690-93.
43. Snijder, M. et al. Adiposity in relation to vitamin D status and parathyroid hormone levels: a population-based study in older men and women. *J Clin Endocrinol Metab*

2005;90:4119-23.

44. National Psoriasis Foundation web site Oct. 2005.
45. Basler, R. et al. Psoralen and sunlight for psoriasis in the Southwest. *Cutis* 1979;24:386-88.
46. Yelverton, C. et al. Home ultraviolet B phototherapy: a cost-effective option for severe psoriasis. *Manag Care Interface* 2006;19:33-36, 39.
47. Holick, M. The UV advantage. Ibooks Inc. New York, 2003. pp 118-19.
48. Reynolds, N. et al. Narrow-band ultraviolet B and broad-band ultraviolet A phototherapy in adult atopic eczema: a randomized controlled trial. *Lancet* 2001;357:2012-16.
49. Valkova, S. et al. UVA/UVB phototherapy for atopic dermatitis revisited. *J Dermatolog Treat* 2004;15:239-44.
50. Myerson, A. Influence of ultraviolet radiation on excretion of sex hormones in the male. *Endocrinology* 1939;25:7-12.
51. Sood, S. et al. Effect of vitamin D deficiency on testicular function in the rat. *Ann Nutr Metab* 1992;36:203-08.
52. Inpanbutr, N. et al. Effect of vitamin D on testicular CaBP28K expression and serum testosterone in chickens. *Biol Reprod.* 1996 Jan;54(1):242-8.
53. Kwiecinski, G. et al. Vitamin D is necessary for reproductive functions of the male rat. *J Nutr* 1989;119:741-44.
54. Rojansky, N. et al. Seasonality in human reproduction: an update. *Hum Reprod* 1992;7:735-45.
55. Gammack, J. Quoted in *Medical News Today,* April 10, 2005.
56. Downes, A. Researches on the effect of light upon bacteria and other organisms. Proc Roy Soc Med 1877;26:488. Cited in Kime, Z. sun*light Could Save Your Life*. World Health Publications, Penryn, CA 1980:126-30.
57. Miley, G. The Knott technic of ultraviolet blood irradiation in acute pyogenic infections. *New York J Med* 1942;42:38.
58. Rebbeck, E. Ultraviolet irradiation of autotransfused blood in the treatment of puerperal sepsis. *Amer J Surg* 1941;54:691.
59. Rebbeck, E. Ultraviolet irradiation of autotransfused blood in the treatment of postabortal sepsis. *Amer J Surg* 1942;55:476.
60. Rebbeck, E. Ultraviolet irradiation of the blood in the treatment of escherichia coli septicemia. *Arch Phys Ther* 1943;24:158.
61. Rebbeck, E. The Knott technic of ultraviolet blood irradiation as a control of infection in peritonitis. *Amer J Gastroenterol* 1943;10:1-26.
62. Hancock, V. Irradiated blood transfusions in the treatment of infections. *Northwest Med* 1934;33:200.
63. Barrett, H. Five years experience with hemo-irradiation according to the Knott technic. *Am J Surg* 1943;61:42.
64. Barrett, H. The irradiation of autotransfused blood by ultraviolet spectral energy: results of therapy in 110 cases. *Med Clin N Amer* 1940;24:723.
65. Miley, G. The present status of ultraviolet blood irradiation. *Arch Phys Ther* 1944;25:357.
66. Hollaender, A. The inactivating effect of monochromatic ultraviolet radiation on influenza virus. *J Bact* 1944;48:447.
67. Heding, L. et al. Inactivation of tumor cell-associated feline oncornavirus for preparation of an infectious virus-free tumor cell immunogen. *Cancer Res* 1976;36:1647.
68. Hart, D. Sterilization of the air in the operating room by special antibacterial radiant energy. *J Thorac Cardiovasc Surg* 1936;6:45.
69. Gameson, A. et al. Field studies on effect of daylight on mortality of coliform bacteria. *Water Res* 1967;1:279.
70. Calkins, J. et al. The role of solar ultraviolet radiation in natural water purification. *Photochem Photobiol* 1976;24:49.
71. Centers for Disease Control 2004.
72. University of Pennsylvania Center for Health Transformation 2006.
73. Zhang, L. et al. Contribution of Human -Defensin 1, 2, and 3 to the Anti-HIV-1 Activity

of CD8 Antiviral Factor. *Science* 2002;298:995-1,000.

74. Daher, K. et al. Direct inactivation of viruses by human granulocyte defensins. *J Virol* 1986 Dec;60(3):1068-74. *J Virol* 1986 Dec;60(3):1068-74.

75. Nizet, V. et al. Innate antimicrobial peptide protects the skin from invasive bacterial infection. *Nature* 2001;414:454-57.

76. Gantz, T. et al. Defensins: antimicrobial peptides of innate immunity. *Nat Rev Immunol* 2003 Sep;3(9):710-20.

77. Wang, T. et al. Cutting edge: 1,25-dihydroxyvitamin D3 is a direct inducer of antimicrobial peptide gene expression. *J Immunol* 2004;173:2909-12.

78. Liu, P. et al. Toll-like receptor triggering of a vitamin D-mediated human antimicrobial response. *Science*. 2006;311:1770-73.

79. Gombart, A. et al. Human cathelicidin antimicrobial peptide (CAMP) gene is a direct target of the vitamin D receptor and is up-regulated in myeloid cells by 1,25-dihydroxyvitamin D3. *FASEB J* 2005;19:1067-77.

80. Wang, T. et al. Cutting edge: 1,25-dihydroxyvitamin D3 is a direct inducer of antimicrobial peptide gene expression. *J Immunol* 2004;173:2909-12.

81. University of Pennsylvania Center for Health Transformation 2006.

82. Ikeda, K. Evaluation of vitamin D metabolism in patients with bilateral sensorineural hearing loss. *Am J Otol* 1989;10:11-13.

83. Brookes, G. Vitamin D deficiency and deafness: 1984 update. *Am J Otol* 1985;6:102-7.

84. Bertone-Johnson, E. et al. Calcium and vitamin D intake and risk of incident premenstrual syndrome," *Arch Intern Med* 2005;165:1246-52.

85. Thys-Jacobs, S. et al. Vitamin D and calcium dysregulation in the polycystic ovarian syndrome. *Steroids* 1999;64:430-35.

86. Stern, R. et al. The carcinogenic risk of treatments for severe psoriasis. Photochemotherapy Follow-up Study. *Cancer* 1994;73:2759-64.

87. Muller, K. et al. 1,25-Dihydroxyvitamin D3 inhibits cytokine production by human blood monocytes at the post-transcriptional level. *Cytokine* 1992;4:506-12.

88. Canning, M. et al. I-alpha,25-Dihydroxyvitamin D3 (l,25(OH)(2)D(3)) hampers the maturation of fully active immature dendritic cells from monocytes. *Eur J Endocrinol* 2001;145:351-57.

89. Cannell, J. et al. Epidemic Influenza and vitamin D. *Epidemiol Infect* 2006;134:1129-40.

90. Aloia, J. et al. Colds and Flu. Letter to the editor. *Epidemiol Infect* Jan 15, 2007.

91. Botella-Carretero J. et al. Vitamin D deficiency is associated with the metabolic syndrome in morbid obesity. *Clin Nutr* 2007 Jul 9; [Epub ahead of print].

92. Smotkin-Tangora, M. et al. Prevalence of vitamin d insufficiency in obese children and adolescents. *J Pediatr Endocrinol Metab* 2007;20:817-23.

93. Autier, P. et al. Vitamin D supplementation and total mortality: a meta-analysis of randomized controlled trials. *Arch Intern Med* 2007;167:1730-37.

94. Richards, J. et al. High serum vitamin D concentrations associated with longer leukocyte telomere length in women. *Am J Clin Nutr* 2007;86:1420-25.

95. Valdes, A. et al. Telomere length in leukocytes correlates with bone mineral density and is shorter in women with osteoporosis. *Osteoporosis International* 2007;18:1203-10.

96. Camargo, C. et al. Maternal intake of vitamin D during pregnancy and risk of recurrent wheeze in children at 3 y. *Am J Clin Nutr* 2007;85:788-95.

97. Hart, P. et al. sunlight may protect against asthma. Perth (Australia) Telethon institute for child health research. Quoted in Australian AP Oct 24, 2006.

98. Xystrakis, E. et al. Treatment of Steroid-Resistant Asthma. *J Clin Invest* 2006;116:146-55. Epub.

99. Devereux, G. et al. Maternal vitamin D intake and early childhood wheezing. *Am J Clin Nutr* 2007;85:853-59.

100. Jefferson, T. et al. Influenza vaccination: policy versus evidence. *BMJ*. 2006;333::912-15.

101. Mutter, J. et al. Side effects of mercury containing vaccines like influenza, *bmj.com*, 22 Nov 2006.

102. Simonsen, L. et al. Impact of influenza vaccination on seasonal mortality in the USA elderly population. *Arch Intern Med* 2005;165:265-72.

239

103. Simonsen, L. et al. Mortality benefits of influenza vaccination in elderly people: an ongoing controversy. *Lancet Infect Dis* 2007;7:658-66.

104. Rajapakse, R. et al. 1,25(OH)2D3 inhibits in vitro and in vivo intracellular growth of apicomplexan parasite *Toxoplasma gondii*. *J Steroid Biochem Mol Biol* 2007 Mar;103(3-5):811-4.

105. Bodnar, L et a. Maternal vitamin D deficiency increases the risk of preeclampsia. *J Clin Endocrinol Metab* 2007;92:3517-22.

106. Camargo, C. et al. Regional differences in EpiPen prescriptions in the United States: the potential role of vitamin D. *J Allergy Clin Immunol* 2007;120:128-30

107. Camadoo, L et al. Maternal vitamin D deficiency associated with neonatal hypocalcaemic convulsions. *Nutr J* 2007;6:23.

108. American Epilepsy Society 61st annual meeting: Abstract 3.337. November 30-December 4, 2007.

109. Litonjua, A. et al. Is vitamin D deficiency to blame for the asthma epidemic? *J Allergy Clin Immunol* 2007;120:1031-35.

110. Grant, W. Solar ultraviolet-B irradiance and vitamin D may reduce risk of septicemia. Unpublished manuscript furnished to author Dec 28,2007.

111. Mookherjee, N. et al. Cathelicidins and functional analogues as antisepsis molecules. *Expert Opinions on Therapeutic Targets* 2007;11:993-1004.

112. Wang, H. et al. National estimates of severe sepsis in United States emergency departments. *Crit Care Med* 2007;35:2461-2.

113. Danai P. et al. Seasonal variation in the epidemiology of sepsis. *Crit Care Med.* 2007;35:410–15.

114. Danai P. et al. The epidemiology of sepsis in patients with malignancy. *Chest.* 2006;129:1432–40.

115. Montague M, et al. Slip! Slop! Slap! and SunSmart, 1980-2000: Skin cancer control and 20 years of population-based campaigning. *Health Educ Behav.* 2001;28:290–305.

116. Giacometti, A. et al. Cathelicidin peptide sheep myeloid antimicrobial peptide-29 prevents endotoxin-induced mortality in rat models of septic shock. *Am J Respir Crit Care Med* 2004;169:187-94.

117. Giacometti, A. et al. The antimicrobial peptide BMAP-28 reduces lethality in mouse models of staphylococcal sepsis. *Crit Care Med.* 2004;32:2485–90.

118. Cirioni O. et al. LL-37 protects rats against lethal sepsis caused by gram-negative bacteria. *Antimicrob Agents Chemother.* 2006;50:1672–9.

119. Grant, W. Personal communication with author, Dec 31, 2007.

120. Parekh, N. et al. Association between vitamin D and age-related macular degeneration in the Third National Health and Nutrition Examination Survey, 1988 through 1994. *Arch Opthalmol* 2007;125:661-69.

121. Morgan, I. et al. Report to Australasian Ophthalmic and Visual Sciences Meeting, Canberra, Australia, December 2007.

122. Cutolo, M. et al. Review: vitamin D, immunity and lupus. *Lupus* 2008;17:6-10.

123. Tomazic, J. Prevalence and risk factors for osteopenia/osteoporosis in an HIV infected male population. *Wein Klin Wochenschr* 2007119:639-46.

124. Corbett, S. et al. Vitamin d receptor found in human sperm. *Urology* 2006;68:1345-49.

125. Zittermann, A. et al. Vitamin D and vascular calcification. *Curr Opin Lipidol* 2007;18:41-46.

126. Palmer, B. et al. Sexual dysfunction in men and women with chronic kidney disease and end-stage kidney disease. *Adv Ren Replace Ther* 2003;10:48.

127. Guan, J. et al. Sexual dysfunction in female patients with chronic renal insufficiency. *Sichuan Da Xue Bao Yi Xue Ban* 2005;36:555-58.

128. Kinuta, K. et al. Vitamin D is an important factor in estrogen biosynthesis in both female and male gonads. *Endocrinology* 2000;141:1317-24.

129. Sood, S. et al. Effect of vitamin D deficiency on testicular function in the rat. *Ann Nutr Metab* 1992;36:203-8.

130. Sood, S. et al. Effect of vitamin D repletion on testicular function in vitamin-D deficient rats. *Ann Nutr Metab* 1995;95-98.

131. Visser, M. et al. Low serum vitamin concentrations of 25 hydroxyvitamin D in older persons and the risk of nursing home admission. *Am J Clin Nutr* 2006;84:616-22.

132. Gordon, C. et al. Nutrient status of adults with cystic fibrosis. *J Am Diet Assoc* 2007;107:2114-19.

133. Rovner, A. et al. Vitamin D insufficiency in children , adolescents and young adults with cystic fibrosis despite routine oral supplementation. *Am J Clin Nutr* 2007;86:1694-99.

134. Martineau, A. Effect of vitamin D supplementation on anti-mycobacterial immunity: a double-blind randomized placebo-controlled trial in London tuberculosis contacts. *Int J Tuberculosis Lung Dis* 2005;9:S173.

135. Martineau, A. et al. Vitamin D status of tuberculosis patients and healthy blood donors in Samara City, Russia. *Int J Tuberculosis* Lung Dis 2005;9:S225.

136. Martineau, A et al. A single dose of vitamin D enhances immunity of mycobacteria. *A J Respir Crit Care Med* 2007;176:208-13.

137. Liu, P. et al. vitamin D mediated human antimicrobial activity against mycobacterium tuberculosis is dependent on the induction of cathelicidin. *J Immunol* 2007;179:2060-63.

138. Liu, W. et al. A case-control study on the vitamin D receptor gene polymorphisms and susceptibility to pulmonary tuberculosis. Zhonghua Liu Xing Bing Xue Za Zhi 2003;24:389-92.

139. Gibney, K. et al. vitamin D deficiency is associated with tuberculosis and latent tuberculosis infection in immigrants from sub-Saharan Africa. Clin Infect Dis 2008'46:443-46.

140. Selvarj, P. et al. Regulatory role of promoter and 3' UTR variants of vitamin D receptor gene on cytokine response in pulmonary tuberculosis. *J Clin Immunol* 2008; January 30. Epub ahead of print.

141. Vidyarani, M. et al. 1, 25 Hydroxyvitamin D3 modulated cytokine response in pulmonary tuberculosis. *Cytokine* 2007;40:128-34.

142. Thys-Jacobs, S. Alleviation of migraines with therapeutic vitamin D and calcium. *Headache* 1994;34:590-92.

143. Cann, B. Vitamin D supplementation and the risk of postmenopausal weight gain. *Arch Intern Med* 2007167:893-902.

144. Smotkin-Tangora, M. er al. Prevalence of vitamin D insufficiency in obese children and adolescents. *J Pediatr Endocrinol Metab* 2007;20:817-23.

145. Herr, C. et al. The role of cathelicidin and defensins in pulmonary and inflammatory diseases. *Expert Opin Biol Ther* 2007;7:1449-61.

146. Grant WB. Hypothesis-Ultraviolet-B Irradiance and Vitamin D Reduce the Risk of Viral Infections and thus Their Sequelae, Including Autoimmune Diseases and some Cancers. *Photochem Photobiol* 2008 Jan 7; [Epub ahead of print]

147. Ascherio, A. et al. Environmental risk factors for multiple sclerosis. Part I: the role of infection. *Ann. Neurol 2007;*61:288-99.

148. Holmoy, T. Vitamin D status modulates the immune response to Epstein-Barr virus: synergistic effect of risk factors in multiple sclerosis. *Med. Hypotheses* 2007 Jun 13; [Epub ahead of print]

149. Tenconi, M. et al. Major childhood infectious diseases and other determinants associated with type 1 diabetes: a case–control study. *Acta Diabetol* 2007;44:14-19.

150. Proud, D. and C. W. Chow (2006) Role of viral infections in asthma and chronic obstructive pulmonary disease. *Am. J. Respir. Cell. Mol. Bio 2006;*35:513-18.

151. Traves, S. et al. Viral-associated exacerbations of asthma and COPD. *Curr Opin Pharmacol* 2007;**7**:252-258.

152. Karatekin, G. Association of subclinical vitamin d deficiency in newborns with acute lower respiratory infections and their mothers. *Eur J Clin Nutr* 2007 Nov 21. [Epub ahead of print]

153. Wayse, V. et al. Association of subclinical vitamin D deficiency with severe acute lower respiratory infection in Indian children under 5 y. *Eur J Clin Nutr* 2004;58:563-67.

154. Hiemstra, P. The role of epithelial beta-defensins and cathelicidins in host defense of the lung. *Exp Lung Res* 2007;33:537-42.

155. Laaksi, I. et al. An association of serum vitamin d concentrations < 40 nmol/L with acute

respiratory tract infection in young Finnish men. *Am J Clin Nutr* 2007;86:714-17.

156. Yorifuji J. et al. Craniotabes in normal newborns: the earliest sign of subclinical vitamin D deficiency. *J Clin Endocrinol Metab* 2008 [Epub]
157. Roth, D. et al. vitamin D receptor polymorphisms and the risk of acute lower respiratory tract infection in early childhood. *J Infect Dis* 2008, Feb 11 [Epub ahead of print].
158. Zou, J. et al. Progressive hearing loss in mice with a mutated vitamin D receptor gene. *Audiol Neurootol* 2008;7:219-230.
159. Kong, J. Molecular mechanism of 1,25-dihydroxyvitamin D3 inhibition of adipogenesis in 3T3-L1 cells. *Am J Physiol Endocrinol Metab* 2006;290:E916-24.
160. Wood, R. Vitamin d and adipogenesis: new molecular insights. *Nutr Rev* 2008;66:40-46.
161. Nnoaham, K. et al. Low serum vitamin D levels and tuberculosis: a systematic review and meta-analysis. *Int J Epidemiol* 2008;37:113-19.
162. Kumar, R. Urbanites More Prone to Leprosy. *Merinews* April 14, 2008. (available at http://www.merinews.com/catFull.jsp?articleID=132447)
163. Shoben, A. et al. Association of Oral Calcitriol with Improved Survival in Nondialyzed CKD. *J Am Soc Nephrol* May 7, 2008 [Epub ahead of print]
164. Belostotsky, V. et al. Vitamin D deficiency in children with renal disease. *Arch Dis Child* 2008. Published online May 7,2008.
165. Kovesdy, C. et al. Association of activated vitamin D treatment and mortality in chronic kidney disease. *Arch Intern Med*. 2008;168:397-403.
166. Kendrick, J. et al. Report to the conference of the National Kidney Foundation, Spring Clinical Meetings. May 16, 2008.
167. Ng, K. et al. Circulating 25-hydroxyvitamin d levels and survival in patients with colorectal cancer. *J Clin Oncol*. 2008;26:2984-91.
168. Dobnig, H. et al. Independent association of low serum 25-hydroxyvitamin d and 1,25-dihydroxyvitamin d levels with all-cause and cardiovascular mortality. *Arch Intern Med*. 2008;168:1340-9.
169. Illinois Dept. of Public Health. Health beat. Accessed July 4, 2008. Available online at http://www.idph.state.il.us/public/hb/hbmening.htm
170. Dowell, S. et al. Seasonal patterns of invasive pneumococcal disease. *Emerg Infect Dis* 2003;9:573-9.
171. Vlaminckx, B. et al. Long-term surveillance of invasive group A streptococcal disease in The Netherlands, 1994-2003. *Clinical Microbiology and Infection* 2005;11:226-31.
172. Schroth, R. et al. Influence of Maternal Vitamin D Status on Infant Oral Health. Presentation at the General Session of the International Association for Dental Research, Toronto, Canada, July 4, 2008.
173. Elter K, et al. Exposure to low outdoor temperature in the midtrimester is associated with low birth weight. *Aust N Z J Obstet Gynecol* 2004;44:553-7
174. Murray, L. et al. Links Season and outdoor ambient temperature: effects on birth weight. *Obstet Gynecol*. 2000 Nov;96(5 Pt 1):689-95.
175. Melamed, M. et al. 25-Hydroxyvitamin D Levels and the Risk of Mortality in the General Population. *Arch Intern Med*. 2008;168(15):1629-1637.

Chapter 15. Solar Power fights depression and other mental disorders.

1. Nielsen Media Research 2000.
2. Golden, R. et al. The Efficacy of Light Therapy in the Treatment of Mood Disorders: A Review and Meta-Analysis of the Evidence. *Am J Psychiatry* 2005;162:656-62.
3. Tuunainen, A. et al. Light therapy for non-seasonal depression. *Cochrane Database Syst Rev* 2004;2:CD004050.
4. USA Food and Drug Administration web site, updated July 12, 2005.
5. Lambert, G. et al. Effect of sunlight and season on serotonin turnover in the brain. *Lancet* 2002;360:1840-42.
6. Holick, M. et al. *The UV Advantage* 2. Ibooks 2003, New York.
7. Warthan, M. et al. UV light tanning as a type of substance-related disorder. *Arch Dermatol* 2005;141:963-96.

8. Feldman, S. et al. Ultraviolet exposure is a reinforcing stimulus in frequent indoor tanners. *J Am Acad Dermatol* 2004;51:45-51.

9. Kaur, M. et al. Induction of withdrawal-like symptoms in a small randomized, controlled trial of opioid blockade in frequent tanners. *J Am Acad Dermatol* 2006;54:709-11.

10. Lansdowne, A. et al. Vitamin D3 enhances mood in healthy subjects during winter. *Psychopharmacology* (Berl) 1998;135:319-23.

11. Vieth, R. et al. Randomized comparison of the effects of the vitamin D3 adequate intake versus 100 mcg (4,000 IU) per day on biochemical responses and the wellbeing of patients. *Nutr J* 2004;3:8.

12. Brenner, A. et al. Season of birth and risk of brain tumors in adults. *Neurology* 2004;63:276-81.

13. Heuch, J. et al. Risk of primary childhood brain tumors related to birth characteristics: a Norwegian prospective study. *Int J Cancer* 1998 Aug 12;77(4):498-503.

14. McNally, R. et al. An infectious aetiology for childhood brain tumors? Evidence from space-time clustering and seasonality analyses. *Br J Cancer* 2002;86:1070-77.

15. Eyles, D. et al. Vitamin D3 and brain development. *Neuroscience* 2003;118:641-53.

16. Feron, F. et al. Developmental vitamin D3 deficiency alters the adult rat brain. *Brain Res Bull*. 2005 Mar 15;65(2):141-8.

17. Benedetti, F. et al. Morning sunlight reduces length of hospitalization in bipolar depression. *J Affect Disord* 2001;62:221-23.

18. Beauchemin, K. et al. sunny hospital rooms expedite recovery from severe and refractory depressions. *J Affect Disord* 1996;40:49-51.

19. McGrath, J. et al. Long-term trends in sunshine duration and its association with schizophrenia birth rates and age at first registration—data from Australia and the Netherlands. *Schizophr Res* 2002;54:199-212.

20. McGrath, J. et al. Hypothesis: Is low prenatal vitamin D a risk-modifying factor for schizophrenia? *Schizophr Res* 1999;40:173-77.

21. McGrath, J. et al. A systematic review of the incidence of schizophrenia: the distribution of rates and the influence of sex, urbanicity, migrant status and methodology. *BMC Med* 2004;2:13-35.

22. Sato, Y. et al. High prevalence of vitamin D deficiency and reduced bone mass in elderly women with Alzheimer's disease. *Bone* 1998;23:555-57.

23. Burne, T. et al. Transient prenatal Vitamin D deficiency is associated with hyperlocomotion in adult rats. *Behav Brain Res*. 2004;154:549-55.

24. Becker, A. et al. Transient prenatal vitamin D deficiency is associated with subtle alterations in learning and memory functions in adult rats. *Behav Brain Res* 2005;161:306-12.

25. Grant, W. Personal communication with author, June, 2006.

26. McGrath, J. et al. Vitamin D3-implications for brain development. *J Steroid Biochem Mol Biol* 2004;89-90:557-60.

27. Levins, P et al. Plasma beta-endorphin and beta-lipoprotein response to ultraviolet radiation. *Lancet* 1983;2:166.

28. Hillhouse, J. et al. Association of frequent indoor UV tanning with seasonal affective disorder. *Arch Dermatol* 2005;141:1465

29. Wilkins C. et al. Vitamin D Deficiency Is Associated With Low Mood and Worse Cognitive Performance in Older Adults. *Am J Geriatr Psychiatry;*2006;14:1032–1040).

30. Muller, K. et al. 1,25-Dihydroxyvitamin D3 inhibits cytokine production by human blood monocytes at the post-transcriptional level. *Cytokine* 1992;4:506-12.

31. Nagpal S. et al. Noncalcemic actions of vitamin D receptor ligands. *Endocr Rev* 2005;26:662– 87.

32. Tan, Z. et al. Inflammatory markers and the risk of Alzheimer disease: the Framingham Study. *Neurology* 2007;68:1902-08.

33. Richards, J. et al. High serum vitamin D concentrations are associated with longer leukocyte telomere length in women. *Am J Clin Nutr* 2007;86:1420.

34. Kalueff, A. et al. Increased anxiety in mice lacking vitamin D receptor gene.

Neuroreport 2004;15:1271-74.

35. Diem, S. et al. Use of antidepressants and rates of hip bone loss in older women; the study of osteoporotic fractures. *Arch Intern Med* 2007:167:1231-32.

36. Kalueff, A. et al. Behavioral anomalies in mice evoked by Tokyo disruption of the vitamin D receptor gene. *Neurosci Res* 2006;54:254-60.

37. Stewart, R. et al. Dental health and cognitive impairment in an English National survey population. *J Amer Geriatr Soc.* 2007;55:1410-14.

38. Kunningas, M. VDR gene variants associate with cognitive function and depressive symptoms of old age. *Neurobiology of Aging* 2007. Manuscript accepted for publication July 2007.

39. Autism Society of America web site, accessed January 29, 2008.

40. Cannell, J. Autism and vitamin D. *Med hypothesis* Oct 24, 2007. Epub ahead of print.

41. Ganz, M. The lifetime distribution of the incremental societal costs of autism. *Arch Pediatr Adolesc Med* 2007;161:343-39.

42. *JAMA* 1989;262:380-84. (No authors listed)

43. Ashwood, P. et al. The immune response in autism: a new frontier for autism research. *J Leukoc Biol* 2006;80:1-15.

44. Cantorna, M. . Vitamin D status, 1,25-dihydroxyvitamin D3, and the immune system. *Am J Clin Nutr.* 2004 Dec;80:1717S-20S.

45. Hibbeln, J. *et al.* Maternal seafood consumption in pregnancy and neurodevelopmental outcomes in childhood (ALSPAC study): an observational cohort study. *Lancet.* 2007 Feb 17;369(9561):578-85.

46. Gillberg, C. Et al. Autism in immigrants: children born in Sweden to mothers born in Uganda. *J Intellect Disabil Res.* 1995;39:141-4.

47. Cannell, J. Vitamin D newsletter, May 2007.

48. Fighting Autism web site: http://www.fightingautism.org/idea/autism.php. Accessed January 31, 2008.

49. Grant, W. Epidemiological evidence for supporting the role of maternal vitamin D deficiency as a significant risk factor for the development of infantile autism in those born prior to 1985. Unpublished manuscript.

50. Centers for Disease Control and Prevention. Prevalence of autism spectrum disorders–autism and developmental disabilities monitoring network, 14 sites, United States, 2002. *MMWR Surveill Summ* 2007;56:12–28.

51. Stevens, M. Season of birth effects in autism. *J Clin Exp Neuropsychol* 2000;22:399–407.

52. Williams, J. et al. Systematic review of prevalence studies of autism spectrum disorders. *Arch Dis Child* 2006;91:8-15.

53. Windham, M. et al. Autism spectrum disorders in relation to hazardous air pollutants in the San Francisco Bay area. *Environ Health Perspect* 2006;114:1438-44.

54. Agarwal, K. et al. The impact of atmospheric pollution on vitamin D status of infants and toddlers in Delhi, India. *Arch Dis Child.* 2002;87:111-13.

55. Gambichler, T. et al. Impact of UVA exposure on psychological parameters and circulating serotonin and melatonin. *BMC Dermatol* 2002;2:6.

56. Waldman M, et al. Does television cause autism? *National Bureau of Economic Research Working Paper* 12632, 2006. http://www.econ.cudenver.edu/mocan/data%20for%20 courses/Autism%5B1%5D.w12632.pdf (accessed Feb 2, 2008.).

57. Wang, H. Quoted by Dan Olmsted in *The Age of Autism: One in 15,000 Amish.* UPI June 8, 2005. Available online at http://pittsburgh.indymedia.org/news/2005/06/18948.php. (accessed Feb 2, 2008.

58. Gloth, F. et al. Vitamin D vs. broad spectrum phototherapy in the treatment of seasonal affective disorder. *J Nutr Health Aging* 1999;3:5-7.

59. Byrne, M. Obstetric conditions and risk of first admission with schizophrenia: a Danish national register based study. *Schizophr Res* 2007;97:51-59.

60. Cannell, J. et al. Epidemic Influenza and vitamin D. *Epidemiol Infect* 2006;134:1129-40.

61. Aloia, J. et al. Colds and Flu. Letter to the editor. *Epidemiol Infect* Jan 15, 2007.

62. Atladottir, H. *et al.* Time trends in reported diagnoses of childhood neuropsychiatric disorders: a Danish cohort study. *Arch Pediatr Adolesc Med* 2007;161:193-8.

63. MacNeal, R. et al. Update on sun protection and tanning in children. *Curr Opin Pediatr* 2007;19:425-29.

64. Kirsch, I. et al. Initial severity and antidepressant benefits: a meta-analysis of data submitted to the Food and Drug Administration. *PLoS Medicine* 2008;5:e45. doi:10.1371/journal.pmed.0050045 Accessed March 11, 2008. ?

65. Carlson, A. et al. Is vitamin D deficiency associated with peripheral neuropathy? *The Endocrinologist* 2007;17:319-25.

66. Oudshoorn C. et al. Higher Serum Vitamin D(3) Levels Are Associated with Better Cognitive Test Performance in Patients with Alzheimer's Disease. *Dement Geriatr Cogn Disord* 2008;25:539-543.

67. Edwards MJ. Hyperthermia in utero due to maternal influenza is an environmental risk factor for schizophrenia. *Congenit Anom (Kyoto);*2007;47:84-9.

68. McGrath J, et al. Vitamin D supplementation during the first year of life and risk of schizophrenia: a Finnish birth cohort study. *Schizophr Res.* 2004;67:237-45.

69. Badian, N. Reading Disability in an Epidemiological Context: Incidence and Environmental Correlates. *J Learn Disabil.* 1984;17:129-36.

70. Martin, R. Season of birth is related to child retention rates, achievement, and rate of diagnosis of specific LD. *J Learn Disabil* 2004;37:307-17.

71. Livingston, R. et al. Season of birth and neurodevelopmental disorders: summer birth is associated with dyslexia. *J Am Acad Child Adolesc Psychiatry.* 1993;32:612-6.

Chapter 16. Solar Power and African Americans

1. Nesby-O'Dell, S. et al. Hypovitaminosis D prevalence and determinants among African American and white women of reproductive age: third National Health and Nutrition Examination Survey, 1988-1994. *Am J Clin Nutr* 2002;76:187-92.

2. Plotnikoff G. et al. Prevalence of severe hypovitaminosis D in patients with persistent, nonspecific musculoskeletal pain. *Mayo Clin Proc.* 2003;78:1463-70.

3. Liu, P. et al. Toll-like receptor triggering of a vitamin D-mediated human antimicrobial response. *Science.* 2006;311:1770-73.

4. Prabhala, A. et al. Severe myopathy associated with vitamin D deficiency in western New York. *Arch Intern Med* 2000;160:1199-1203.

5. Grant, W. Lower vitamin-D production from solar ultraviolet-B irradiance may explain some differences in cancer survival rates. *JNMA* 2006;98:364.

6. USA Department of Health and Human Services 1998. *Tobacco Use Among USA Racial/ Ethnic Minority Groups — African Americans, American Indians and Alaska Natives, Asian Americans and Pacific Islanders, and Hispanics: A Report of the Surgeon General.* Atlanta: USA Department of Health and Human Services, Centers for Disease Control and Prevention.

7. Giovannucci, E. et al. Cancer Incidence and Mortality and Vitamin D in Black and White Male Health Professionals: *Cancer Epidemiol Biomarkers Prev* 2006;15:2467–72.

8. Egan, K. et al. Vitamin D insufficiency among African Americans in the southeastern United States: implications for cancer disparities (United States). *Cancer Causes Control* 2008;19:527-35

Chapter 17 Tanning beds (tanning beds) as health-promoting devices

1. Tangpricha, V. et al. Tanning is associated with optimal vitamin D status (serum 25-hydroxyvitamin D concentration) and higher bone mineral density. *Am J Clin Nutr* 2004;80:1645-49.

2. Kaur, M. et al. Indoor tanning relieves pain. *Photodermatol Photoimmunol Photomed* 2005;21:278.

3. Bataille V, et al. A multicentre epidemiological study on tanning bed use and cutaneous melanoma in Europe. *Eur J Cancer* 2005;41:2141-49.

4. Grant, W. Personal communication with author.

5. International Smart Tan Network 2006. Research shows no connection between tanning and melanoma: Why this is misunderstood..

6. Autier, P. et al. Cutaneous malignant melanoma and exposure to sunlamps and tanning beds: a descriptive study in Belgium. *Melanoma Res* 1991; 1:69-74

7. Autier, P. et al. tanning bed use and risk of melanoma: results from a large multicentric European study. Poster at the XVIII International Pigment Cell conference held 9-13 September 2002 at Egmond The Netherlands.

8. Clough-Gorr, K. et al. Exposure to sunlamps, tanning beds and melanoma risk. *Cancer Causes Control* 2008, February 14. [Epub ahead of print]

9. International Agency for Research on Cancer Working Group on artificial ultraviolet light (UV) and skin cancer. The association of use of tanning beds with cutaneous malignant melanoma and other skin cancer: a systematic review. *Int J Cancer* 2007;120:1116-22.

10. Grant, W. Insufficient evidence exists to link tanning bed use to risk of melanoma for other than those with skin phenotype 1. Sunlight, Nutrition and Health Research Center (SUNARC). March 9, 2007. www. SUNARC org.

11. Autier, P. Perspectives in melanoma prevention: the case of tanning beds. *Eur J Cancer* 2004;40:2367-76.

12. Holick, M. et al. Boston University. "Effects Of Vitamin D And Skin's Physiology Examined." *Science Daily* 21 February 2008 <http://www.sciencedaily.com / releases/2008/02/080220161707.htm>.

13. Grant, W. Personal communication,, February 27, 2008.

14. Bukhari, M. et al. Quoted in London Times April 27, 2008.

15. Garland, C. et al.. Epidemiologic evidence for different roles of ultraviolet A and B radiation in melanoma mortality rates. *Ann Epidemiol.* 2003;13:395-404.

16. Gorham, D, et al. Do sunscreens increase risk of melanoma in populations residing at higher latitudes? *Ann Epidemiol.* 2007 Dec;17(12):956-63.

17. Moan, J. et al. Epidemiological support for an hypothesis for melanoma induction indicating a role for UVA radiation. *Photochem Photobiol.* 1999;70):243-7.

18. Moan, J. et al. Addressing the health benefits and risks, involving vitamin D or skin cancer, of increased sun exposure. *Proc Natl Acad Sci* U S A. 2008;15;105(2):668-73.

Glossary

Actinic keratosis (AK): a slightly raised scaly area that forms on the surface of the epidermis. AK's are considered precursors to some skin cancers.

Alveolar ridge: the ridgelike border of the upper and lower jaws containing the sockets of the teeth.

Anaphylaxis: an extreme allergic reaction to a foreign substance resulting from previous exposure to it.

Angiogenesis: the formation of new blood vessels; in the case of cancer, angiogenesis is necessary to bring nutrients to cancer cells in order to keep them alive, growing and multiplying.

Antioxidant: a substance, such as a vitamin or mineral that protects the cells of the body from the damaging effects of free-radical attack.

Apoptosis: the process by which a cell dies after it has lived long enough to serve its purpose; it is normal, programmed cell death.

Arteriosclerosis: a thickening, hardening, and loss of elasticity of the arterial walls that results in impaired blood circulation.

Atherosclerosis: the deposition of fatty plaques containing cholesterol and lipids on the innermost layers of the walls of arteries.

Autism: a developmental disorder of children, characterized by impaired communication and emotional detachment.

Autoimmune disease: a disease in which the immune system attacks the body's own tissue, mistaking that tissue for a foreign invader.

Basal cell carcinoma: a cancer that occurs in the lower layers of the epidermis, which is the outer layer of the skin.

Bipolar disorder: a psychological disorder characterized by periods of mania alternating with periods of depression.

Body mass index: A measurement of the relative percentages of fat and muscle in the human body.

Calcidiol or 25-hydroxycholecalciferol: the form of vitamin D produced in the liver, and the form that should be measured when one has a blood test for vitamin D. It is also known as 25(OH)D.

Calcification: Impregnation of arterial plaque with calcium.

Calcitriol or 1,25-dihydroxycholecalciferol: the potent, active form of vitamin D produced in the kidneys and in many other tissues of the body. It is also known as 1,25(OH)D.

Cathelicidin: a peptide protein that acts as an internal bactericide.

Cognitive: pertaining to the mental processes of perception, memory, judgment, and reasoning.

Common skin cancer, also known as non-melanoma skin cancer (NMSC): the most common, yet least dangerous of all cancers. It is composed to two forms: basal cell carcinoma and squamous cell carcinoma.

C-reactive protein (CRP): a protein that is a product of inflammation and a predictor of heart disease.

Crohn's disease: A type of autoimmune, inflammatory bowel disease (IBD).

Cytokine: a small protein released by cells that has a regulating influence on cell interactions, communications and behavior.

Dermis: the layer of the skin located below the epidermis. It contains nerve endings, sweat and sebaceous glands, blood and lymph.

Differentiation: the process by which cells take on the characteristics of the surrounding tissue.

DNA: the molecules inside cells that carry genetic information.

Dopamine: a neurotransmitter in the central nervous system that acts to help regulate movement and emotion.

Dyslexia: A learning disorder marked by impairment of the ability to recognize and comprehend written words.

Eczema: a skin disorder primarily occurring in younger people. It is characterized by redness and itching, and may result in lesions that discharge pus and become scaly and crusty.

Endorphin: A "feel-good" chemical that also raises the pain threshold.

Endotoxin: a toxic substance liberated when a microorganism dies.

Epidermis: the outer, protective layer of skin.

EpiPen: a drug that is prescribed to treat or prevent anaphylaxis

Epithelium: a tissue composed of one or more layers of cells, which forms the covering of most internal and external surfaces of the body and its organs.

Essential fatty acid: A fat that is essential for proper functioning of the body, and which cannot be constructed within the body.

Etiology: the cause or origin of a disease or disorder.

Experimental autoimmune encephalomyelitis (EAE): a chemically induced disease of laboratory animals that is similar to multiple sclerosis (MS) and is used as a model to study MS.

Fibromyalgia: a common ailment that is characterized by chronic muscle and joint pain as well as fatigue and tenderness in some parts of the body.

Free radical: any atom, capable of independent existence, with at least one unpaired electron in its outermost shell. Free radicals are unstable and are damaging to cells of the body.

Glycemic response: the change in blood glucose concentration induced by ingested food.

Hodgkin's lymphoma: A progressive, sometimes fatal cancer marked by enlargement of the lymph nodes, spleen, and liver.

Hypertension: high blood pressure.

Hypocalcaemia: an abnormally low level of calcium in the blood

Immunosuppressant: An agent that reduces the body's immune response.

Inflammation: a reaction of tissue to irritation such as oxidative stress, sometimes characterized by pain, redness, swelling, and loss of function.

Inflammatory bowel disease (IBD): an autoimmune disease characterized by inflammation of the intestine and chronic diarrhea.

Intermittent claudication: A peripheral artery disease that causes leg pain due to inadequate blood supply to the legs.

International Unit (IU): a unit of measurement of vitamin D consumed in food or supplements. One IU is equal to .025 micrograms (mcg) of vitamin D as calcidiol.

Invasiveness: the tendency of cancers to spread into surrounding healthy tissue.

Leprosy: A chronic, mildly contagious disease characterized by ulcers of the skin, bone, and gut and leading to loss of sensation, paralysis, gangrene, and deformation.

Libido: sexual drive or instinct.

Lipid peroxidation: the oxidative deterioration of fats.

Lipid peroxidation: the process whereby the lipids in cell membranes become oxidized by free radicals, resulting in cell damage.

LL-37: the cathelicidin that is produced in the human body.

LOAEL: Lowest Observed Adverse Effect Level.

Lupus (see systemic lupus erythematosus)

Macular degeneration (AMD): deterioration of vision in the central area of the visual field.

Mammography: x-ray photography of a breast for the detection of cancer.

Melanin: a naturally occurring dark pigment found in skin.

Melanocyte: a cell of the epidermis that produces melanin.

Melanoma: a very dangerous skin cancer that attacks the melanin (skin pigment) producing cells of the skin (melanocytes).

Melatonin: a hormone produced by the pineal gland. It causes drowsiness and plays a role in sleep. It works in concert with serotonin to regulate sleep cycles.

Metabolic Syndrome (Met S): a group of factors (high blood pressure, abdominal obesity, high triglyceride levels, low HDL levels, insulin resistance) that are linked to increased risk of cardiovascular disease and type 2 diabetes.

Metastasis: the spreading of cancer cells from the initial location of disease to another location, usually by way of the blood vessels or lymphatic systems:

Monounsaturated fatty acids: a class of fats whose carbon chains have one double or triple valence bond per molecule. They are found chiefly in olive oil, almonds, peanuts, avocados and canola.

Multiple sclerosis (MS): an autoimmune disease of the central nervous system in which gradual destruction of the myelin sheath occurs, interfering with the nerve conductivity and causing muscular weakness, loss of coordination, and speech and visual disturbances.

Mutation: a change in a gene or a chromosome that causes a sudden departure from the parent type in a heritable characteristic.

Myelin sheath: the covering or insulation that surrounds nerve fibers in the brain and spinal cord.

Myopathy: a disease of muscle tissue.

Myopia: a condition in which objects can be seen distinctly only when near the eye; nearsightedness.

Nanogram (ng): one billionth of a gram.

Nanomole (nmol): one billionth of a mole, which is the amount of a substance that contains as many atoms, molecules, ions, or other elementary units as the number of atoms in 0.012 kilogram of carbon 12

Necrotizing fasciitis: An infectious disease caused by a virulent strep bacteria also known as "flesh-eating bacteria."

Neuroblastoma: a cancerous tumor of immature nerve cells that most often affects young children.

Neuropathy: any disease condition that causes deterioration of the nerves.

Neurotransmitter: a chemical that transmits nerve impulses to another nerve, gland, or muscle.

Ng/ml: the number of nanograms of a substance contained in one milliliter of blood. It is one of two common methods of expressing the quantity of vitamin D in blood serum.

Nmol/l: a second method of expressing the quantity of vitamin D in serum—1 ng/ml=2.5 nmol/l.

Non-Hodgkin's lymphoma: a cancer that may develop in any organ associated with the lymphatic system.

Nosocomial: relating to any disease contracted by a patient while under medical care.

Omega-3 fatty acids: polyunsaturated fatty acids whose carbon chains have their first double valence bonds three carbons from the beginning. Omega-3 fats are anti-inflammatory and considered to have health benefits.

Omega-6 fatty acids: polyunsaturated fatty acids whose carbon chains have their first double valence bonds six carbons from the beginning. These fats are the type usually used in frying and produce inflammatory chemicals in the body.

Osteoblast: a bone-forming cell

Osteoclast: a cell that breaks down and reabsorbs bone tissue.

Osteomalacia: a bone disease that results from vitamin D or calcium deficiency. It is characterized by a softening of the bones and accompanying pain and weakness, and is sometimes known as "adult rickets."

Oxidation: the combination of oxygen with another substance, leading to a loss of electrons and the formation of free radicals.

Oxidative stress: a condition of increased oxidation in animal cells that results in the release of free radicals and results in cellular degeneration.

Oxybenzone: a chemical used in sunscreens.

Pandemic: prevalent throughout an entire country, continent, or the whole world, widespread.

Parasite: an organism that lives on or in another organism, from which it obtains food.

Parathyroid hormone (PTH): a hormone produced by the parathyroid glands. It works with calcitriol to regulate the amount of calcium and phosphorus in the blood and bones.

Parkinson's disease: a progressive disease of the nerves of the brain and/or spinal cord, characterized by weakness and the inability to control some muscular movements, as well as an unusual gait, partial facial paralysis and tremors.

Peptide: an organic compound composed of amino acids linked together chemically.

Periodontal disease (PD): a disease that attacks the gum and bone around the teeth, causing inflammation, bone loss and subsequent loss of teeth

Peripheral artery disease (PAD): a type of vascular disease which results in occlusion of the arteries of the limbs.

Peripheral artery disease (PAD): a type of vascular disease which occludes arteries of the limbs.

Plaque (arterial): a deposit of fatty material on the inner lining of an arterial wall.

Plaque (dental): a sticky film attached to tooth surfaces, formed by bacteria growth.

Plaque (skin): a flat, often raised, patch on the skin.

Polycystic ovary disease: a disorder in which there are many small cysts in the ovaries, which can affect a woman's ability to become pregnant.

Polyp: a benign (non-cancerous) growth in the colon that is often a precursor to colon cancer.

Polyunsaturated fatty acid: A fat or oil found primarily in fish, corn, soybeans and safflower, and that is usually liquid at room temperature.

Polyunsaturated fatty acids (PUFA): a class of fats that are liquid at room temperature and are found primarily in corn, soybean, safflower, nut, flax and fish oils.

Pre-eclampsia: a pregnancy disorder characterized by hypertension, fluid retention, and excessive protein in the urine.

Proliferation: the uncontrolled growth and reproduction of cancer cells.

Pro-oxidant: a substance that produces oxygen free radicals that damage cells.

Prostate specific antigen (PSA): a protein produced by the prostate gland. A test for PSA is used to screen for prostate cancer and to monitor its progression.

Psoralen: a medication used to increase sensitivity to the sun as a means of controlling psoriasis.

Psoriasis: a skin disease in which cells in the affected area begin to proliferate rapidly, rather than in a controlled manner. This rapid growth of skin cells causes raised patches of skin called plaques, which are scaly and cause extreme itching.

PubMed: the National Library of Medicine's database of scientific journal articles.

Pulmonary: pertaining to the lungs.

Rheumatoid arthritis: an autoimmune disease in which the immune system attacks joint tissue and destroys proper joint function.

Rickets: a crippling, deforming bone disease of children resulting from insufficient sunlight exposure and/or vitamin D deficiency.

Saturated fatty acids: a class of fats whose carbon chains cannot absorb any more hydrogen atoms. They are solid at room temperature and come primarily from animal sources and also from coconuts.

Schizophrenia: a mental disorder sometimes characterized by intellectual deterioration, disorganization, delusions, social isolation, and hallucinations.

Seasonal affective disorder (SAD): A form of depression occurring especially in winter, characterized by depression, irritability, weight gain, fatigue, and inability to concentrate.

Selective serotonin re-uptake inhibitors (SSRI's): a class of antidepressant drugs that inhibit the inactivation of serotonin.

Sepsis: the presence of various infectious organisms or their toxins in the blood or tissues.

Septicemia: a type of sepsis of the blood also known as "blood poisoning."

Serotonin: a hormone that acts as a neurotransmitter in the brain. It is produced by the pineal gland in response to sunlight, and causes feelings of alertness, happiness and wellbeing.

Seven (7)-dehydrocholesterol: a type of cholesterol that is contacted by sunlight to begin vitamin D production in skin.

Squamous cell carcinoma: a cancer that occurs in the upper layers of the epidermis and is characterized by rough, scaly patches.

Sunscare: relating to the effort by the medical profession and government to frighten people out of the sun.

Systemic lupus erythematosus (SLE): an autoimmune disease commonly known as "lupus." It is a disease that principally affects the skin and joints but can attack almost any system of the body.

Telomere: the segment of DNA that occurs at the ends of chromosomes.

Ultraviolet light (UV): light that is invisible because its wavelength is shorter than the violet part of the sunlight spectrum. There are three main varieties of UV: UVA, UVB and UVC.

UVA: light with a wavelength of 380-315 nanometers, which can penetrate beyond into a lower layer of skin called the dermis.

UVB: light has a wavelength of 315-290 nanometers (nm) that penetrates only the epidermis when it contacts the skin. Actually UVB extends to 280 nm, but solar UVB stops at 290 nm due to atmospheric absorption.

Vitamin D receptor (VDR): a vitamin D receptor found in most tissues of the body. It specifically links with and binds calcitriol.

Vitamin D Winter: the time of year in temperate climates in which the sunlight is not sufficiently direct to stimulate vitamin D production by the skin.

Vitamin D2 or ergocalciferol: a form of supplemental vitamin D derived from vegetable sources. It is not a form that functions well as a supplement and is not recommended.

Vitamin D3 or cholecalciferol: a form of vitamin D that is produced by the skin and is the preferred form for supplementation.

INDEX

A

Acid 53, 79, 110-1, 118, 137, 144
  haze 79
Actinic keratosis (AK) 52, 55, 132
Acute lower respiratory infections (AlRI) 173
Adenoma 96
African American 6, 23, 93-5, 122, 125, 143, 147, 169-71, 193-4, 200,
African Canadians 28
Aging 3, 34, 49, 53, 68, 70, 112, 179-80, 197, 204
Agrarian 63
AIDS 169-70, 174
Ainsleigh, Dr. Gordon 4, 46, 63, 105, 207
Air travel 65
AK, *see* Actinic keratosis
Alcohol 63, 101
AlRI, *see* Acute lower respiratory infections
Altitude 43, 80, 98, 132, 151-2, 164, 198
Alveolar ridge 160-1
Alzheimers 115, 187, 192
AMD, *see* Macular degeneration
American academy of pediatrics 32, 190
American cancer society 58, 79
American Indian 23
American Medical Association 189
Amino acid 144
Amish 191
Anaphylaxis 168, 182
Anemia 169
Angiogenesis 77, 91-2, 103, 105
Animal fats 50-1, 59, 142
Antibiotic 8, 19, 177-9, 181
Antidepressant 6, 119, 184, 192, 200
Antifungal 8
Antioxidant 44, 46-7, 49, 72, 77-8, 92, 186
Antiseptic 8, 177, 179, 181, 200
Anxiety 173, 189, 192

Apoptosis 76, 91-2, 98, 101-2, 105
Apperley, Dr. Frank 20
Argentina 134, 162
Arizona 24, 43, 151, 162, 165
Arthritis 11, 16, 108, 127-8, 130-1, 137, 140, 179, 195
Asia 2, 126
Asquith, Pamella 4
Asthma 175-6, 178, 181
Atherosclerosis 141, 150, 157
Athletic 26, 120, 128
Atom 45-6
Attachment loss 160-1
Australia 2, 64, 132-3, 139, 167, 171, 174, 176
Autier, Dr. Philippe 196
Autism 189-92
Autoimmune disease 127, 131, 140, 147-8

B

Bacteria 18, 160, 169-70, 173-4, 177-9, 181
Baggerly, Carole 4
Balance 45-6, 48, 50, 108, 110, 123-4, 128, 130-1, 179, 184, 197
Basal cell carcinoma 52
Bax 98
Berwick, Dr. Marianne 60
Beta-carotene 63
Bile duct 104, 106
Bipolar disorder 189, 192
Bischoff-Ferrari, Dr. Heike 118
Black American 27, 102, 104, 193
Black, Dr. Homer 20, 54
Black men 27-8, 91, 159, 194
Black physicians 194
Black women 23-4, 27-8, 32, 159, 193
Bladder cancer 101
Blood
  level 26, 83-5, 97, 112
  levels 6, 24-6, 30-2, 83, 87, 96-7, 99, 106, 112-3, 115, 122, 127, 129, 156, 176, 187
Blunt, Thomas 18

Body mass index 151, 162, 176
Bone 2, 16, 25-6, 32, 76-7, 110-21, 124, 129, 156, 160-1, 185, 199
Boston 4, 26, 28, 42, 125, 141
Botella-Carretero, Dr. Jose 176
Brain 102, 104, 106, 131, 148, 150, 161, 174, 183, 185-92
  cancer 102
Breast 6, 16, 27, 32, 57, 60-1, 76-85, 87, 89, 90, 93, 96, 101, 119-22, 144
  cancer 6, 16, 27, 60, 77-85, 87, 93, 119-21, 126, 170
Britain 23, 162
Bukhari, Dr. Marwan 116

C
Calcidiol 3, 34-5, 122, 157
Calcification 156-7, 159, 161
Calcitriol 16, 34-5, 111, 118, 135, 137, 148-9, 156-7, 168-9, 182
Calcium 2, 35, 78, 86, 109-11, 117-8, 120-1, 123, 129-30, 156-7, 163-4
Campbell, Dr. T. Colin 100
Canada 26, 42, 146
Canadian 33, 79
Cancer, *see* special kind; breast, colon, etc.
Cannell, Dr. John 26, 30, 128, 164, 171, 189, 204
Carotenoid 63, 72
Cartilage 127, 130
Castelli, Dr. William 150
Cathelicidin 2, 169, 171, 174, 193
Caucasian 161
CDC, *see* Center for Disease Control
Centenarians 28, 123
Center for Disease Control (CDC) 69
C-Fos 113
Chaplin, Dr. George 22
Chemotherapy 6, 84, 120
Cholecalciferol 29, 34
Cholesterol 7, 11, 15, 34, 49, 94, 137, 150-1, 159, 162-3, 176, 194
Christophers, Dr. Warren 61
Cigarette 47, 56
Clark, Dr. John 4, 144, 161
Clothing 17, 22, 28, 64, 89, 121-2, 130, 154, 164, 183
Cloud cover 44, 198
Cod liver oil 15, 145

Cognitive 180, 186-7, 192
Cold 10-2, 22, 171-2, 183, 187
Colds 11, 16, 171, 181
Colon cancer 4, 7, 16, 60, 79, 90, 94, 96-100, 104-6, 170
Colorectal cancer 96-7, 101, 179
Common skin cancers 53-4, 58-9, 70, 82, 94, 111, 132, 198
Conception 166, 187
Cooper, Dr. Ken 120
C-reactive protein (CRP) 157, 169
CRP, *see* C-reactive protein
Cummings, Colleen 4
Cummings, Todd 4
Cuzco 164
Cystic fibrosis 177, 241
Cytokine 155, 157

D
Dark-skinned 12, 21, 23-4, 27, 31, 71, 125-6, 147, 155, 187, 190, 200
Davenport, Dr. Charles 134
Denmark 109, 188
Dental 11, 16, 160-1, 181, 187
  caries 161, 237
Depression 6, 9, 10, 16, 155, 167, 173, 180, 183-6, 192, 206
Dermatologist 4, 62, 165, 197
Dermatology 62, 70
Dermis 14, 64
Diabetes 8, 9, 16, 23, 27, 57-8, 127, 131, 140-6, 149, 162-3, 175-6, 194-5, 206
DNA 48-9, 51, 56, 179, 197
Dopamine 168, 185, 192
Downes, Arthur 18
Duhamel, Madame 18

E
EAE, *see* Experimental autoimmune encephalomyelitis
Eclampsia 168, 182
Economic 8, 10, 21, 61
  burden 8, 10, 21, 61
Eczema 165, 181, 199
Electron 45-6, 51
Endometrial cancer 85
Endorphin 185, 192
Endotoxin 170
England 70, 72, 126, 132-3, 144, 151, 155, 168

Environmental Protection Agency (EPA) 53

EPA, *see* Environmental Protection Agency

Epidermis 14, 52, 64

Epilepsy 169

EpiPen 168

Epstein-Barr 175

Ergocalciferol 24, 34, 200

Eskimo 22

Esophagus 99, 106

Essential fatty acid 52

Estrogen 69, 121

Exercise 10, 12, 47-8, 100-1, 108-9, 111, 114-5, 119, 121, 124, 128, 140-1, 143, 152, 192

Experimental autoimmune encephalomyelitis (EAE) 131, 134-5

Eyles, Dr. Darryl 188

F

Falls 108, 117, 122-4, 179

Fat 11, 15, 32, 49-52, 54-8, 72, 87, 89, 103, 136-41, 143, 149-50, 162-4

Fatigue 122, 124, 154, 169, 184

FDA, *see* Food and Drug Administration

Fertility 166, 181-2, 199

Fibromyalgia 122, 130

Fielder, Dr. John 17

Finland 144

Finsen, Dr. Niels 18

Fish 2, 22-5, 52-3, 55, 59, 69, 92-3, 111, 167

Florence Nightingale 18, 178

Flu

  see Influenza

  shots 172

Fluorescent light 71

FNB, *see* Food and Nutrition Board

Food

  and Drug Administration (FDA) 68, 184-5

  and Nutrition Board (FNB) 33

Fracture 108-12, 114-9, 123

France 2, 18, 155, 196

Frassetto, Dr. Lynda 110-1

Free radical 45-51, 54, 56, 64, 77, 92, 198

Fruit 11, 45, 63, 72, 74, 141, 164

Fungus 169-70, 181

G

Gammack, Dr. Julie 167

Garland, Dr. Cedric 2, 4, 16, 79, 97-98, 207

Garland, Dr. Frank 2, 4, 16, 79, 97-8, 207

Germany 162

Gillie, Dr. Oliver 4

Giovannucci, Dr. Edward 5, 21, 61, 76, 94, 104-5, 153

Goldblatt, Dr. 15

Grant, Dr. William 4, 16, 21, 23, 31-2, 61, 70, 80, 98, 104, 135, 137, 139, 170-1, 174-5, 188, 193, 196-7, 204

Greece 162

Gum 16, 160

H

Hanley, Dr. David 26

Hart, Dr. Prue 176

Harvard 21, 62, 176

Hawaii 24, 120, 168

HDL 94, 176, 250

Headache 241

Heaney, Dr. Robert 33, 118

Hearing 167, 182

Heart

  attack 150-3

  disease 9, 11, 16, 27-8, 48, 50-1, 53, 57-8, 69, 73, 150-1, 158-9, 162-4, 194-5

  failure 154-6, 159, 171, 194

Heidrich, Dr. Ruth 119, 121

Heliotherapy 17-9

Hess, Dr. 15

Hippocrates 18, 37

Hispanic 27-8

HIV 169, 174, 181

Hobday, Richard 204

Hodgkin's lymphoma 60, 175

Holick, Dr. Michael 4, 10, 15, 25, 72, 122, 130, 165, 185, 204, 207

Hollis, Dr. Bruce 4, 26, 113, 202

Hospital 113, 115, 120, 125-6, 155, 157, 159, 170, 177-8, 181, 189, 207

Howard, Robbie 4

HRT 121

Hughes, Dr. 57

Hydrogenated fats 50

Hyperactivity 189-90

Hypercalcemia 30
Hypertension 57, 69, 153-4, 159, 162, 175, 194, 199
Hypocalcaemia 155-6

I
IBD, *see* Inflammatory bowel disease
Immune 2, 3, 8, 48, 52, 56, 127, 131, 140, 144, 155, 160, 169, 176, 181
Immunosuppressant 131
India 44, 175
Infection 157, 170, 173-4, 178, 182, 195, 207
Inflammation 147, 155, 157, 159-61, 174, 181, 190, 194
Inflammatory bowel disease (IBD) 131, 147, 149
Influenza 3, 6, 11-2, 16, 171-2, 178, 181, 187-8, 192
Insomnia 9, 167
Insulin 94, 131, 140-3, 149, 176
Intensity 13, 36, 43, 105, 152, 177-8, 198
International Unit (IU) 29, 30, 123, 134, 171, 176, 195
Inuit 23
Invasiveness 77, 91-2
IU, *see* International Unit

J
Jablonski, Dr. Nina 22
Japan 93, 99, 144, 162
John, Dr. Esther 31, 81, 88

K
Ketone 50
Kidney 15-6, 34, 102, 104, 106, 118, 164, 166
  cancer 102
  disease 16, 164, 166
Kime, Dr. Zane 88, 96, 161, 177
Koch, Robert 18, 177

L
Lappe, Dr. Joan 86
Latitude 20, 22-3, 38, 42, 70, 72, 91, 98, 132, 136, 146, 151, 166, 191, 197-9
Lawsuit 7, 68
Leprosy 175
Leukemia 16, 102, 104, 106, 170

Libido 166
Light therapy 6, 178, 183-4, 192
Lipid peroxidation 49-51, 54, 56-7
Lipids 49, 52
Liver 15-6, 30, 34, 92, 100, 103, 112, 145
LL-37 2, 3, 169, 174-5
LOAEL 26
Longevity 34, 136, 147, 179, 204
Los Gatos Longevity Institute 34, 204
Lung 16, 62, 94, 102-4, 106, 155
  cancer 16, 94, 102-3
Lupus 18, 131, 147, 149
Lutein 63
Lycopene 63, 72
Lymphoma 8, 16, 60, 74, 103-4, 106, 175

M
Macular degeneration (AMD) 167
Malta 162
Mammography 85
Massachusetts 42, 150, 168
McCollum, Dr. E.V. 15
McDougall, Dr. John 12, 120, 137
Meat 100, 106, 110-1, 137, 141, 165
Melamed, Dr. Michal 152
Melanin 52
Melanocyte 64
Melanoma 2, 3, 7, 8, 21, 32, 52, 54, 58, 60-72, 74, 82, 94, 196, 198-9
Melatonin 84, 184
Mellanby, Sir Edward 15
Menstrual 166
Menstruation 166
Met S, *see* Metabolic Syndrome
Metabolic Syndrome 94, 175-6, 182
Metastasis 77, 91-2, 103, 105
Mexican American 143
Mexico 85, 152, 162, 178, 202
Microgram 29
Micronesia 162
Migraine 177, 181
Milk 11, 15, 32, 100, 103, 117-8, 122, 137, 139, 143-6, 149, 165, 199
Miller, Dr. Phillip 4, 34, 204
Mineral 119, 135
Minnesota 23, 193
Mizoue, Dr. 99, 101
Mole 62, 64

Molecule 26, 122, 202
monomers 50
Mookherjee, Dr. N 170
Moon, Dr. S 90
MS, *see* Multiple sclerosis
Multiple sclerosis (MS) 3, 7, 9, 11, 16, 53, 57-8, 67, 73, 131-7, 139-40, 175, 199
Muscle 8, 9, 16, 117, 123-4, 128, 155-6, 162, 179, 193, 199
Mutation 49
Myelin sheath 131
Myeloma 103-4, 106
Myerson, Dr. Abraham 166
Myopathy 124, 193
Myopia 167-8, 182

N
Nanogram 24-30, 32-3, 78, 83-4, 96-7, 104-6, 112-3, 115-6, 118, 123-8, 135, 147, 152-3, 155-6, 202
Nasopharyngeal cancer 175
National Cancer Institute 60, 80, 86, 214
Native Americans 125, 163, 193
Nauru 162
Necrotizing fasciitis 173
Neuropathy 127, 143
Neurotransmitter 184
Nevada 11, 101, 183
New England 144, 168
New Mexico 152
New York 100, 177
New Zealand 109, 119, 152, 162
Ng, *see* Nanogram
NHANES 27
Nightingale, Florence
Nmol 3, 25-7, 29, 32, 125, 192, 202
NMSC, *see* common skin cancers
Non-Hodgkin's lymphoma 60, 75
Non-melanoma skin cancer, *see* common skin cancers
Nonspecific musculoskeletal pain 125-6
Norway 70, 109, 133, 135, 145
Norwegian 90, 163
Nosocomial 178, 181
Nursing 32, 122, 124, 167, 178-80, 182
Nutrition 12, 26, 33, 45, 70, 87, 100, 111, 118, 120-1, 128, 137, 140, 165

O
Obesity 6, 16, 63, 94, 140, 149, 153, 161-4, 176, 181, 199, 200
Omega-3 fatty acids 53
Omega-6 fatty acids 53
Oral 33, 160, 164-5, 175, 181
Osteoblast 113
Osteomalacia 11, 25, 112, 121-2, 125, 130, 199
Osteoporosis 32, 108-10, 113, 129, 160
Ovarian cancer 7, 85-6
Oxidation 47-8, 50-1, 57
Oxidize 53, 92
Oxybenzone 69
Ozone 44, 69, 70, 98

P
PAD, *see* Peripheral artery disease
Pain 8, 9, 11, 16, 23, 108, 122, 124-7, 130, 137, 143, 147, 150
Pancreatic cancer 101, 221, 223
Pandemic 19, 27, 32, 63, 108, 124-5, 161, 172, 183, 189
Papua New Guinea 109
Parasite 168
Parathyroid hormone (PTH) 26, 35, 112-3, 116, 121, 124, 156
Parkinson's Disease 148-9
PD, *see* Periodontal disease
Peller, Dr. Sigismund 19
Penicillin 19
Pennsylvania Center for Health Transformation 178, 238-9
Peptide 169
Periodontal disease (PD) 3, 92, 160-1, 181, 199
Peripheral artery disease (PAD) 150, 152, 159
Peru 164
Petroleum 48
Pharmaceutical 69, 81, 125, 141, 202
Phobia 10, 54
Pigment 52
Pima 162
Pima Indians 162
Pittas, Dr. Anastassios 142
Plaque 150, 160
Pliny 18
PMS 16, 167, 182, 206
Pneumonia 173, 178, 200

258

Pollutant 44
Pollution 44, 69, 79-81, 98, 154, 191, 198
Polycystic ovary disease 166
Polymers 50
Polyp 96
Polyunsaturated fatty acid (PUFA) 49-53, 56-7, 72, 142
Pre-eclampsia 168, 182
Pregnancies 122, 166, 188
Pregnancy 30, 33, 112, 116, 129, 146, 176, 188
Pregnant 33, 69, 102, 112, 161, 166, 168, 173, 176, 181-2, 187-8, 190-1, 195
Prenatal 102, 122, 188
Pritikin, Nathan 12
Pro-oxidant 77-8
Proliferation 63, 76-7, 84, 91-2, 95, 102, 105, 188
Prostate 6, 16, 27, 30-1, 57, 60-1, 87-96, 101, 104, 124, 175, 199
  cancer 6, 16, 30-1, 60, 87-95, 124
  specific antigen (PSA) 91, 95
PSA, see Prostate specific antigen
Psoralen 165
Psoriasis 165, 181, 199
PTH, see Parathyroid hormone
PubMed 102
PUFA, see Polyunsaturated fatty acid
Pulmonary 177

Q
Queensland 64, 132

R
Rabinowich, Dr. I.M 141
Radiation 2, 19, 48, 54, 72, 82, 88, 99, 104, 120, 200
Rancidity 50
Reaction time 128
Relative risk 24, 82, 146
Retina 104, 167
Rheumatoid arthritis 127, 131, 140
Rhodes, Dr. Arthur 62
Rickets 2, 14-5, 25, 32, 112, 121-3, 168, 191, 199
Rollier, Dr. 18

S
SAD, see Seasonal affective disorder

Samoa 162
Saturated fatty acids 53
Schwartz, Dr. Gary 91-3
Seafood 190
Seasonal affective disorder (SAD) 183-4, 189, 192
Selective serotonin re-uptake inhibitors (SSRI) 119, 184-5
Sepsis 170-1
Septicemia 3, 170, 182
Serotonin 116, 119, 184-6, 192
Seventh-Day Adventist 100
Sexuality 166
Shift work 84-5, 87
Singapore 167
Skin cancer 2, 3, 7, 9, 19-21, 45, 48-59, 63, 68-9, 74, 82, 103, 197-8
SLE, see Systemic lupus erythematosus
Smedby, Dr. Karin 103
Smoking 48, 102, 105, 115, 194
Solarium 18
Sonicare 178
Sorenson, Vicki 4, 12, 105, 137, 171, 202
South Africa 133, 162
Spain 115, 155, 159
Speed 128
Sperm 69, 166
Squamous cell carcinoma 52, 57, 165
SSRI, see Selective serotonin re-uptake inhibitors
Steenbock, Dr. 15
Steroid 176
Strength 7, 8, 16, 110, 112-3, 116-7, 123-4, 128-30, 178-9, 199
Stroke 7, 150-3, 157, 159-60, 162, 199
Suicidal 184, 192
Suicide 76
Sulfanilamide 19
Sulfur amino acids 110, 129
Sun phobia 10, 54
SUNARC 2, 4, 80, 86, 99, 204
Sunbathing 6, 12, 18-9, 23, 72, 88-90, 92, 95, 100, 105, 133, 163, 177
Sunblock 68
Sunburn 60, 63, 65, 70, 72, 89, 197, 199
Sunscare 32, 68, 82, 190
Sunscreen 7, 10, 17, 21, 23, 54, 63-70, 74, 79, 121, 132, 183, 202

Supplementation 8, 30, 32, 34, 98, 117-8, 121, 123, 147, 156-7, 167, 172
Surface reflection 43
Swank, Dr. Roy 136
Sweden 109, 191, 196
Sweeney, Dr. J.S. 141
Switzerland 132
Systemic lupus erythematosus (SLE) 131, 147

T
Tanning bed 7, 24, 31-2, 87, 103, 116, 119, 171, 185, 195-8
T cell 131
Telomere 179
Testicular function 166
Testosterone 69, 166
Toll-like receptor 169
Tomato paste 72
Tourette's syndrome 190
Toxic 25, 29-31, 33, 49, 56-7, 73, 172
Tropic of Cancer 38
Tropic of Capricorn 38, 40-1
Tuberculosis 2, 18, 33, 169, 174, 181, 193
Tumor 54, 77, 84, 98, 104, 106
Type-1 diabetes 8, 131, 140, 143-6, 149, 175, 206
Type-2 diabetes 29, 69, 140-3, 149, 176, 206

U
UK, *see* United Kingdom
Ultraviolet light 8, 14-5, 20, 22, 54, 61, 128, 149, 159, 176-8, 185, 196
United Kingdom (UK) 109-10, 133, 139
Utah 11, 23, 38, 101, 120, 127, 143, 183, 202
UV 2-4, 14-5, 18-9, 44, 54-5, 72, 88, 165-6, 178-9, 181, 197
UVA 7, 14, 32, 64-5, 68, 70-2, 74, 165, 197, 199
UVB 2, 3, 14, 16, 21, 32-4, 37, 41-4, 68, 98-9, 134-5, 151-4, 164-6, 171-2, 191, 199, 200

V
Vaccination 19, 172
VDR, *see* Vitamin D receptor (VDR)

Vegetable 49, 55-6, 63, 100, 106, 110-1, 118, 121, 129, 198
Vegetarian 120, 128, 137, 165
Vieth, Dr. Reinhold 5, 26, 29-30, 105, 112
Vieth, Dr. Walter 50
Viral 3, 171, 174-5, 178, 182
Vitamin A 15, 31, 92, 145
Vitamin D2 24, 34, 200
Vitamin D3 or cholecalciferol 3, 23-4, 26, 28-9, 34 78, 84, 86, 112, 122, 127, 143, 176, 200
Vitamin D deficiency 24, 26-9, 123-6, 147, 155-6, 166-7, 169-71, 173-4, 181-2, 186-94, 199
Vitamin D-deficient 98, 106, 112, 122, 124, 128, 166, 168, 189
Vitamin D receptor (VDR) (VDR) 34-5, 76, 147-8, 156, 166, 169, 173-4, 187
Vitamin D Winter 23, 42, 79, 91, 98, 133-4, 152, 173, 195

W
Wagner, Carol 122
Walking 100, 123, 127, 141, 150
Wang, Dr. Heng 191
Wang, Dr. Thomas 153
Weakness 9, 124, 131, 148, 169
Webb, Dr. Ann 72
West Indies 133, 139
Wheelchair 125, 193
World Health Organization 162

X
X-rays 48

Z
Zitterman, Dr. Armin 151, 152

A Tribute to William Grant, PhD

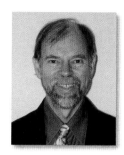

As Dr. Grant's work has been quoted extensively throughout this book, and because he went far beyond the call of duty in assisting me with research, it is only appropriate to let the reader know more about the background of this brilliant scientist. His help was beyond what I could have expected, but it only shows his dedication to promoting optimal health for all human beings.

Dr. Grant is Founding Director, Sunlight, Nutrition and Health Research Center (SUNARC), an entity devoted to research, education, and advocacy relating to the prevention of chronic disease through changes in diet and lifestyle. His primary mission is to identify and quantify risk-modifying factors for chronic diseases. He is particularly interested in UVB, cancer and infectious diseases, but also studies the role of diet in disease risk.

After an extensive career devoted to developing and applying laser remote sensing systems for the measurement of atmospheric trace species, primarily aerosols and ozone with NASA, in the 1990s, Dr. Grant undertook a project for the Sierra Club to determine the effect of acid rain and ozone on eastern hardwood forests. Upon reading that Japanese men in Hawaii had 2.5 times the risk of developing Alzheimer's disease (AD) than native Japanese, he made the connection between acid rain and AD and increased uptake of aluminum by trees and humans, and hypothesized that dietary factors played a very important role in the etiology of AD. He quickly determined that total energy (calories) and total fat were primary risk factors, while fish and cereals/grains were risk reduction factors. This paper was published in *Alzheimer's Disease Review* on June 17, 1997. The results were confirmed in 2002 and 2003 in case-control studies. After this discovery, he began studying dietary and environmental risks for other diseases including heart disease and cancer. That led to his current primary interest of studying the role of solar ultraviolet-B (UVB) and vitamin D in reducing the risk of cancer and other diseases.

Since he began his work on UVB/vitamin D and cancer in 2000, the list of vitamin D-sensitive cancers has grown from 5 to over 20. His findings interested Harvard University in including solar UVB in their cohort studies, and subsequent findings by Dr. Edward Giovannucci and coworkers did much to convince many other scientists of vitamin D's importance for cancer and other diseases. During 2006, the health community awakened to the fact that vitamin D is required for optimal health, and that at least 1000--4000 I.U. of vitamin D3 per day is indicated.

More recently, he has turned some attention to the role of vitamin D in reducing the risk of diseases linked to viral infections. He was a coauthor on a paper hypothesizing that the annual cycle of influenza is due, in part, to the annual cycle of solar UVB. This paper was supported by experimental results from a randomized controlled trial shortly thereafter. This finding should have profound consequences. He has also submitted manuscripts showing how solar UVB and vitamin D very likely reduce the risk of septicemia and pneumonia. He is currently working on developing the hypothesis that vitamin D in winter reduces the risk of autoimmune diseases and cancers linked to viruses such as the Epstein Barr virus by reducing the risk of viral infection. He has a background in environmental issues, and is also examining the roles of air pollution and agricultural herbicides in cancer risk. Here are just a few more of the many contributions Dr. Grant has made to the increasing pool of knowledge that contributes to optimal human health for those willing to follow his lead.

1. He identified dietary sweeteners (added sugar) as a significant risk factor for acute myocardial infarction (heart attack) for women below the age of 65 years.

2. He reported that animal products are a significant risk factor for prostate cancer and confirmed an earlier report that onions and other allium family vegetables significantly reduce the risk of prostate cancer.

3. He helped reestablish the ecologic approach as an important tool for identifying and quantifying risk-modifying factors for chronic and infectious diseases.

4. He led studies to estimate the reduction in total (direct plus indirect) economic burden of disease through higher vitamin D intake and production.

He is motivated by being able to use his scientific abilities to make important findings regarding human health and seeing his results used by others in their research programs or policy decisions. He is also motivated by the desire to help people realize that being healthy is up to them. For more about Dr. Grant, see www.sunarc.org and the list of references at www.grassrootshealth.org/references/htm or search www.pubmed.gov using Grant WB.

About the author

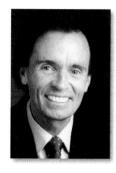

Dr. Marc Sorenson and his wife, Vicki, founded and operated one of the top health resorts in the world. During the time of their ownership of the health institute, known as National Institute of Fitness (NIF) their clients lost one hundred ten tons of fat. Two-thirds of diabetic guests were free of all medication in less than two weeks and many others recovered from high blood pressure, high cholesterol, lupus, arthritis, migraines and allergies.

Dr. Sorenson received his doctorate in education and health education from Brigham Young University, where he graduated with honors as a member of the Phi Kappa Phi honor society.

His book *Megahealth* was a selection of the Literary Guild, Doubleday Book Club and Doubleday Health Book Club. It was Book of the Month for the Doubleday Health Book Club.

He has spoken on health in many states in the USA and in many cities in Canada and Japan.

He was named an honorary Kentucky Colonel by Kentucky's Governor.

A popular speaker in the field of preventive health, he has appeared on scores of radio and TV programs.

A flag has been flown over the United States Senate building in honor of his contributions to the health and fitness of the citizens of the USA.

He was given the Money School of Boston award for Excellence in Nutrition writing—the only person so honored by the school.

Dr. Sorenson's favorite activities include time with family, reading medical and nutritional journals, speaking Spanish and hiking with Vicki in the alpine areas near their Nevada ranch. Marc and Vicki also enjoy listening to classical music, attending concerts and theater, and traveling in Mexico and Europe.

He and his colleagues will soon be building a new health institute/resort and will also be building a web site. Information may be obtained on these and other projects by email: drmarcsorenson@hotmail.com

Fiat lux. I read this book as an affirmation of an ancient truth, that all terrestrial life is dependent on the sun. Only recently have we seen the increasing value and vitality of the multiple roles of Vitamin D as a mediator of solar energy. This book is a compelling call to arms.

Philip Lee Miller, MD, Founder, Los Gatos Longevity Institute, www.antiaging.com

I have known Dr. Marc Sorenson for over two decades and have witnessed the success of his books, lectures and health spa in improving my life and health and the lives and health of many thousands of persons over the years. Marc is a scrupulously honest educator and tirelessly researches the medical literature for truth and wisdom. He is able to analyze the data and come up with simple, yet profound ideas that can be used by all persons who quest for health and vitality. All the while, he leaves nothing to guesswork; each statement is meticulously and fully documented.

Humans have neglected the environment that nurtured them for all of mankind's history, moving out of the sunlight and substituting fractured and depleted foods for healthful whole foods, thereby becoming the weakest and fattest Homo Sapiens to ever inhabit the Earth. People would do themselves a valuable service to read and apply the wisdom of *Vitamin D3 and Solar Power* and Dr. Sorenson's other books in their lives.

Maurice Henry Van Strickland, MD, F.A.A.A.A.I., F.A.C.A.A.I., F.A.A.P., A.C.P. A.M.A.A. Clinical Associate Professor of Medicine, University of Kansas School of Medicine, Wichita, Kansas

Dr. Sorenson does not hesitate to swim against a swift current. His meticulous research corroborates his extensive and intensive observations in the health-enhancing professions. Any one chapter in *Vitamin D3 and Solar Power*, when prefaced by the dedication and foreword, would be a magnificent solo treatise. A quick inspection of chapter 10, for example, displays how contemporary are (most of) his scientific references. This book cuts a broad swath counter to many modern institutions and lifestyles. The reader who resists common sense and tenaciously adheres to customary habits does so at his own misguided peril.

John Clark, MD, Neurosurgeon, FACS

So what is so new about *Vitamin D3 and Solar Power*? From the 1920's when I began general practice in Chicago we did everything to heal our patients. This included prescribing ozone lamps in the winter to get our patients the sunlight they needed to boost their vitality and immunity."

Russell B. Clark, MD (At 107, the oldest man in Utah)